AF183275

A History of the Moncton Hospital

A proud past—a healthy future

(1895–1995)

Dr. Donald I. MacLellan
M.D., C.M., F.R.C.S. (C)

NIMBUS
PUBLISHING

Nimbus Publishing Limited
PO Box 9301, Station A
Halifax, NS B3K 5N5
(902) 455-4286

The Department of Community Relations and Education
Southeast Health Care Corporation
135 MacBeath Avenue
Moncton, New Brunswick E1C 6Z8
Tel. (506) 857-5390
Fax (506) 857-5386

Design: Joan Sinclair
Page layout: Terri Strickland
Front cover photo: The Moncton Hospital.
Back cover photos: see pages 34, 39, 303.
Printed and bound in Canada

Canadian Cataloguing in Publication Data
MacLellan, D.I. (Donald I.)
A history of The Moncton Hospital
Includes index.
ISBN 1-55109-278-6
1. Moncton Hospital—History. I. Title.
RA983.M58M66 1998 362.1'1'091715235 C98-950252-X

Nimbus Publishing acknowledges the financial support of the Canada Council and the Department of Canadian Heritage.

Dedication

This book is dedicated to all those Friends of The Moncton Hospital in the broadest sense—the members of the board, the volunteers, the individuals and the organizations who have devoted time and money to ensure the best possible health care to the citizens of greater Moncton and beyond.

Once, when I was being interviewed for a residency position, I made some comments about the nice, brand-new facility that this hospital had just moved into and the man interviewing me remarked that the success of a hospital depended not so much on bricks and mortar as on the people who worked there. This book is also dedicated to all those physicians, nurses and other health care workers who have dedicated their lives over the past one hundred years to the care of the health of their fellow citizens.

FOREWORD

When a committee was formed in 1994 to plan for the centennial celebrations of The Moncton Hospital, I was appointed as the medical staff representative on that committee. When sub-committees for the celebration were being set up I found myself appointed to the history committee. There were no archives for The Moncton Hospital, but some of the old annual reports were available and there were various materials of historical value scattered around numerous rooms in the hospital and the former nurses' residence. As I started looking at this material it was evident that there were great gaps in the information that was available. Fortunately, the microfilms of the *Moncton Times* and the *Moncton Transcript* are available at the Albert-Westmorland-Kent Regional Library in Moncton. For the use of the Monctonian Room and for the assistance given to me in this research, I wish to thank the library staff.

The focus of this book is primarily on the medical staff but I have tried to cover major events in the administration and nursing aspects of the hospital. The book proceeds in chronological sequence with the major events of each year occurring at the hospital discussed first, followed by short biographical sketches of members admitted to the medical staff in that year. Statistics for that year are then given in a final paragraph for each year.

Like the hospital, this book took three years from its conception before the final draft was produced. I would like to thank Dr. Ginette Gagné-Koch and the medical staff for allowing me access to the personnel records of the medical staff. I also must thank Margaret Gladbois and Ruth Jenson of the medical staff office who patiently pulled the files and sorted out the necessary biographical material from the files. My wife, Alberta, Dr. Arthur Oatway and Dr. James Noonan read my first draft of the manuscript, made helpful suggestions and encouraged me to proceed with a second draft. Dr. Robert Caddick was the source for most of the material on the abortion issue of 1982. Stephen Herc, The Moncton Hospital photographer, has been most helpful in supplying me with photos from the hospital collection as well as making copies of photos from the annual reports. Vaughn MacLellan, my son, carried out editing of my first draft. I am indebted to the late J. Edward Belliveau who then read the second draft and felt that the manuscript would be of interest beyond the hospital confines and encouraged me to proceed with publication. I must also thank Mrs. Geraldine Dayton who has reviewed and edited the third draft of the book. I appreciate the action taken by Dr. Ginette Gagné-Koch, Carroll Ann O'Leary and James Quick of the administration staff of The Moncton Hospital that has made possible the publication of this book. Last but not least I must thank the publisher and my editor, Elizabeth Eve at Nimbus Publishing for putting the finishing touches on the manuscript and bringing the book to fruition.

As far as possible the place names in Europe and Asia have been verified but some inaccuracies may arise principally because of the inability to interpret the doctor's writing in their personnel records.

Table of Contents

Chapter One

The Beginning

In 1895 the population of Moncton was more than 8,000. Although there were several doctors, there was no hospital. It was Dr. James Duncan Ross who was instrumental in bringing the need for a hospital to the attention of the community.

For many years there had been discussions in the columns of the city's newspapers, the *Moncton Times* and the *Moncton Transcript*, concerning the need for a local hospital. Now, because of Dr. Ross's initiative, the interest grew and the city's clergy along with several prominent citizens, took up the challenge. Many women in the community were especially active in promoting this project. One non-sectarian group—The King's Daughters—voted at a September 1894 meeting to devote their energies toward the establishment of a medical facility for the city.

On the morning of Monday, December 31, 1894, a meeting was held in the parlour of the YMCA. It was well attended and supported by the clergy. J.S. Benedict, U.S. Counsel, was called to the chair, and Dr. A. Myers served as secretary. Those attending unanimously supported the establishment of a hospital and discussed various ways of bringing about the objective. A committee was formed, consisting of J.S. Benedict, Mrs. C.T. Purdy, wife of Dr. C.T. Purdy, Rev. Weeks, Rev. Green, Rev. Father Meahan, Rev. Hopper, Dr. J.D. Ross and Merv Flemming. The duty of this committee was to gather information concerning the probable cost of the facility and to consider methods of raising the necessary funds. Local clergymen took an active interest in the movement, promising to promote the plans through their congregations.

On January 26, 1895, a public meeting was held at the Opera House attended by 300 of the city's leading citizens. The proposal for the establishment of a hospital was accepted. A group consisting of Alfred E. Chapman, Israel L. Miller, Andrew H. Jones, John H. Harris, Murray Flemming, Peter McSweeney, Henry A. Whitney, Charles W. Bradley, Hugh Hamilton, Frederick W. Givan, Frederick P. Reid and Henry C. Hannington was entrusted with applying for and obtaining incorporation of the hospital. It is interesting to note and perhaps reflective of the time, that, although much effort to propose the idea of a hospital was expended by women of the community and by the clergy, it was left to the businessmen of the city to do the legwork resulting in the passing in the provincial legislature of the act of incorporation of the hospital. This took place on March 5, 1895.

Although the idea of a hospital for the city had been easily conceived, there was a three-year gestation period before the facility became a reality. Queen Victoria's Diamond Jubilee celebrations were to be held in 1897, and, as she had been voicing her desire that her subjects do what they could to better the lives of the sick and the poor, the hospital's supporters proposed their plans as the city's Diamond Jubilee project. This, however, was defeated by the city council as being too expensive. The municipality finally agreed instead to spend $600 to renovate the second and third floors of the almshouse at Leger's Corner (now Dieppe) for which the provincial government provided an additional grant of $300. A citizens' hospital committee was formed at a meeting of February 19, 1898, with Dr. Ross, Dr. Myers and Dr. McCully as the medical society representatives. G.B. Willett was elected chairman of the hospital committee with A.H. Jones as treasurer, H.F. Hamilton as secretary and Dr. McCully as vice-president. The hospital committee was composed of 12 men, including two medical men. The question of putting medical men on the committee aroused some debate. Dr. Botsford reported that the latest medical journals reporting on the operation of hospitals indicated that the majority of Boards of Managers were medical men and he argued unsuccessfully that it should be so with the new Moncton hospital.

At a meeting in city council chambers on February 21, 1898, the hospital committee met with the almshouse committee to arrange for the accommodation of hospital patients in the almshouse. Necessary renovations were carried out to the almshouse with Miss M.C. Grant appointed as matron on May 11, 1898.

The hospital first opened its doors on Saturday afternoon, June 11, 1898, with the ceremony presided over by Mayor E.C. Cole. All the members of the Board of Trustees were present for the occasion: G.B. Willett, president; Dr. O.J. McCully, vice-president; Hugh Hamilton, secretary; A.H. Jones, treasurer; L.I. Miller, Peter McSweeney, Dr. J.D. Ross, C.W. Robinson, Dr. A.R. Myers, J.M. Ross. J.H. Wran, J.S. Marmie, E. Girouard and B. Toombs. On June 13, 1898, the *Moncton Times* reported: "The opening was attended by an auspiciousness that reflects credit on the citizens of Moncton and more specifically on the Board of Trustees who have undertaken on behalf of the city to manage the institution." At this meeting, tribute was paid to Dr. J.D. Ross who was regarded as the father of the hospital movement. For twenty years he had been agitating for a medical facility, more so to accommodate the sick poor, than for any other reason. This first hospital consisted of five small private rooms, a matron's room and reception room on the second floor and an eight-bed female ward and a six-bed male ward on the third floor, as well as a kitchen, washroom and operating room. It was situated on a hill, with the women's ward looking out on the Petitcodiac River.

On the afternoon of June 10, 1898, a meeting was held in the YMCA

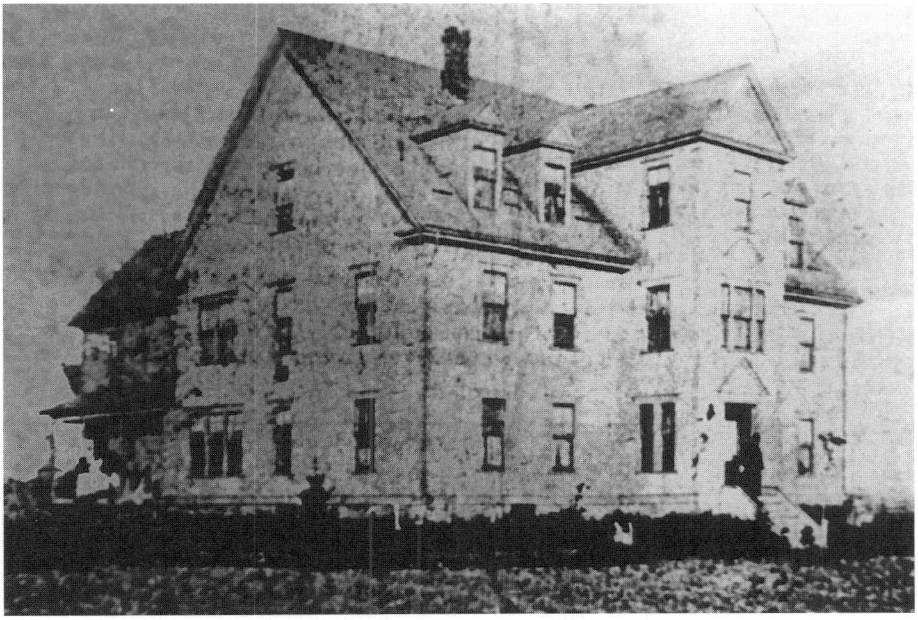

The almshouse—site of the first Moncton Hospital, opened in 1898.

parlours for the purpose of forming a Ladies' Auxiliary in connection with the hospital. A large and representative number of women from the community were present. A nominating committee consisting of Mrs. G.B. Willet, Mrs. J.C. Abbott, Mrs. W.B. Chandler and Mrs. George McSweeney was chosen and at a subsequent meeting brought in the first slate of officers: Mrs. Henry C, Hannington, president; Miss Hennigar, first vice-president; Mrs. F.W. Sumner, second vice-president and Miss Agnes McSweeney, secretary-treasurer.

In order to look after the public wards, doctors took turns serving without pay for a month at a time. The roster for the first year was as follows:

1898

June	Dr. Louis Bourque
July	Dr. C.T. Purdy
Aug.	Dr. F.J. White
Sept.	Dr. J.D. Ross
Oct.	Dr. O.J. McCully
Nov.	Dr. A.R. Myers
Dec.	Dr. Gaius Smith

1899

Jan.	Dr. Henry Hicks Coleman
Feb.	Dr. E.O. Steeves
Mar.	Dr. Leverett Price
Apr.	Dr. William Cruise
May	Dr. A. Henry Chandler
June	Dr. Robert Botsford

Although Canada at this time was thirty years old as a country, the Maritimes still took its trade with the Yankees. It is therefore not surprising to note that many of these pioneer doctors practising in the Maritimes had taken their training in the United States.

As has been previously noted, Dr. James Duncan Ross was one of the leading lights in the medical profession seeking the establishment of a medical facility and is regarded as the "Father of The Moncton Hospital." In his obituary in the *Moncton Times* it was noted that he "held a large place in the hearts of the people in consequence of his genial and friendly nature and charitable deeds for the poor." Born in Pictou in October 1839, he was the son of Rev. Jas. Ross, DD, a former principal of Dalhousie College and the grandson of Rev. Duncan Ross, one of the earliest Presbyterian missionaries sent out from Scotland to Nova Scotia. His mother was a daughter of William Matheson, a wealthy Nova Scotian merchant who, in his will, left $70,000 for educational and religious work. Dr. Ross was educated in Pictou and West River seminary and then took undergraduate studies in Philadelphia before going to Harvard where he received his MD in 1862. His diploma from Harvard is preserved in the archives of The Moncton Hospital and is signed by Oliver Wendell Holmes, Professor of Anatomy and Physiology at Harvard. He later took a course in medicine and surgery at Edinburgh University. Returning to his native province, he practised in Dartmouth where he aided in the establishment of the Halifax Medical School, at which he was Demonstrator in Anatomy during the first two years of its existence. He moved to Moncton where he continued to practise until he died, in his sleep, on March 31, 1911.

Dr. Louis Napoleon Bourque was the first Acadian to practise medicine in Moncton, after having graduated from Victoria College (McGill) in 1876 and practising in Richibucto for two years. He was very active in the community outside his medical practice, serving on the city council for many years and being a member of the school board for 40 years. He was an accomplished musician and for several years served as organist at Saint Bernard's Church. He was made a Grand Knight of the Knights of Columbus in 1906.

Dr. Clinton Tramline Purdy received his MD from the University of New York in 1884. He served as president of the New Brunswick Medical Society in 1911-12 and also was active in civic affairs. Like Dr. Bourque, he served on the School Board and City Council. He was mayor of Moncton in 1908. Active in his church, he served on the Board of Trustees of St. John's Presbyterian Church when it reopened in 1915 after being destroyed by fire in the year before.

Frederick Job White was born in Greenspan, Newfoundland, and after attending Mount Allison, received his MD, CM from McGill in 1866. After spending some time in the Grenfell Mission Field he took postgraduate training in London, receiving his Licentiate of the Royal College of Physicians in 1888. He first practised in Shediac for seven years before coming to Moncton. While in McGill he was one of the medical students who formed the McGill unit of stretcher bearers in the army under General Middleton in the Riel Rebellion in 1885. He later served in the Boer War and remained active in the militia all his life serving regularly as Surgeon Major in the 70th battery of volunteer militia attending camp in Sussex. During the First World War, he served as Chief Medical Inspector for recruiting in the Moncton area. He always remained a strong supporter of a national policy and an even stronger supporter for a British connection. An avid sportsman, he boxed in his youth and later refereed boxing matches. He was a supporter of the Victorias, a local hockey team that competed for the Stanley Cup in 1912. He was a curler and was vice-president of the rifle club in 1899. He was also active in civic politics, serving as mayor in 1907, and was responsible for the opening of Bore Park. The eastern end of the city had supported such a park but the western end of the city was opposed. As mayor, he cast the deciding vote in favour of "Bend View Square." Along with Drs. Bourque and Ferguson he was among the first automobile owners in Moncton. He died on April 10, 1921. His daughter, Marion White, became a well-known music teacher in Moncton.

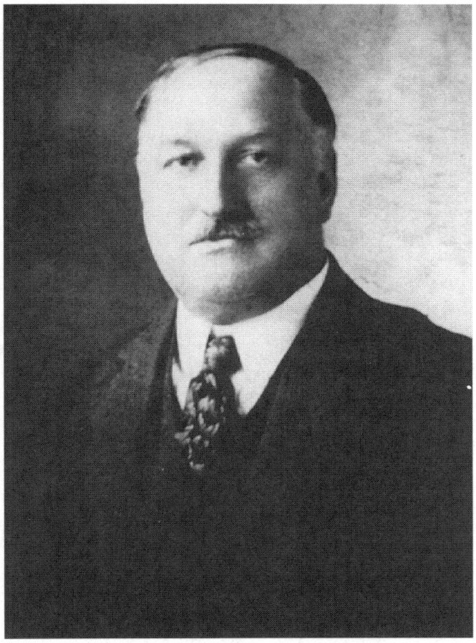

Dr. F.J. White, member of the first hospital staff, and mayor of Moncton in 1907.

After receiving an MA from UN in 1875, Oscar J. McCully attended McGill, receiving an MD, CM degree in 1879. Further postgraduate work in England resulted in his becoming a Master of the Royal College of Surgeons of England in 1885. After practising in Baie Verte, he settled in Moncton where he resided until his death in 1911. He wrote several articles for the medical journals of both the Maritime and Canadian Medical Societies and served as president of the New Brunswick Medical Society in 1896-1897.

Dr. Ambrose Richard Myers was a native of Ontario and received his MD from Queen's University in 1894. He started a practice in Moncton shortly after graduation but in 1905 he took a year's sabbatical to do postgraduate work in Berlin, Paris and London. He soon gained an excellent reputation as a surgeon and, along with Dr. Ferguson, captured the bulk of the surgical practice in Moncton. The rivalry between them must have been fierce and, it would appear, not too friendly. When his son, Dr. Ralph Myers, had appendicitis in his youth, he sent to Saint John to have a surgeon come to Moncton to perform the appendectomy rather than entrust him to Dr. Ferguson. He became a Fellow of the American College of Surgeons and reportedly performed the first bone graft of the spine in Moncton. He was active in first aid work and was awarded a Fellowship by the Order of St. John of Jerusalem. He served as president of the New Brunswick Medical Society in 1904-05 and was a vice-president of the Canadian Medical Society. For his work as a surgeon, he was awarded an Honorary Doctorate from St. Joseph's

University and the King George V Silver Jubilee Medal. He married the daughter of Senator Peter McSweeney, a well-known Moncton merchant. After the senator's death he had a falling out with A.R. McSweeney, his brother-in-law, with whom he had been appointed an executor of the estate. McSweeney assumed the presidency of the late senator's department store and refused to open the books to Dr. Myers, who finally had to take him to court on behalf of the estate. His lawyer was F.P. Murphy, the father of Drs. Pat and Fred Murphy. McSweeney was represented by Ivan C. Rand who later became a supreme court justice. Eventually a settlement was reached between the litigants with McSweeney and Myers resigning as executors and being replaced by a trust company. When everything was settled it proved the financial ruination of A.R. McSweeney and within ten years the department store failed. Dr. Myers died in August 1949. His two sons became doctors. His son, Ralph, who had joined him in practice, is now retired but is on the honorary staff of the hospital. The name "Myers" has thus been on the medical staff roster for one hundred years.

Dr. Gaius Smith received his MB, Chb degree from Edinburgh in 1887 and continued further studies there receiving an MD degree in 1890, a degree only awarded to those who had shown great skill and competence. He was the first specialist in eye, ear, nose and throat at the Moncton Hospital.

Henry Hicks Coleman was born in Sackville on March 2, 1853, the son of Rev. W.B. Coleman. After graduating from Harkens Academy in Newcastle, he went to the University of New York obtaining his MD degree in 1878. After graduation, he established his medical practice in Lower Cape, Albert County, and then moved to Sackville before coming to Moncton shortly before incorporation of the hospital. He remained on staff until his death on November 22, 1937. He established a reputation as an anaesthetist and the esteem in which he was held by his medical colleagues is attested to by the fact that he served on the Board of Trustees of the hospital for over 20 years as the representative of the Moncton Medical Society. He also served as coroner for a time, was medical director for the Port of Moncton and doctor in charge of Indian medicine in this district. Raised in a manse, he remained dedicated to the Baptist Church throughout his life, serving as a deacon and church clerk at the First Baptist Church for over 25 years. He was also active in the British and Foreign Bible Society, serving as president of both the Moncton Branch and the Provincial Branch and at the

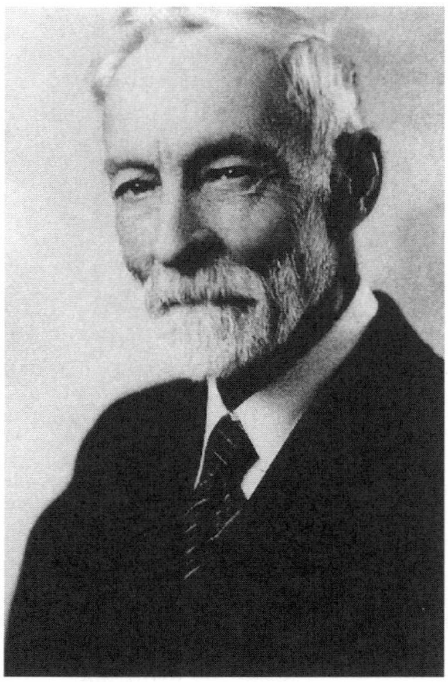

Dr. H.H. Coleman, member of the first medical staff and long-serving representative of medical staff on the Board of Trustees.

time of his death was the honorary president of the provincial society. His son, Dr. William Coleman, rose to prominence among educators, becoming Professor of English and later dean and vice-president of academic affairs at Bucknell College in Lewisburgh, Pennsylvania.

Dr. Edward Omar Steeves graduated from the University of New York in 1885 and moved to Moncton in 1886. In addition to his medical practice, he was active in civic politics, serving on the city council and as mayor in 1906. He was one of the founding members of the volunteer Moncton Salvage Corps and Fire Police organized in 1913. He owned a drugstore and one of its advertisements for Swiss Buttermilk Soap at ten cents a box can be found in the Moncton Transcript of April 22, 1899. In 1919 he sold the drugstore to W.B. Rodd when Rodd returned from service in the war. Rodd's Drugstore continued in business under Mr. Rodd and later his daughter, Marjorie, for many years. Its last location was in the Brunswick Hotel block. By 1995 all the individually owned drugstores, with one exception, had been absorbed into the large retail chains.

Dr. Leverett Herbert Price was born in Havelock on February 14, 1868, and graduated from Bellevue Hospital Medical School in 1892. He practised in Grand Manan for a short period of time and then returned to New York to pursue postgraduate work at Bellevue. He then practised in New York before returning to his native New Brunswick and Moncton where he resided until his death on March 1, 1933. He was a past president of the New Bruns-wick Medical Society and a former president of the Moncton Horticultural and Improvement Society. He designed and successfully operated the Lakeside Golf Club. At the outbreak of the Boer War in 1899, he tried unsuccessfully to become a member of the Canadian contingent but his request was denied and, instead, he went to South Africa as a medical officer on a steamer running to Cape Town. There he was offered a position as medical officer for the British government in charge of the Boer prisoners confined on the Island of St. Helena, including the famous General Cronje. He remained on St. Helena for two years, returning to Canada when the war ended.

Dr. William Cruise graduated from Harvard in 1867, and practised in Buctouche until 1890, when he moved to Moncton continuing to practise medicine until his death in 1905.

Dr. Amos Henry Chandler was the son of Judge W.B. Chandler and the grandson of E.C. Chandler, a prominent lawyer and governor of New Brunswick before Confederation and lieutenant-governor after Confederation. Doctor Chandler graduated from the University of Pennsylvania in 1857 and then spent three years studying in Europe, including a stint as a private pupil of the Queen's physician in London. On returning to Canada, he practised in Salisbury before moving to Moncton. He served on the school board and was chairman in 1874. A well educated and cultured man, he was a poet of considerable talent and, with a collaborator, published a book of poems. One of his poems, "Sad and Low," is recorded in Dr. W.B. Stewart's

Medicine in New Brunswick. It is surmised that this may have been written in his later years when he divorced his wife and the Anglican Church refused to recognize it. He left Moncton and settled in Cocaine where he hunted for gold unsuccessfully. It was his theory that Joseph Gueguen, the fur trader, scholar and linguist, reputed to be the richest Acadian of his time, had buried his gold when privateers raided his properties during the American Revolution.

Dr. Robert L. Botsford came from another prominent Moncton family, being the son of Judge Bliss Botsford, for whom Botsford Street is named. He graduated from Jefferson Medical College in 1869 and came back to New Brunswick in 1870. He served on the city council in 1905. In 1912 he served as chairman of the board of health.

Some of the doctors were considered wealthy at the time and could not pretend otherwise because the *Transcript* on June 15, 1899, printed the names of all those citizens of Moncton who paid more than $50.00 in taxes. Included among those names were: Dr. L.N. Bourque, Dr. A.H. Chandler, Dr. C.T. Purdy, Dr. E.O. Steeves and Dr. William Cruise.

Within four months of the hospital's opening in the old almshouse its beds were filled. By the end of the first year of operation, the need for a larger facility was evident. Indeed, several times during that first year every bed had been occupied and admission refused to some, showing the great need for a larger building.

In the first annual report to the hospital, dated June 30, 1899, it is reported that 70 patients were admitted to the hospital with an average stay of 28.2 days. Forty-one patients were discharged as cured, 13 as improved, 3 untreated, 9 under treatment and 3 deaths. Among the admission diagnoses were 8 patients with neurasthenia and 10 with typhoid fever. There were 14 operations performed in the first year, all reported as successful. These included two thigh amputations, one excision of a knee joint, one osteomyelitis of the radius, two necrosis of femur, one strangulated hernia, one drainage of bulla, one circumcision, 3 D&Cs, one repair of a lacerated cervix and perineum and one enucleation of an eye.

The budget for the hospital's first year was $1,730.42. With expenses of $1,947.17, this resulted in a deficit of $216.75. It is noted that pharmacists donated drugs free of charge to the poor. With $212.22 of the budget coming in the form of gifts, the foundation of the Friends of the Moncton Hospital was already being laid. Private patients were charged $4.00 a week. Fifty-one of the patients came from the city of Moncton with the remainder from the county. Only ten of these were private patients, with 9 paying patients in the wards, and 32 public patients.

In 1899 Dr. W. Ferguson came to the hospital and soon gained fame as one of the finest surgeons in New Brunswick. Born in Richibucto on April 30, 1864, he received a BA from McGill in 1881 and then his MD, CM from McGill in 1884, where he studied under Sir William Osler. He served as house surgeon at the Montreal General Hospital under Dr. F.J. Sheppard and then went west where he was employed by Canadian Pacific Rail as a medical officer among their construction crews. Returning east, he practised for several years in Rexton and Newcastle. After postgraduate work in New York, he returned to New Brunswick and to Moncton. He performed the first abdominal and thyroidectomy operations at the Moncton Hospital and the first caesarean section in the Moncton area, done in a private residence, on the kitchen table. As related in Dr. Brent Stewart's *Medicine in New Brunswick*, a pregnant Mrs. Anderson of Hopewell Hill was seated at a large roll-top desk when her three-year-old son, playing with a revolver, shot his mother in the abdomen. Dr. Ferguson rushed the 30 miles to Hopewell Hill in his new Packard. Both mother and the baby survived, although the baby had been shot in both legs. Dr. Ferguson was noted for his phenomenal memory and was described as a plain man who abhorred all public show. He served as Regional Medical Officer for the Canadian National Railway and remained active in practice until he died from pneumonia on October 2, 1935.

At the end of the second year of the hospital's operation, it was evident that the almshouse facilities were totally inadequate. At a meeting of the hospital board in May 1900, the treasurer, Mr. Jones, moved a resolution that the board procure a site in the city for the purpose of erecting a more suitable hospital building. The operation of the hospital in 1899-1900 showed operating revenues of $1,766.12 with expenses of $1,788.48. There was an overdraft at the bank of $22.56 and donations to the hospital during the year totalled $150.

The annual meeting for the year ending May 31, 1901, was held in the office of Alderman Jones, treasurer of the board, on June 24. The president, George Willett, was in the chair, and Hugh Hamilton served as secretary. Once again, the need for a new facility was stressed. The president noted that many cases were going to Saint John and Montreal that could have been treated in Moncton had adequate facilities been available. The treasurer's report showed operating expenses of $1,652 with $441.55 cash on hand. It is noted in the report that collections were taken, or were to be taken, for the benefit of the hospital at St. Bernard's Church, the Central Methodist Church, St. George's Episcopal Church and St. John's Presbyterian Church. The matron reported that 76 patients were admitted during the year with 74 discharged with an average length of stay of 27.69 days. Fifty-seven patients were discharged as cured, and one improved. There were 2 deaths, 23 patients were private, 9 paying on the ward and 44 free patients. There were 43 medical cases and 42 surgical cases. It was reported that 35 operations were performed, all successfully. This unblemished record of successful operations was preserved, albeit in an unfortunate manner. On November 16, 1900, an elderly man, William MacFarlane, was being assisted to the operating room by Doctors Ross, McCully and Myers and died before surgery could be performed.

Chapter Two

A New Beginning

As it has been noted, within two years it had become apparent that the almshouse facilities were totally inadequate to serve the community, and the hospital board commenced planning the construction of a new facility. Once again community support for this cause was strong and the Ladies' Hospital Sewing Circle, under its president Mrs. W.F. Humphrey, raised money to support the purchase of land. This was done principally by having bazaars at the Victoria Rink in 1902 and 1903. As a result of their efforts, land was purchased at the corner of King St. and Mountain Road for the sum of $2,000.00., and construction of the new hospital began in the summer of 1902. The money for the new construction was to be raised by grants from the city, county and province as well as public subscription. The board appointed a building committee consisting of G.B. Willett, H.F. Hamilton, A.H. Jones, Mr. J.M. Ross, F.W. Givan and B. Toombs. F. Neil Brodie of Saint John was the architect and the contract for construction of the exterior walls was given to Messrs. T.B. and Morris LeBlanc. The exterior work was finished before Christmas 1902. Construction resumed in the spring with the contract for the interior work being given to Philip N. LeBlanc. The handsome hardwood veneer with which the building was finished was donated by Mrs. George Prescott of West River, Albert County. The plumbing contract was awarded to F.W. Sumner.

The cornerstone of the new facility was laid by Lieutenant-Governor Snowball on October 29, 1903, and the new hospital opened on November 11, with great fanfare. A ceremony was held that afternoon, with addresses to the guests by the Hon. L.J. Tweedie, premier of New Brunswick; Hon. H.R. Emmerson, MP; Senator Ward; Rev. J.E. Brown; Rev. Father Meahan; Dr. J.D. Ross; L.M. Legere, MPP; and Sheriff J.A. McQueen. In addition, an evening program and musical were held, presided over by Mayor F.W. Givan. This facility, with further additions, would continue to serve the citizens of Moncton for the next fifty years. The members of the board at the time of this inaugural event were: G.B. Willett, president; J.S. Rayworth, vice-president; H.F. Hamilton, secretary; A.H. Jones, treasurer; Sen. P. McSweeney; Edward Girouard; Hon. C.W. Robinson; J.M. Ross; J.S. Marnie; F.W. Givan;

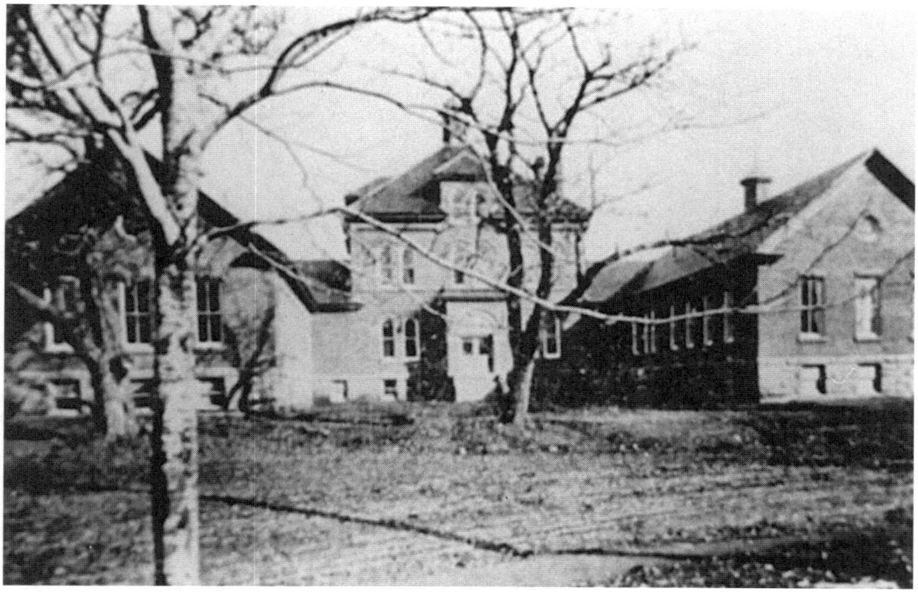

The new hospital was built on King Street in 1903.

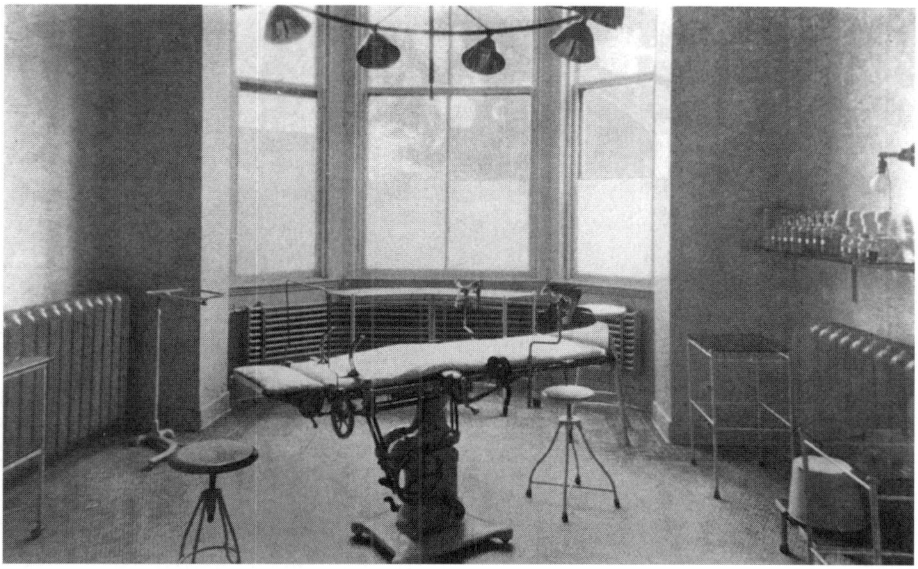

The operating room in the new hospital.

B. Toombs; F.W. Sumner; Dr. A.R. Myers and Dr. J.D. Ross. On December 9, 1903, the first medical staff was appointed to the new hospital and included the following: Dr. A.H. Chandler, Dr. Gaius Smith, Dr. A.R. Myers, Dr. L.I. Bourque, Dr. William Ferguson and Dr. F.J. White. Dr. J.D. Ross and Dr. L.H. Price were appointed as consultants. Again, the doctors took turns in attending to non-paying patients in the public wards, with two doctors serving for a two-month period. This was indeed a banner year for

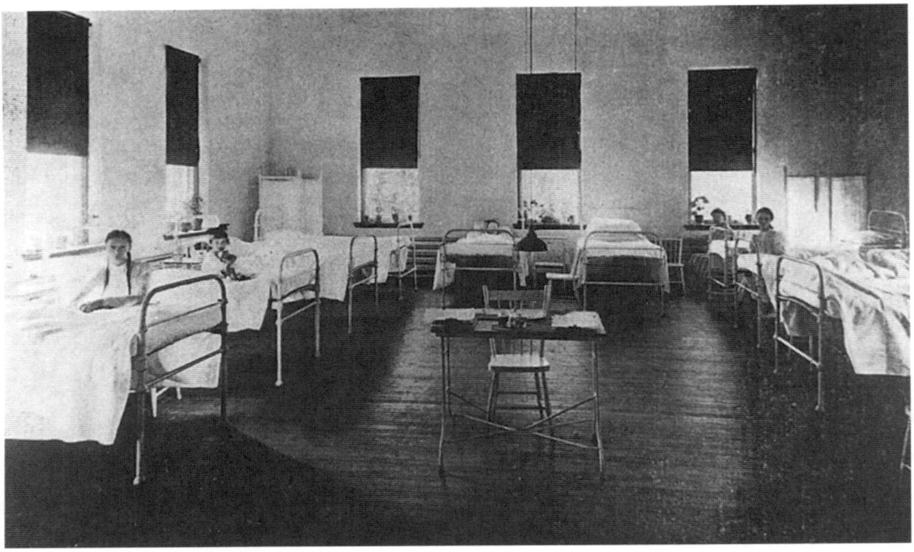

A typical ward in the new hospital.

Moncton as the prime minister, Sir Wilfrid Laurier, announced that Moncton would be the eastern terminus of the National Transcontinental Railway, which would extend from Moncton to Winnipeg.

At the annual meeting of the hospital board held on June 8, 1904, with the president, G.B. Willett, in the chair, thanks were extended to C.F Harris for donating land at the rear of the new building. At this meeting, a resolution was passed that the hospital would only use pasteurized milk although one trustee voiced his disapproval. The treasurer, A.H. Jones, reported that income during the year was $9,423.61, of which $5,929.72 was transferred to the building fund. The matron, Miss Magee, indicated in her report that 131 patients had been admitted with 81 discharged as cured, 19 as improved, one left against advice, and 10 as incurable. There were 2 deaths in hospital. There were 82 private patients and 48 free public. There were 88 surgical cases and 42 were classified as medical cases.

The medical staff was divided into three categories. First, there was visiting staff consisting of six doctors: Dr. L.N. Bourque, Dr. A.R. Myers, Dr. A.H. Chandler, Dr. F.J. White, Dr. L.H. Price and Dr. R. Botsford. Secondly, there was consulting staff consisting of two doctors: Dr. J.D. Ross and Dr. C.T. Purdy. The visiting and consulting staff looked after the free public patients. Finally, there was a general staff, consisting of all licensed practitioners in the city, who would have the privilege of attending to patients in any of the private wards.

In March 1904 Miss M.C. Grant resigned as superintendent and in December was replaced by Miss Janet MacEachern. Miss Magee served as interim superintendent between March and December. Miss MacEachern was to prove instrumental in setting up the Moncton Hospital School of Nursing in 1906.

At the 1905 annual meeting of the hospital board, Mr. Willett, the president, summing up the first full year in the new hospital, noted that it was able to operate with a deficit of $266.73 on operating expenses of $6,128. It was hoped that the debt in the building account could be paid off with greater donations in the coming year. In his report, he noted that a diphtheria epidemic had nearly put the hospital out of business for two months. The Ladies' Hospital Aid continued to play a prominent role in assistance to the hospital and during the year raised enough money for the purchase of a sterilizer and the installation of a tile floor in the operating room. For the ensuing year, J.S. Rayworth was elected president of the hospital board with Mr. Willett remaining on the executive as vice-president. The secretary was Mr. Hamilton and the treasurer, Mr. Jones.

The year 1905 marked the beginning of an ambulance service at the hospital when the Ladies' Hospital Aid purchased a horse-drawn, rubber-tired ambulance fitted with ball bearing axles, from the Marks Carriage Works for $500.

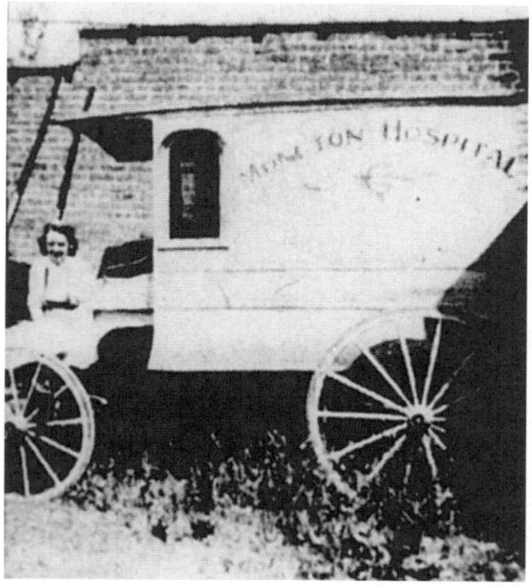

The first horse-drawn ambulance for the hospital, purchased in 1905.

During the year 1904-05, 238 patients were admitted to the hospital, 137 male and 181 female, of which 175 were paying and 67 were non-paying patients; 110 of the patients came from the city, 61 from Westmorland County, 29 from Kent County, 17 from Albert County and 18 from other counties and cities. There were 61 patients who received medical treatment and 177 who underwent surgical treatment; 157 operations performed. In all, 188 patients were discharged as cured, 18 improved, one incurable and two not treated.

Medical staff selected for the next year were: Dr. White, Dr. Price, Dr. McNaughton, Dr. Myers, Dr. Purdy and Dr. Ferguson. At this time there occurs the first appearance of a new category of staff, the "specialist," with the listing of Dr. Sherman W. Burgess as a specialist in eye, ear, nose and throat.

Although Dr. Gaius Smith had been recognised as the first eye, ear, nose and throat specialist on the staff, it was only in 1905 with Dr. Burgess's arrival that the medical staff recognised EENT as a speciality and established this specialist category in the staff roster. EENT thus has the distinction of being the oldest speciality service in the hospital's history. Dr. Burgess was born in 1866, near Apohaqui, graduated from provincial Normal School and taught in Westmorland and other parts of the province before entering medical school at Bellevue, from which he graduated in 1891. He served as a general practitioner in greater Shemogue and then took a specialist's course before setting up practice in Moncton as an eye, ear, nose and throat specialist. In 1922, he was made a Fellow of the American College of Surgeons. Outside his medical practice he was a keen golfer and curler. He died on December 13, 1943.

A new name that appeared on the attending staff list for 1905 was that of Dr. James Arthur McNaughton. Born on December 13, 1874, McNaughton graduated from McGill in 1902 and interned at the Royal Victoria Hospital in that year. He then practised in Salisbury before coming to Moncton. He soon established a reputation as a good obstetrician and delivered many babies over the years, including myself and several older members of the hospital's present medical staff. He also served many years on the anaesthetic staff before retiring in May 1950. My mother related to me that he never sent a bill and his patients eventually had to go to his office to find out how much they owed him.

The big news in 1906 was the laying of the cornerstone for the new Intercolonial Railway Shops by Hon. H.R. Emmerson on August 14. The big news for the hospital that year was the establishment of the School of Nursing. During the annual meeting in June, the president of the board had brought up the idea of opening a nursing school and nurses' house in connection with the hospital and a committee was appointed to examine the matter. F.W. Sumner suggested that a building be purchased rather than going to the extra expense of construction. The board subsequently exercised an option to purchase from William Marks, for the price of $2,400. a property opposite the hospital which would serve as a nurses' residence. The board had until January to come up with the money and once again the Ladies' Hospital Auxiliary came to the rescue, raising $2,000 toward the purchase. At this time we see the first evidence of an organization taking on the task of the upkeep of a room in the hospital when the women of Shediac furnished the "Shediac Room." At the annual meeting held on June 14, 1906, the president, J.S. Rayworth, was happy to report increased revenues for the year resulting from an increase in the number of paying patients. Expenses for the year were $8,352.34, with an over expenditure of $711.88 due to capital expenditures.

Visiting staff appointed for the 1906-07 year were Dr. Ferguson, Dr. White, Dr. Purdy, Dr. Price, Dr. Myers and Dr. McNaughton. Dr. Burgess was appointed as specialist staff and Dr. Ross and Chandler as consulting staff.

During the year, 312 patients were admitted, of which 223 were paying and 89 non-paying. There were 78 medical cases and 234 surgical cases with 218 operations performed; 258 patients were discharged as cured with 10 improved, 7 not treated, and 5 incurable. There were 12 deaths. There were 162 patients from the city, 71 from Westmorland County, 39 from Kent County, 11 from Albert County and 26 from other counties and towns.

At the annual meeting of the hospital board on January 12, 1907, the treasurer reported operating expenses of $11,591.29. One member of the board, F.W. Sumner, raised the point that the banks being established in the city should become subscribers to the hospital as part of their civic duty. In his remarks, the president, J.S. Rayworth, noted that the nurses' residence had been purchased during the year with the help of $2,000 raised by the Ladies' Auxiliary. During 1907, 307 patients were admitted to hospital, 76 as medical patients and 231 as surgical cases. The average length of stay was 17.77 days and 255 patients were discharged as cured, 8 improved, 4 not improved, 4 incurable, and 2 left against advice. There were 21 deaths in hospital that year. There were 212 paying and 95 non-paying patients.

The medical staff appointed for the coming year were Dr. Ferguson, Dr. White, Dr. Bourque, Dr. Harris, Dr. L.H. Price with Dr. S.W. Burgess as specialist. Consultants appointed were Dr. J.D. Ross and Dr. J.A. McNaughton. Dr. O.B. Price was appointed dentist on the staff. With the exception of 1906, when Dr. C.A. Murray was the dentist, it appears that Dr. Price had served as dentist to the hospital since its inception. Dr. Price subsequently became a member of Parliament, the only member of the hospital staff to obtain this position. The secretary at the annual meeting was instructed to advise the medical staff that they had the privilege of electing a physician to represent them on the board.

At the annual meeting of June 10, 1908, held in city council chambers, a communication was read from Miss Agnes McSweeney, president of the Ladies' Hospital Auxiliary, requesting that they have representation on the board consisting of the president of the group and one other representative. The matter was postponed until the next meeting, but when Mr. Harris tried to bring the subject up again at the meeting it was pointed out that the bylaws at present would not permit these appointments. Mr. Jones gave his treasurer's report, which showed expenditures during the year of $10,285.62 with an overdraft at the bank of $867.56. It was noted that Kent County Council had voted $200 as a grant to the hospital, but the treasurer of Kent County informed the hospital that there was no money in the treasury to pay this amount. After serving faithfully as treasurer for ten years, Mr. Jones submitted his resignation at this meeting. The new executive elected was: F.W. Sumner, president; James Doyle, vice-president; H.F. Hamilton, secretary; and J.H. Harris, treasurer. At the conclusion of this annual meeting the outgoing president, J.S. Rayworth, entertained the board members by treating them to ice cream at Miss McGee's Restaurant.

Statistics for the year show a dramatic decrease in the length of stay to 7.52 days. During the year, 386 patients were admitted, of which 301 were surgical and 82 medical cases. There were 228 private and 158 public patients and the patients discharged were classified as 320 cured, 11 improved, 3 not treated, 3 incurable, and 2 left against advice. Among the medical cases admitted were 82 cases of typhoid fever, one resulting in death. Among the surgical operations performed were 92 appendectomies.

The medical staff appointed for the 1908-09 year were: Dr. W.B.

Ferguson, Dr. F.J. White, Dr. L.H. Price, Dr. L.C. Harris, Dr. J.A. McNaughton and Dr. C.T. Purdy. Dr. S.W. Burgess was appointed as specialist, Dr. J.D. Ross and Dr. F.A. Richard as consultants, and Dr. C.A. Murray as dentist.

In 1908, the Isolation Hospital on North Street was sold and planning was begun to convert the old Albert Street residence of Christian Trites, built around 1800, into a new Isolation Hospital facility with a capacity of forty beds. Following its completion, this remained as a separate hospital until the Moncton Hospital opened its own isolation ward in a separate building, the Dunlop House, in 1921.

The annual meeting for 1909 was held at the usual location, city council chambers, with the following trustees present: F.W. Sumner, president, George B. Willett, W.D. Martin, J.M. Lyons, B. Toombs, Dr. O.J. McCully, J.H. Harris, James Doyle, J.S. Rayworth, J.S. Geary and H.F. Hamilton. A Mr. Saulnier from Harcourt and a Mr. C. Campbell from Sackville attended the meeting as representatives of the counties. The president pointed out that the number of patients treated over the past year had increased by 25 percent from 311 to 497. He also noted that a large number of outpatients were treated at the hospital. At the rear of the hospital, on land donated by L.H. Harris, an ice house had been built. It was reported that a sterilizer was supplied by the nursing staff. Other work done during the year included painting of the hospital's walls. The treasurer reported expenditures during the year of $12,656.15 with a bank balance of $282.03.

Of the 497 admissions that year 292 were private patients and 205 were public patients. 395 surgical and 102 medical cases were treated with 428 discharged as cured, 9 improved, 6 not treated, 6 incurable and 2 left against advice. There were 26 deaths.

Miss MacEachern stayed on as superintendent of the hospital long enough to see the first class of nurses graduate from the School of Nursing in 1909 at a public ceremony in the Pythian Temple. Although subsequently resigning her post to marry Dr. Ferguson, she always remained a strong supporter of the hospital, serving on the board of Trustees. She was prominent in all aspects of welfare and community work, being one of the organizers of the Canadian Red Cross Society in Moncton and its first president. She was also the first president of the Moncton Council of Women, which was organized after the first World War. Mrs. Ferguson served as president of the VON for many years and was honorary regent of the Bonar Law Chapter of the IODE. She was interested in children's welfare and was one of those instrumental in having the Children's Aid Shelter built in Moncton. After the death of her husband, Mrs. Ferguson resided in Charlottetown and died there on October 2, 1960, at the age of 85 years. Her remains were brought to Moncton to be interred beside her husband's in Elmwood cemetery.

When Miss MacEachern resigned as superintendent, the position was filled by Miss Sophie MacDonald, formerly the assistant superintendent.

The first two nurses to graduate from the School of Nursing were Miss

Lillian Barnes and Miss A.J. MacMaster, who later would play a dominant role in the history of the hospital. In 1909 there were twelve nurses in training and one probationer at the school and it had no trouble obtaining students since there were 30 applications on its file. The medical staff of the hospital participated in the education of the student nurses by giving lectures, a practice that continued until the school closed in 1975. The lecturers in 1909 were as follows:

Dr. L.C. Harris	Anaesthetics
Dr. F.J. White	Anatomy and Physiology
Dr. F.A. Richard	Materia Medica
Dr. L.N. Bourque	Obstetrics
Dr. J.A. McNaughton	Medical Diseases
Miss Janet MacEachern	Anatomy, Materia Medica & Nursing
Miss S.G. MacDonald	Theory of Obstetrics and Practical Nursing

The medical staff appointed at the hospital for the 1909-10 year were: Dr. W.B. Ferguson, Dr. F.J. White, Dr. L.C. Harris, Dr. L.H. Price, Dr. L.N. Bourque and Dr. J.A. McNaughton, with Dr. O.J. McCully listed as a specialist and Dr. F.A. Richard and Dr. Gaius Smith as consulting staff.

During the first decade of the century it is apparent that doctors were quite active in civic politics and community affairs. Dr. E.O. Steeves, Dr. F.J. White and Dr. C.T. Purdy all served as mayors of Moncton and Dr. G.T. Smith and Dr. L.N. Bourque served as aldermen. Dr. Bourque was obviously the most politically minded, serving twelve terms on city council at various times until his last term in 1921. No doctor on the medical staff has sat on the city council since then, except for Dr. J.A. Gaudet, who served as an aldermen in 1931 and 1932. Dr. F.J. White, Dr. E.B. Chandler, Dr. L.C. Harris, Dr. L.H. Price and Dr. W.B. Ferguson were all charter members of the Moncton Club which was incorporated in 1909. Dr. Leverett H. Price was an avid golfer and owned the Lakeside Golf Club. Dr. L.H. Price and Dr. White were both gun enthusiasts having served as president and vice-president respectively of the Moncton Rifle Club in 1899.

Chapter Three

The Teens— Growing Pains and the Great War

Moving into the second decade of this century, F.W. Sumner, president of the board, noted at the annual meeting of January 13, 1910, held in city council chambers, that the number of patients treated during the year had decreased. This decrease was attributed to the fact that the Grand Trunk Pacific Railway was not employing nearly as many men as it had previously with the construction of the new shops being nearly complete. A decrease in the number of public patients admitted from the city of Moncton was reported, a sign of the positive employment prospects in the city at the time, but there was an increase in the number of public patients from Westmorland and Kent counties. A considerable increase in the number of outpatients treated was recorded. Mr. Sumner pointed out that there had been no complaints from patients treated on the public wards. Work carried out on the hospital's facilities during the year consisted of repainting all the private rooms and painting and papering of all the rooms in the nurses' residence. Expenditures by the hospital during the year were $11,227.87 with a balance in the bank at the end of the year of $255.91.

Three issues were brought forward at this 1910 meeting, two of which would be resolved in the next few years while the other, the opening of a maternity service, would not be resolved until 1923. Dr. L.C. Harris proposed to the board that an X-ray machine be obtained and a committee was appointed to meet with him to negotiate the procurement of a machine for installation. The different lodges of the Intercolonial Railway (ICR) had pledged to the hospital board that they would raise sufficient funds to install an X-ray machine, but at this time there was not sufficient room to do that so the board was again faced with the necessity of enlarging the hospital. Mr. Sumner also drew the board's attention to the need of a maternity ward. The need in the community, he stated, was apparent at this time and he felt some action was necessary in the next year. Mr. Sumner also noted that, although two nurses had been presented with their diplomas at a graduation ceremony, three more nurses, Mildred Fraser, Alice Dalton and Katherine Scott had finished their training and some public recognition and presentation of diplomas would be arranged for them shortly. With the increasing number of students at the School of Nursing, he stated that the enlargement of the nurses' residence would also have to be given present consideration.

Until this time, all the doctors who were permitted to treat public patients in the hospital were appointed by the board, apparently in an arbitrary manner, although all the doctors in the community could treat private patients in the hospital. A new by-law was passed prior to the annual meeting, providing that all duly-registered medical practitioners in Moncton should have the opportunity of attending to patients in the public wards. The secretary of the hospital accordingly wrote to all physicians in the city informing them of the proposed changes and requesting applications for positions on the hospital medical staff. It was proposed that there be three divisions of staff: visiting, consulting and specialist. J.H. Harris moved and J.S. Rayworth seconded a resolution that the visiting staff consist of six members. Dr. McCully made an amendment to the motion, seconded by Mr. Toombs, that the visiting staff consist of eight members but the amendment was defeated and the visiting staff was set at six. A motion was passed that the consulting staff consist of four members. Applications to join the staff were received from Dr. J.A. McNaughton, Dr. H.H. Coleman, Dr. F.J. White, Dr. S.W. Burgess, Dr. R.L. Botsford, Dr. L.C. Harris, Dr. G.T. Smith, Dr. C.T. Purdy, Dr. A.R. Myers, Dr. O.J. McCully, Dr. L.N. Bourque, Dr. L.H. Price and Dr. W.B. Ferguson. All of these were appointed, making up the following staff:

Visiting:	Dr. White, Dr. Bourque, Dr. Price, Dr. Ferguson, Dr. McNaughton and Dr. Myers.
Specialists:	Dr. McCully, Dr. Smith and Dr. Burgess.
Consulting:	Dr. Purdy, Dr. Harris, Dr. Botsford and Dr. Coleman.

There were 436 patients admitted to hospital in 1910, of which 327 were classified as surgical cases and 108 as medical. Of the patients, 241 were private and 195 public; 361 patients were discharged as cured, 19 improved, 4 not treated, 5 incurable and 2 left against advice. There were 25 deaths with 8 of them occurring within 48 hours of admission. Religion and the churches played a large role in the community in these days and, although the hospital was non sectarian, it recorded in its reports each year the religions of the patients. In 1910, these included: Adventist (1), Baptist (105), Episcopal (32), Hebrew (1), Jewish (1), Methodist (54), Presbyterian (51), Roman Catholic (181) and Salvation Army (7).

In 1911, all legally qualified medical practitioners resident in the city continued to be eligible to treat private patients in the hospital and for appointment to the medical staff for the care of the public ward patients. The staff was divided into visiting staff, a consulting staff consisting of two or more and a specialist staff of one or more for EENT. The medical staff had restrictions on the patients to be admitted to the hospital. Psychiatry had not yet been integrated into the hospital system, as no insane or lunatic person was to be admitted. Moreover, no incurable patients were to be admitted without the permission of the board and it was decreed that any patient who had been admitted who was proven to be incurable was to be removed. In these days, people obviously expected to die at home in their own beds. Finally, no patient with any contagious disease was to be admitted. All professional services at the hospital were to be gratuitous, except in the case of private patients.

At the annual meeting on June 14, 1911, the staff appointed for 1911-12 were as follows:

Visiting:	Dr. White, Dr. Myers, Dr. Ferguson, Dr. Price, Dr. Bourque and Dr. Harris
Specialists:	Dr. McCully, Dr. Smith and Dr. Burgess
Consulting:	Dr. Purdy, Dr. Steeves, Dr. McNaughton, Dr. Coleman and Dr. Richard.

In 1911, rules for the patients were quite strict by today's standards. Back then, all ward patients were required to be in their proper place at meal times and during the visits of physicians and surgeons. In the evening they were to be in their own place by 8 o'clock and actually in bed at 9 o'clock. Male patients were not permitted to enter the female ward and vice versa. No food or liquor was to be brought in by visitors and if this were done, the items had to be handed over to the superintendent. Patients admitted free of charge were allowed to have visitors only from 2 to 4 on Tuesday and Friday and 3 to 5 on Sunday. Visitors for private patients, however, were permitted at any time during the day but had to have permission from the superintendent to remain at night. Any patient bringing liquor into the hospital or found intoxicated was to be discharged. It is interesting to note that in Mr. Sumner's annual report he stated that there were no complaints of any kind from any patients.

In 1911, admissions increased to 458 patients with 281 paying and 177 public patients. There were 338 surgical patients and 120 medical patients, with 287 operations performed. Among the operations performed were: 30 T&As, 38 appendectomies, 4 cholecystectomies, 10 circumcisions, 1 caesarean section, 5 D&C's, 5 enucleation of eye, 8 inguinal hernia, 7 hysterectomies, 6 prostatectomies, 20 I&D's and one operation for a submerged clitoris! We often seem to think that we are living in a more violent society today, but in 1911 there were 6 operations performed for gunshot wounds. Twenty-one deaths occurred during the year. Out of a budget of $11,246.32, paying patients provided revenues of $6,291.35, leaving $4,954.97 to be covered by the public purse.

Miss Sophie MacDonald resigned as superintendent in this year and was replaced in February 1912 by Miss Blanche MacDonald.

The annual meeting for 1912 was held as usual, in the city hall, with the full board in attendance. In his report, the president, Mr. Sumner, stated that the hospital would buy the Dunlop house for a nurses' residence and pay the

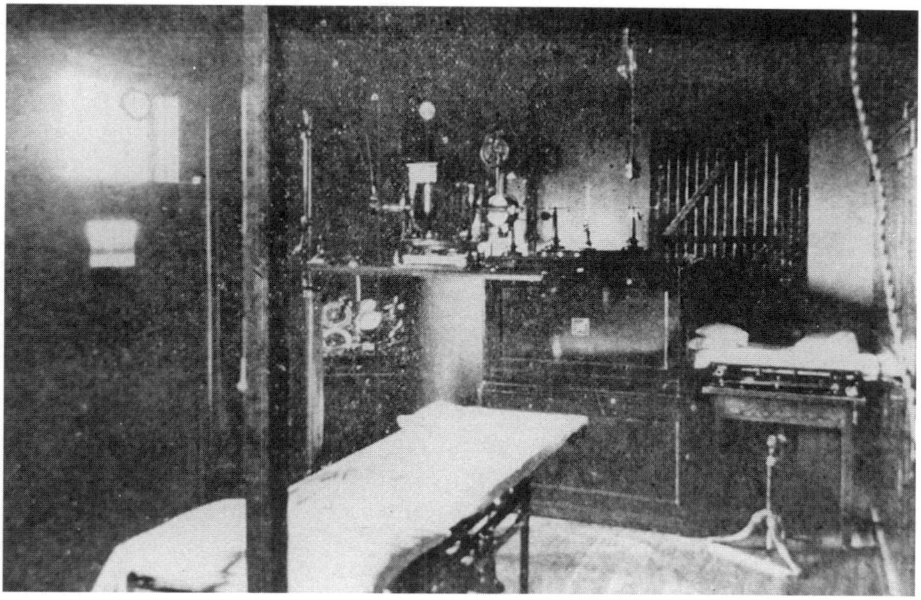

The first X-ray equipment at The Moncton Hospital.

difference in value if the owner, Mr. Fergus, would take the present nurses' residence in trade. For the hospital proper, Mr. Sumner advocated that it be supplied with an up-to-date electric elevator. At the regular monthly meeting, held just prior to the annual meeting, Dr. Taylor had reported to the board that, following the proposal of Dr. Harris at the previous year's annual meeting to purchase one, he had visited the leading hospitals in Boston and New York and looked into X-ray machines. He was of the opinion that the Coil machine was a better machine compared to the Transformer machine. A committee consisting of Dr. H. Coleman as chairman, James Geary, James Doyle and H. Hamilton were selected to investigate the purchase of a machine. It is not recorded which machine they bought, but, true to their word, the railway brotherhoods contributed $750 towards its purchase. The treasurer reported a good year with receipts of $12,910.44 with a bank balance of $822.37.

The question of increasing the visiting staff from six to eight again became an issue with a motion by Dr. Coleman, but Mr. Harris moved an amendment that the visiting staff consist of six doctors and the amendment carried. The visiting staff, then appointed for the coming year, consisted of Dr. White, Dr. Ferguson, Dr. Price, Dr. Bourque, Dr. Myers and Dr. Purdy. The specialists (EENT) were Dr. G. Smith and Dr. Burgess while the consulting staff were Dr. Coleman and Dr. F.A. Richard. In previous years the superintendent had appointed the lecturers to the School of Nursing but this year the superintendent felt that this task should be assumed by the board and a committee consisting of Dr. Coleman, Mr. Sumner and Mr. Harris was appointed to name the lecturers for the coming year. When the X-ray machine was purchased, Dr. George Taylor left Moncton to take a special course in its operation and on returning, was appointed as the hospital's first radiologist. Dr. Taylor held the job for only about two years, however, before it was taken over by Dr. F.A. Richard, who continued in that position for the next 30 years.

There were 581 admissions that year, with 489 patients discharged as cured, 21 improved, 11 incurable, 7 not treated, 1 left against advice and 33 patients died. There were 411 private patients and 171 public. The average length of stay was 11.2 days.

On June 11, 1913, a long and protracted annual meeting of the hospital board was held in council chambers with the president, F.W. Sumner, in the chair. Other members of the board present included the secretary, Mr. H. Hamilton, the treasurer, Mayor W.K. Gross, Mr. J.H. Harris, E. Girouard, A.H. Jones, J.A. Geary, J.S. Rayworth, Dr. H.H. Coleman, Sheriff Willett, Dr. M.A. Oulton, councillor for the parish of Westmorland, and Albenie Bourque, councillor for the parish of Moncton. In his remarks, Mr. Sumner stated his wish that more county councillors would attend the meetings of the board and also visit the hospital and see what they were contributing their money towards. "Not enough visit the hospital and have no conception of the great work carried on there," he said. He stated that he believed the hospital was equal to any in Lower Canada, if not the whole Dominion. All of this served as a prelude to his noting that the number of patients had increased in the last year and that the board would have to ask for larger grants from the city and counties, suggesting $3,000 from the city and $5,000 from the counties. The budget in the 1911-12 fiscal year was $20,256.08 with a bank overdraft of $3949.20. It was reported that the Ladies' Auxiliary had donated $1,000 worth of linen in the past year and Mr. Sumner stated that he had a conversation with Mrs. S.L. Shannon and Mrs. F.C. Jones and he felt that, with a little encouragement, they would undertake to raise the funds for a new nurses' residence. At the time, there were 9 nurses in training and 5 probationers and as the nurses' residence only had 7 bedrooms and 1 bath, it was thought that a residence with 12 bedrooms and 4 baths would be needed.

During 1912-13, 679 patients were admitted to hospital of which 523 were surgical cases and 156 medical. There were 447 private and 232 public patients; 555 patients were discharged as cured, 38 improved, 4 not improved, 4 incurable and 16 not treated. 30 patients died, with 10 of the deaths occurring within 48 hours of their admission and 8 out of the 10 within 24 hours.

At the annual meeting held on June 12, 1914, Dr. Oulton, the county councillor for Westmorland, reported that at the last county meeting a motion was passed that the hospital be asked to appoint two doctors from the county to the consulting staff of the hospital. The board agreed to this request and appointed Dr. M.A. Oulton from Shediac and Dr. J.O. Calkins of Sackville to the consulting staff. The remaining staff continued as in the previous year except for the appointment of Dr. George Taylor as Operator of X-ray.

Appointments to the staff at the annual meeting of June 10, 1914, with the vice-president, James Doyle, in the chair included:

Visiting:	Dr. Ferguson, Dr. Myers, Dr. J.A. McNaughton, Dr. White, Dr. Bourque and Dr. Price
ENT Specialists:	Dr. G. Smith and Dr. S.W. Burgess.
Consultants:	Dr. Coleman and Dr. Purdy, and from the county, Dr. J.O. Calkins (Sackville) and Dr. H. H. Jones (Salisbury).

The only applicant not elected was the new man on the block, Dr. Paul Atkinson, who only moved to Moncton from Salisbury that year.

During this meeting it was moved by Dr. Coleman, and seconded by Mr. Harris, that Dr. F.A. Richard be reelected as X-ray operator. Sometime during the past year, Dr. Richard must have replaced Dr. Taylor, who later appears on the staff listing as a pediatrician.

In the year ending May 31, 1914, the statistics show use of the hospital growing by a fair amount with 747 patients admitted, 422 male and 325 female. Of these, 482 were private patients and 265 were public patients. There were 191 admissions to the medical service with 10 admissions for alcoholism, 15 cases of syphilis and 31 patients with typhoid fever resulting in 3 deaths. The surgical service remained the busiest service with 556 surgical cases admitted and 463 operations being performed. Surgery carried considerable risk in these days as may be attested to by the fact there were 53 appendectomies performed with 2 deaths and 8 prostatectomies with 3 deaths. Operative treatment of fractures was coming into vogue about this time and 3 platings of the femur and one of the humerus were recorded this year. The operating budget for the year was $21,362.33. The hospital announced at this time that it was prepared to supply private duty nurses at $10 a week or $1.50 a day.

There were no changes in the medical staff in 1915, except for the dental staff appointment, which usually changed yearly, and that year's appointment was Dr. O.B. Price. The mortality rate with surgery showed an improvement this year with 50 appendectomies performed with no deaths and 11 prostatectomies with only one death. T&A's were becoming the operation of the day with 120 performed. There were only 2 cholecystectomies and 2 caesarean sections performed and 1 cataract operation. Gunshot wounds remained a problem with 3 admissions, one of which was a fatal gunshot wound to the abdomen. Typhoid fever remained a medical problem, accounting for 24 admissions. There were also 24 admissions for tuberculosis.

The year 1916 saw the addition of two new members to the medical staff who would continue to serve the hospital until past the halfway mark of the century, Dr. A. Raymond Landry and Dr. Paul McL. Atkinson. Dr. Landry, the son of Sir Pierre Landry, a chief justice of New Brunswick, was born in Dorchester. He obtained his BSc from St. Joseph's College in 1903 and graduated from McGill Medical School in 1907. He then pursued an internship and postgraduate work at the Royal Victoria Hospital in Montreal and subsequently studied surgery in Paris for two years. When the Royal College of Physicians and Surgeons was formed, he was the only Moncton doctor made a Fellow of the Royal College of Surgeons. He died in 1957.

Paul McL. Atkinson was born in Amherst, Nova Scotia, on October 17, 1886. In 1903 he graduated from the New Brunswick Normal School. Leaving the teaching profession after a few years, he graduated from McGill Medical School in 1909. He interned at the Montreal General Hospital in 1909-10 and, after practising in Petitcodiac, moved to Moncton in 1914. He received his FACS in 1931. Dr. Brent Stewart in his *Medicine in New Brunswick* relates a humorous anecdote. Dr. Atkinson and Dr. L.H. Price were delegated to get a supply of liquor for a New Brunswick Medical Society Convention in Moncton. This being prohibition days, they left after dark with a $100 to seek out their supplier in Cocaine. They returned home to Moncton after midnight, sampling some of their wares on the return journey. As a consequence, Paul managed to drive his car straight through his garage into the neighbour's yard resulting in an upset wife along with recriminations from his neighbours. Dr. Stewart also mentions an incident that I can recall personally, that occurred to Dr. Atkinson in his later years. He suffered from diabetes then, and one day took a weak spell while driving his car on MacBeath Avenue. The car ended up in the centre of the boulevard up the guy wire of a telephone pole.

Dr. Atkinson served as coroner for many years, and was always very stingy in spending the public's money. If a person had died unexpectedly at home it was the doctor's responsibility to notify the coroner. Paul always had one question to ask "Is there any evidence of foul play?" If the answer was "No" Atkinson would deem an autopsy unnecessary. Any unexpected death was just one of those poor unfortunate things!

The annual meeting of the board, held on June 14, 1916, was held in the board of trade room at the YMCA. There was an unusually large attendance and anyone who paid $1 was eligible to vote. The treasurer reported that expenses of running the hospital in 1916 totalled $29,594.35. The board members had been incensed earlier that year when they learned that the provincial government gave a grant of $4,300 to the hospital in Saint John and only $700 to the Moncton Hospital. James S. Rayworth resigned from the board and the terms of office for three of the members, H.F. Hamilton, J.M. Lyons and E. Girouard, had expired. Nine of the members of the previous board were reelected and the new members selected were Reid McManus, Frank P. Murphy and Camille Belliveau. A.H. Jones and Sheriff Willett expressed regret at losing Mr. Hamilton as secretary of the board, and said that he should have the office after having served faithfully since the opening of the hospital. They both offered to resign to make room for him on the board but Mr. Hamilton declined under the circumstances. A new slate was elected to the executive of the board that year composed of James

Doyle, president; C.W. Robinson, vice-president and Reid McManus, treasurer. Mr. Jones and Mr. Willett then submitted their resignations but apparently they were not accepted. Mr. Hamilton must somehow have been elected as secretary again and the squabble was patched over temporarily. As we shall see, Mr. Hamilton, Mr. Jones, Mr. Willett, James Doyle and Hon. C.W. Robinson were all to resign from the board at the regular monthly meeting held just prior to the 1917 annual meeting.

In her report to the board, the hospital superintendent, Miss L.E. Corbett, indicated that 559 private and 240 public patients, for a total of 799, were admitted during the year, of which 580 were surgical and 219 medical; 629 patients were discharged as cured, 47 improved, 19 not improved, 10 incurable, 17 not treated and 45 patients died. While typhoid fever was on the wane, a new condition, "La Grippe," made its appearance and accounted for 20 admissions. The medical service saw 15 admissions for alcoholism and 12 for syphilis. There were 580 surgical admissions with 485 operations performed. Appendectomies again led the list with 69 performed. There were 16 circumcisions, 6 caesarean sections and 16 hysterectomies. There were 7 suprapubic prostatectomies performed and 2 peroneal prostatectomies. The latter could not have become too popular as the procedure is never mentioned again in later years. There were 4 fractured femurs admitted, 2 of which resulted in death. Multiple trauma had a pretty grim prognosis; there was one case of "accident," presumably multiple trauma, admitted in 1916, one in 1915 and two in 1914, all of which resulted in death. One case of an infected foot with tetanus is reported and had a fatal outcome. This year saw the establishment of an outpatient service, although treatments were given in the operating room due to lack of space. There were 100 electrical treatments and 57 bladder irrigations given.

In 1917, we see a change in the board with a lot of the old guard submitting their resignations including James Doyle, Hon. C.W. Robinson, A.H. Jones, G.B. Willett and Hugh Hamilton. Mr. Jones, in his letter of resignation, felt that after twenty years it was time for someone else to replace him on the board. The new executive chosen for the board was as follows: president, A. Cavour Chapman; vice-president, John H. Harris; treasurer, Reid McManus; secretary, F.W.S. Colpitts. Mr. Chapman would continue as chairman of the board until 1943, the longest serving board chairman in the hospital's history.

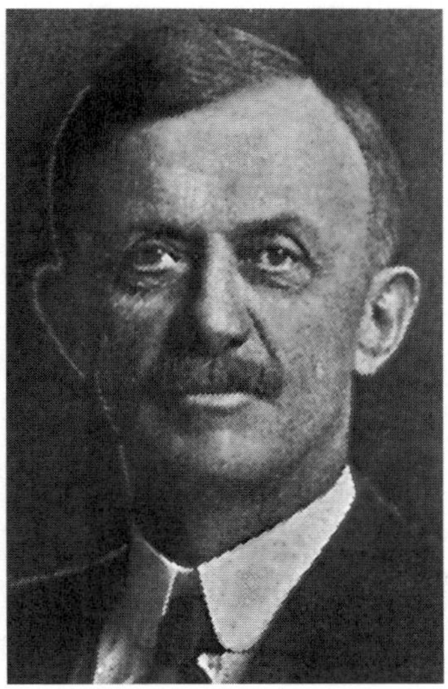

Mr. A. Cavour Chapman—Chairman of the Board from 1917-1943.

The medical staff selected for the 1917-18 year were as follows:

Visiting:	Dr. McNaughton, Dr. Ferguson, Dr. White, Dr. Bourque, Dr. Purdy and Dr. Atkinson
Consulting:	Dr. Botsford, Dr. Coleman, Dr. W.G. King (Petitcodiac) and Dr. J.O. Calkins (Sackville)
Oculist and Aurist	Dr. C.W. Burgess
X-ray Operator	Dr. Richard
Dental Surgeon	Dr. C.A. Murray.

In 1918, a change in the designation of the staff in the by-laws occurred. The consulting staff was to consist of four members, two from the City of Moncton and two from the County of Westmorland. The medical staff was divided into medical and surgical divisions. The medical staff was to consist of six members and the surgical staff of not fewer than three. Two physicians and one surgeon were to serve for two-month periods. Cases were assigned by the superintendent. Patients with private rooms were allowed to employ their own physicians as long as they were legally licensed practitioners residing in Moncton. No major operations were to be performed without giving notice to the consulting staff. Again, the rules forbade admitting any person believed to be incurable or insane. Infectious diseases were to be admitted only to an infected ward. No person suffering from VD or DT's was to be admitted but this rule could not have been strictly enforced as statistics record many admissions for alcoholism and syphilis.

In the annual report for the year ending May 31, 1918, the following staff were appointed for the 1918-19 year:

Surgeons:		
Dr. W.B. Ferguson	July, Aug. 1918	Jan., Feb. 1919
Dr. A.R. Myers	Sept., Oct. 1918	March, April 1919
Dr. F.J. White	Nov., Dec. 1918	May, June 1919
Physicians:		
Dr. McNaughton and Dr. Bourque	July, August 1918	Jan., Feb. 1919
Dr. Coleman and Dr. Landry	Sept., Oct. 1918	March, April 1919
Dr. Jones and Dr. Atkinson	Nov., Dec. 1918	May, June 1919
Eye:	Dr. S.W. Burgess	
Radiologist:	Dr. F.A. Richard	
Consulting Staff:	Dr. E.B. Chandler and Dr. L.H. Price—Moncton Dr. W.G. King—Petitcodiac Dr. J.A. Gaudet—St. Joseph	

Since there was no obstetrical service at The Moncton Hospital in 1918, student nurses were sent to Saint Luke's Hospital in New Bedford,

Massachusetts, for a three-month training period in obstetrics and infant feeding. In the year ending May 31, 1918, there were 856 admissions of which 694 were surgical and 162 medical. There were 574 private patients and 282 public patients. The average length of stay was 11 days. Typhoid fever remained a problem with 31 admissions but with no deaths recorded. There were 25 admissions for La Grippe, 10 for pneumonia, 7 for syphilis and 24 for tuberculosis. T&A was the most popular operation accounting for 149 of the 613 operations performed. Appendectomies came a close second with 112 performed. There were 12 hysterectomies performed and a new gynaecological operation arrived on the scene at this time with 12 operations for shortening of the round ligament recorded. The outpatient service continued to grow with 1,341 dressings, 149 bladder irrigations, 31 rectal exams, 157 vaginal exams, 50 plaster casts, 30 electrical treatments, 94 ear, nose and throat treatments and six cystoscopic exams. 29 deaths occurred this year and 553 patients were discharged as cured, 104 improved, 10 not improved and 7 not treated.

In 1918 the spread of the Spanish Influenza throughout North America was epidemic. The Moncton Hospital could not cope with the number stricken with this disease so on October 1, the Vestry, Brotherhood Hall and the Sunshine Room of the new First Baptist Church were turned into an emergency hospital of 25 beds to care for these patients. Dr. Hinson West, a medical missionary, who was home from India on furlough and who would later at the end of his career, become a staff member of the Moncton Hospital, served as house physician. He was assisted by Dr. L.H. Price. Armistice Day, November 11, 1918, marked the end of the crisis over the influenza epidemic and the temporary hospital was closed.

Two significant events occurred in the hospital in 1919. In August, Miss Alena J. MacMaster became superintendent and remained a dominant force in the hospital until she retired in 1947. The position also included being superintendent of the School of Nursing. Her influence in this role can be attested to by the fact that when the Moncton Hospital School of Nursing ceased to exist in 1975, the new school of nursing was named the A.J. MacMaster School of Nursing. On December 10, 1919, the Ladies' Auxiliary presented a Studebaker ambulance to the hospital, and the hospital said a fond farewell to the old horse-drawn ambulance. The care and maintenance

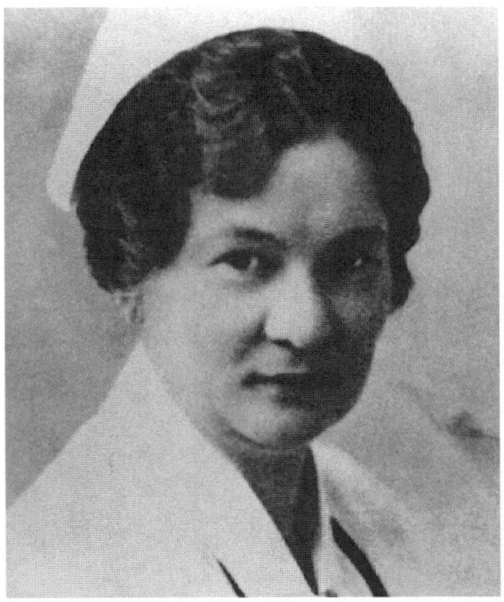

Miss A.J. MacMaster was the superintendent at The Moncton Hospital from 1919 until 1947.

of the ambulance became part of the workload of the Moncton Police Department. At a small cost, the hospital built a garage at Police Headquarters to house the ambulance.

At the annual meeting of the board, on June 12, 1919, a communication received from the Amalgamated Labour Unions was read stating that they believed labour was not sufficiently represented on the board and they submitted four names as candidates. At this time the board consisted of 25 members, 12 elected for two year terms and 13 appointed for one year terms. The annual meeting was open to the public. Moreover all who had contributed $25 since the hospital's opening were life members and those who had contributed $2 per year up to within 30 days of the end of the hospital year were eligible to vote. This year there were six vacancies to fill and after four ballots all the six whose terms were up were reelected. None of the labour candidates were elected and Mr. Chapman pointed out that the union men should have more men attend the meetings to support their candidates. The treasurer reported expenses of $33,530.91 with 77 percent of revenue coming from private patients. Appointments to the medical staff for the 1919-1920 year were as follows:

Surgeons:	Dr. Ferguson, Dr. White and Dr. Myers
Medical:	Dr. Bourque, Dr. Landry, Dr. Atkinson, Dr. Jones, Dr. McNaughton and Dr. Coleman
Consulting:	Dr. Botsford, Dr. Price and Dr. Sormany (Shediac), Dr. Calkins, (Sackville) for the County
EENT:	Dr. S.W. Burgess
X-ray Specialist:	Dr. Richard
Dental Surgeon:	Dr. F.E. Burden

In the annual report dated May 31, 1920, covering the period from June 1, 1919, to May 31, 1920, the number of private patients increased to 784 and the number of public patients decreased to 166, probably indicating some post war prosperity for the city. Post-war prosperity, however, did not bring better health. Typhoid fever reached a new height this year with 45 admissions accounting for four deaths. T&As still led the surgical list with 211, followed by appendectomies with 102. Shortening of the round ligament had lost favour with only one performed but attention was at this time directed towards the kidney as a source of abdominal pain, with 11 operations performed for suspension of the kidney. The outpatient service again showed an increase, especially in EENT, with 486 treatments. During the year, the work of the X-ray department doubled, as new equipment had been added during the year. There were 392 examinations carried out, of which 174 were done for fractures of the upper and lower extremities. There were 128 X-ray treatments carried out, 47 for epithelioma of the face, 26 for post-op cancer of the breast, 19 for Hodgkin's Disease and 5 for sarcoma. The use of the machine was not restricted to treatment of malignancies, moreover, as treatment was given for Banti's disease, TB glands, psoriasis and eczema.

Chapter Four

The Roaring Twenties—A Time to Expand

The period from 1920 to 1925 saw an expansion of the hospital and it is noteworthy that financing during this time was carried out on the personal notes of the board members on many occasions. On May 20, 1920, property adjacent to the hospital was acquired from W.F. Ferguson at a cost of $19,000. In 1921 an annex with twenty beds opened and that September the X-ray department was transferred to the new annex. An adjoining cottage was also remodelled to provide 16 beds for isolation cases. In December a passageway connecting the annex to the main hospital was completed. The pathological department also opened in 1920 but it operated mainly as a laboratory staffed by a technician. The City of Moncton was

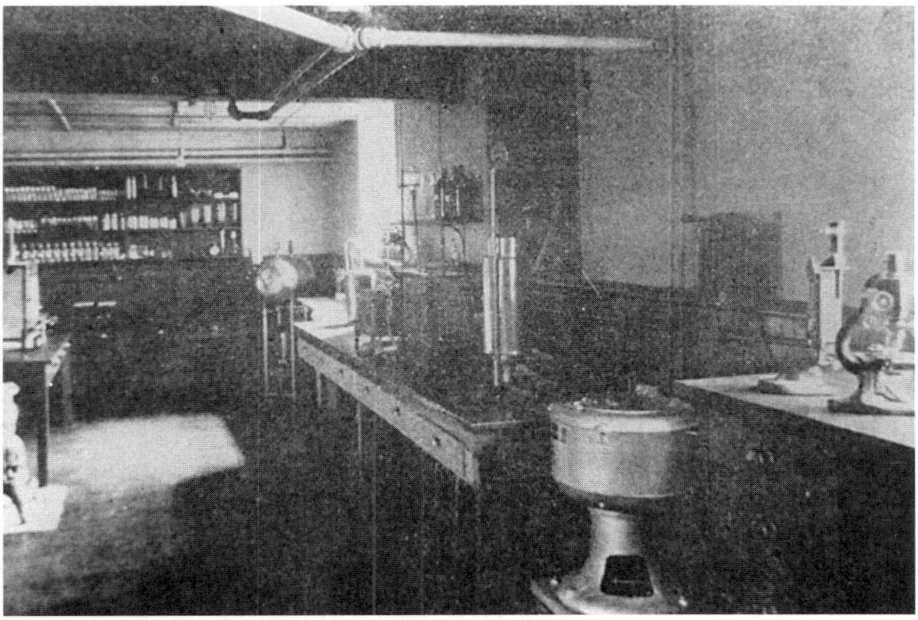

The Moncton Hospital's first laboratory in 1920.

asked to make a yearly contribution to the lab in exchange for which the department would provide free of charge examinations such as Widal for typhoid fever, mouth and throat cultures for diphtheria, sputum for tuberculosis and milk and water analysis.

In July 1921, in order to comply with the requirements of the American College of Surgeons, the attending physicians formed a staff association and began holding monthly staff meetings. In 1922, the hospital qualified as a standardized institution under the requirements of the American College of Surgeons. Dr. W.B. Ferguson, Dr. A.R. Myers, Dr. L.N. Bourque and Dr. S.W. Burgess were all awarded the Fellowship of the American College of Surgeons.

The year 1922 saw many new additions to the medical staff, listed as follows:

Senior Surgeons	Dr. W.B. Ferguson
	Dr. A.R. Myers
Junior Surgeons	Dr. H.A. Jones
	Dr. P.McL. Atkinson
	Dr. A.R. Landry
	Dr. W.P. Kirby
	Dr. H.E. Britton
Senior Physicians	Dr. L.N. Bourque
	Dr. J.A. McNaughton
Junior Physicians	Dr. George Lyons
	Dr. A.R. Forbes
Pediatrician	Dr. George O. Taylor
Anaesthetists	Dr. H.H. Coleman
	Dr. George Lyons (Alternate)
EENT Senior	Dr. S.W. Burgess
	Dr. R.A. Hughes
EENT Junior	Dr. H.C. LeBlanc
Roentgenologist	Dr. F.A. Richard
Consulting Staff	Dr. L.H. Price—City of Moncton
	Dr. H.H. Coleman—City of Moncton
	Dr. George Flemming—County of Westmorland
	Dr. C.E. Gaudet—County of Westmorland
Dental Surgeon	Dr. G.T. Leighton

Dr. Howe Alonzo Jones was a McGill graduate of 1900 and first practised in Salisbury before moving to Moncton.

Albert Ernest Forbes was born in Loch Katrine, Antigonish County, the son of a minister, and graduated from Dalhousie in 1900. He spent some time as senior house surgeon at the Victoria General Hospital in Halifax and later practised in Sydney. He subsequently moved to Upper Stewiacke and practised there for five years, after which he moved to Moncton. Soon after coming to Moncton, he was appointed one of the district coroners, a position he maintained until his death on March 17, 1936.

William B. Kirby, son of the Rev. W.J. Kirby, was born in Bayfield, Westmorland County, on March 20, 1882. He attended Prince of Wales College for one year and then attended business school. A career in business did not prove to be his niche and he subsequently received a BA from Mount Allison in 1904, and an MD from McGill in 1908. He first practised in Elgin and later Hillsborough. He came to Moncton at the urging of Dr. Ferguson, whom he assisted. Under Dr. Ferguson's guidance Dr. Kirby developed his surgical skills, establishing a reputation as a fine surgeon in his own right. His professional career was cut short when, after completing an operation on May 14, 1932, he sustained a stroke. He never regained consciousness and died on May 22, 1932, at the age of 49 years.

Dr. R.A. Hughs graduated from Queen's University in 1908 and came to Moncton after the First World War as a trained specialist in eye, ear, nose and throat surgery.

In 1920, Dr. G.T. Leighton was appointed as the dental surgeon. He was the father of Dr. Claude Leighton, who later became a very popular paediatrician on the hospital's staff and he was the grandfather of Dr. Ross Leighton, who served on the orthopaedic service.

Special mention must be made of the appointment to the staff of Dr. Britton and Dr. Lyons as they both had a long involvement with The Moncton Hospital. Dr. Harry Earl Britton was one of several Pictou County, Nova Scotia, men who sought careers in the medical profession. He was born in Westville on August 31, 1890. He was always known as "Jerry" although I'm not certain where the name came from. He obtained a BA from Dalhousie in 1914 and graduated with his MD, CM from McGill in 1917, after interning at the Montreal General Hospital. He went overseas with the Canadian Army Medical Corps and remained there for two and a half years, spending part of his time in postgraduate work in surgery. He returned to Canada in 1920 and set up practice in Moncton. He became a Fellow of the American College of Surgeons in 1927 and was certified in surgery by the Royal College of Physicians in 1944. He served as president of the Medical Council of New Brunswick and was president of the New Brunswick Medical Society in 1942-43. He was a member of the board of governors of the American College of Surgeons from 1959 to 1962 and was made a senior member of the Canadian Medical Association in June 1964. He was a big handsome man with a gruff manner, who seemed to be very popular with the railway workers and he had a large number of them as patients. Although he was known for his bluntness when giving a patient a poor prognosis, he was equally blunt when it applied to himself. It was discovered that he had an inoperable carcinoma, and during his convalescent period he made a visit to the surgeon's lounge. Someone asked him how he was, and he replied without hesitation that he was dying. This brought the room to complete silence. He died in 1968.

Dr. George Lyons had a personality that was in direct contrast to that of Dr. Britton. He was always soft-spoken and had a compassionate manner. He was born in Moncton on November 17, 1888, graduated from Saint Francis Xavier University, where he had been a star athlete, and received his MD from McGill in 1916. He went overseas with the Canadian Army Medical Corps. During this time with the corps, he survived the torpedoing of his ship in the Mediterranean. After the war he remained in England, doing post-graduate work at London Hospital in 1918-19, and at the Paddington Infirmary in 1919-20. During the Second World War he served as a colonel in the Royal Canadian Army Medical Corps. Dr. Lyons was in charge of the first venereal disease clinic at The Moncton Hospital. He resigned from the active staff in 1950, remaining on the courtesy staff until he retired in 1972. He died soon thereafter, at the age of 83.

There were 1,295 patients admitted to the hospital in 1922 with 64 deaths occurring in hospital. There were 1,027 private patients and 268 public patients. T&A remained the predominant operation with 304 performed, followed by appendectomies at 104. Four deaths were due to appendicitis complicated by peritonitis. There was still no obstetrical service at this time, but 3 births were recorded and these were caesarean sections. There were 445 X-ray exams carried out with 72 X-ray treatments given. The new pathological laboratory carried out 1,263 examinations, of which 812 were urinalysis, 127 blood counts, 92 smears, 24 Wassermanns, 40 cultures and 46 Widal exams. It bears noting that the hospital was a smoke-free environment at this time, with no smoking or chewing tobacco allowed. No unnecessary noise and no profane or vulgar language was to be tolerated in the hospital or, for that matter, on the grounds. National Hospital Day was observed this year for the first time, on May 12, and became a yearly event.

Two new names appear on the medical staff roster in 1923: Dr. R.G. Girvan was appointed as a senior physician and Dr. L.E. Goodridge as a junior specialist in ENT.

Robert Goldie Girvan was born in Rexton on February 7, 1877. He graduated from the Provincial Normal School in 1895 and from McGill in 1907 with his MD, CM degree. He first practised in Harcourt and later Rexton before moving to Moncton. He served on the anaesthetic staff for many years and retired from the staff in 1952, moving back to Harcourt.

L.A. Goodridge, affectionately known as "Speed," was born in Bridgetown, Barbados, on January 25, 1893. After receiving his MD from McGill in 1919, he interned at the Royal Victoria Hospital from 1919 to 1921. He trained in ear, nose and throat surgery at the London Central Hospital and the Hajeck Clinic in Vienna, joined the Colonial Register in 1922 and registered in New Brunswick in the same year. He received his FACS(C) in 1931. His association with The Moncton Hospital was to last for the next 50 years. He was appointed to the consulting staff in 1952 and the honorary staff in 1976. He was a lifelong bachelor and enjoyed sailing as a hobby. He was an astute investor and could be found every day at noon at his stockbroker's office getting the latest stock market quotations. His favourite advice was "Boys, buy bank stocks as the banks make money in both good and bad times." His advice obviously had some merit because when he died on October 20, 1982, he willed $2 million to Mount Allison University to establish the L.A. Goodridge Scholarship Fund for students interested in pursuing careers in the medical field.

Prior to 1923, the hospital, as previously noted, provided no obstetrical service. Babies were either delivered at home or in one of the area's nursing homes which provided obstetrical care. The only case in which a woman was admitted to hospital for childbirth was if a caesarean section was required. This changed in 1923 when the Annex was converted into a maternity department. There was not a great rush to use the new service, however, as there were only seven births recorded for the year and three of them were caesarean sections. Although I can find no record in the annual reports of an obstetrical service before 1923, J. Edward Belliveau, however, tells me that he was born in 1913 and his younger brothers in 1916 and 1919 at The Moncton Hospital and none were caesarean births.

Free laboratory service was started at this time for those examinations which came under the heading of Public Health for the City of Moncton. There was also a marked increase in the laboratory work as all patients admitted were to have a routine blood and urine examination in accordance with requirements of the American College of Surgeons. A flat rate of $5 per private patient and $2.50 per semi-private was charged to cover the service. In the annual report for this year thanks were extended to J.W. Ferguson, who cared for the sheep which were used for the laboratory work in performing Widal tests.

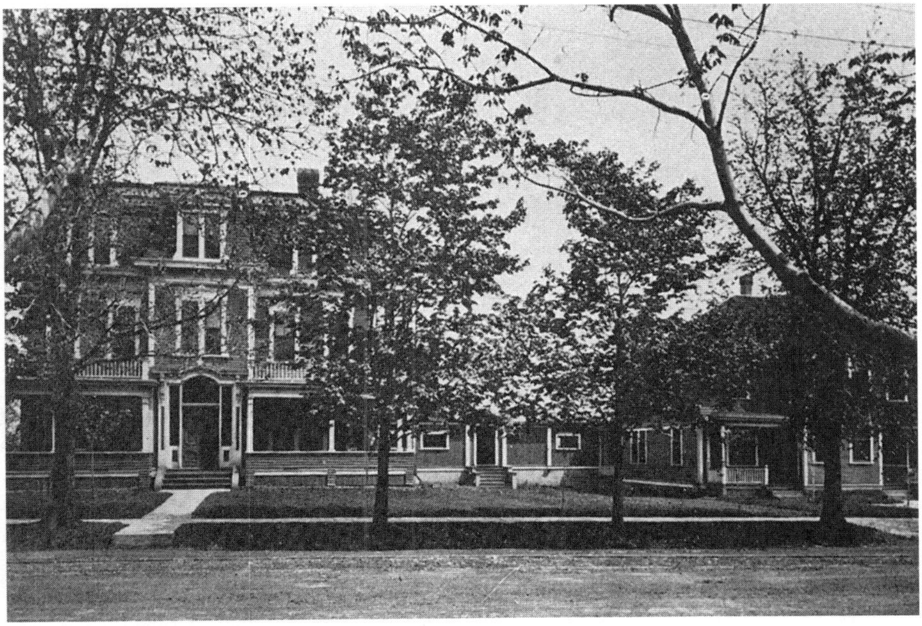

In 1924 the Maternity Annex (left) and the Isolation Unit (right) were connected to the main hospital by a passageway.

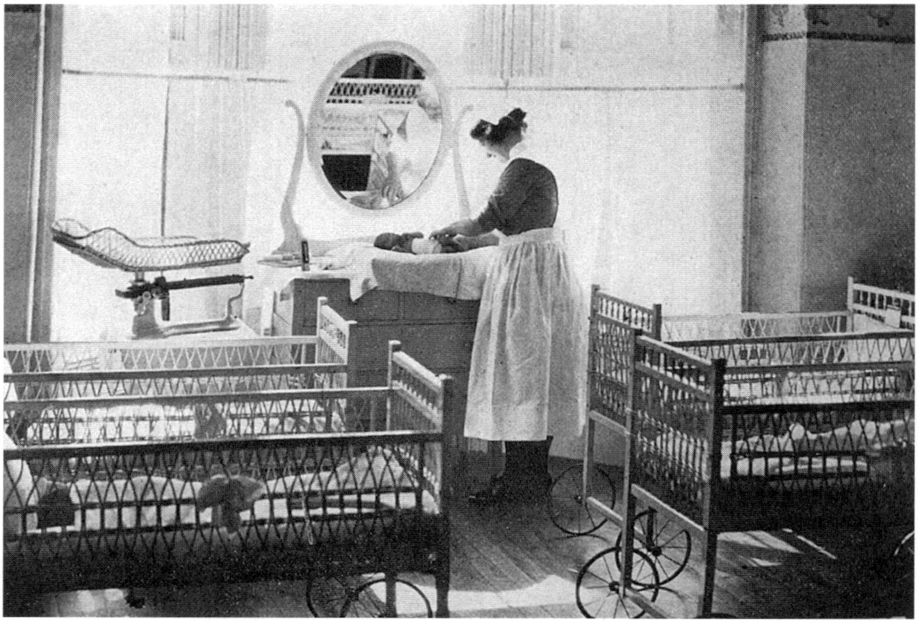

The first nursery at The Moncton Hospital.

During the year ending May 31, 1923, there were 1,118 patients admitted of which 199 of the patients were free patients. Typhoid fever was again on the wane with only 10 admissions. Among the other 150 medical admissions were 14 admissions for neurasthenia, 5 for grippe, 11 for influenza and 2 cases of diphtheria. Among the 937 operations performed were 249 T&As, 97 appendectomies, 12 circumcisions, 3 caesarean sections, 14 D&Cs, 25 herniotomies, 22 hysterectomies and 14 prostatectomies. It is noteworthy that there was 1 thyroidectomy, 1 thoracotomy and 1 transplantation of bone performed. There were 443 X-ray exams and 90 X-ray treatments performed. X-ray was still being used on benign skin lesions at this time with 3 ring worm and 3 dermatitis being treated. There were 61 deaths.

In 1924, Dr. J. Alfred Gaudet's name first appears as a junior physician. Dr. Gaudet was the son of Dr. Edward T. Gaudet of Memramcook. After graduation from the University of Chicago and a period of practice in St. Joseph's, he moved to Moncton. His brother, Camille, graduated from Laval Medical School in 1913 and practised in St. Joseph's for over 40 years.

In 1922, insulin was discovered by Banting and Best and this important development was not long in making its appearance in Moncton with the establishment of an insulin service for diabetics in 1924. New equipment purchased for the hospital during the year included a basal metabolism apparatus, which remained the mainstay for diagnosis of thyroid disease until the advent of nuclear medicine. Since it was considered inappropriate to transport those people with contagious diseases by the regular ambulance, a much needed conveyance (non-motorized) was provided for this purpose at the expense of the hospital. The year also saw the inauguration of free school clinics for T&As for children of parents in poor circumstances. The doctor's services were free and the hospital provided care for 8-12 hours with the child then being sent home under the supervision of the school nurse for the city. Dr. Wherett, a travelling diagnostician for the Department of Health, carried on chest clinics at the hospital. Thirty percent of those examined had either active or quiescent TB. A VD clinic was also being considered at this time. The maternity service was catching on with 82 births recorded in 1924. A semi-private ward of 6 beds was opened up that year increasing the hospital's maternity capacity to 20 beds.

In the annual report for the year ending May 31, 1925, the following staff were appointed for the 1925-26 year:

Senior Surgeons:	Dr. W.B. Ferguson
	Dr. A.R. Myers
	Dr. W.P. Kirby
Junior Surgeons:	Dr. J.A. McNaughton
	Dr. A.E. Forbes
	Dr. P. McL. Atkinson
	Dr. H.E. Britton
Senior Physicians:	Dr. H.A. Jones
	Dr. R.G. Girvan
Junior Physicians:	Dr. G.A. Lyons
	Dr. J. Alfred Gaudet
	Dr. J.E. Leger
Senior EENT:	Dr. S.W. Burgess
	Dr. R.A. Hughes

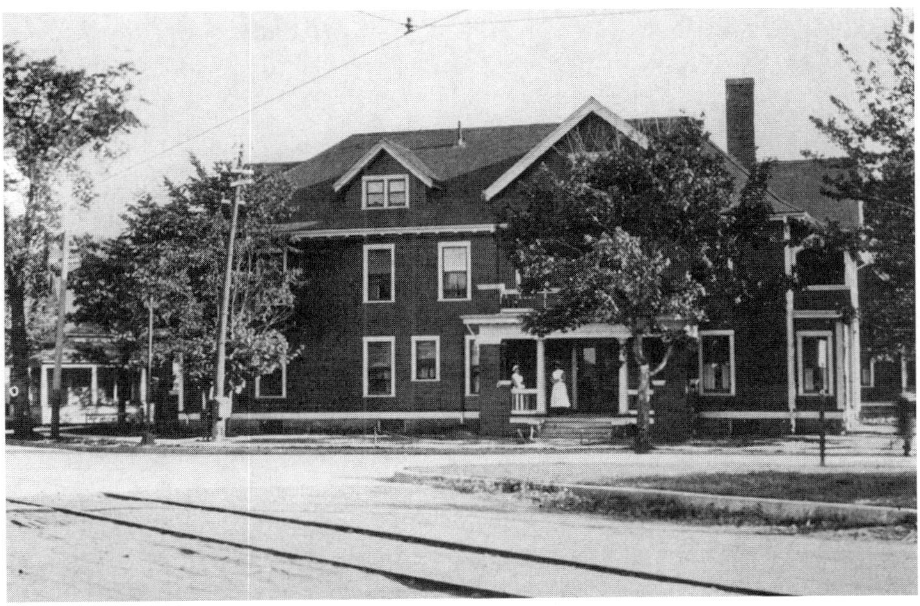

The Moncton Hospital's nurses' residence in 1924.

Junior EENT:	Dr. L.A. Goodridge
Anaesthetist:	Dr. H.H. Coleman
	Dr. G.A. Lyons
Pediatrician:	Dr. G.O. Taylor
Roentgenologist:	Dr. F.A. Richard
Consulting Staff:	Dr. L.H. Price—City of Moncton
	Dr. H.H. Coleman—City of Moncton
	Dr. H. Logan—Salisbury
	Dr. A. Sormany—Shediac

The administrative staff of the hospital consisted of seven people who were also responsible for the School of Nursing:

Superintendent of Hospital and Training School
Executive Secretary
Supervisor—Day
Supervisor—Night
Supervisor—Surgical
Laboratory Technician
House Mother and Housekeeper—
(in charge of nurses' home and housekeeping)

The major workload in the hospital was borne by the student nurses, a practice which was carried on until the 1950s.

The only new face appearing on the list of doctors that year was Dr. J. Euclide Leger, who was born in St. Joseph's in 1898 and graduated from Laval in 1922. He did three years' postgraduate work in surgery in Paris and elsewhere in Europe. Dr. Leger said, "Above the entrance of the Sorbonne in Paris is the inscription which translated from the Latin says, 'First, do no harm,' and that has always been my own motto." Although appearing on the roster for 1925-26 as a junior physician, he is listed as a surgeon in the 1927-28 roster. He enjoyed a long surgical career in Moncton, although he practised mostly at l'Hôtel Dieu after it opened in 1928. His son-in-law, Dr. Joseph Gagnon, served many years as a pathologist at The Moncton Hospital.

During the year ending May 31, 1925, there were 1,419 admissions of which 237 were ward patients. There were 91 births recorded with 7 stillbirths, one set of twins and 5 babies delivered by caesarean section. There were 951 operations performed, of which 388 were classified as major and 563 as minor. 19 were T&As performed on children being treated through the school clinic. There were 436 X-ray exams and 135 X-ray treatments carried out; 2,381 examinations were carried out in the pathology laboratory.

The annual report for the year ending May 31, 1926, records the first appearance on the Moncton scene of another prominent physician, Dr. Charles (Charlie) E. Baxter. Born in Moncton, Charlie spent his boyhood in Stellarton, Nova Scotia. He graduated from Dalhousie in 1925, after interning at the Victoria General Hospital from 1924 to 1925, and established a practice in Moncton. Having been injured in a plane crash in the Royal Flying Corps in the First World War, he always walked with a limp and in later years he used a cane with the wings of the R.C. attached. He could be described as a handsome man with a fine head of wavy white hair. He exuded charm and at any social gathering quickly gathered a crowd around him as he had a great repertoire of stories which he told with charismatic gusto. Dr. Frank Archibald, a long-time friend and minister of St. John's United Church, used to say that Charlie could preach a great sermon and knew all the biblical terms but didn't quite put them in the right context. Anyone caught smoking a cigarette, for instance, was sure to get a lecture from Charlie. He also preached on the evils of alcohol, although his friend, Dr. Kelly MacLean, could always cut the lecture short by saying, "Come off it, Charlie, I knew you when..." One of the staff meetings in the 1950s provides another illustration. The medical director was admonishing the staff for the number of physicians who were delinquent in completing their hospital charts. Dr. Baxter replied by getting up and delivering a lecture on how terrible it was for these doctors to be abusing the system and asked that the names of the culprits be read out. When the names were read out, whose name should appear but Charlie's. Quick as a flash he was on his feet and replied, "And lo, Ben Adams name led all the rest," and sat down to the great amusement of his fellow physicians. I can find no record of his having undertaken any postgraduate training except a course at the British Post-Graduate Medical School in 1937, but he learned surgery by the apprenticeship method, as was the custom in those days, and received his Fellowship in the American College of Surgeons in 1933. He always maintained an interest in aviation and was president of the Moncton Aero Club in 1928. He was an avid curler and past president of the Moncton Curlers Association. Active in community affairs, he was a past president of the YMCA and the Canadian Legion. He died in February 1976.

In May 1926, the hospital became a member of the American Hospital Association. As a requirement for such membership, the hospital was inspected for accreditation and the only recommendation to come out of that inspection was that case histories be more fully written. Miss MacMaster subsequently recommended to the board that efforts be made to obtain an intern. She thought this would be a distinct advantage overcoming the difficulty of securing proper histories. Moreover, ward anaesthetics (for which the hospital paid $550) would be administered by the intern as part of his duties. Emergency cases would receive a doctor's attention until the arrival of the attending physician, and various other duties, such as supervision of obstetrical cases and of very ill patients, dressings and the like, would be shared by the house doctor. This report would seem to indicate that a new policy had arisen so that doctors were now paid for administering anaesthetics to ward patients whereas all other physician's services to ward patients were free.

The major medical purchases for the hospital during the year were a HeidLink Nitrous-Oxide-Oxygen-Ether apparatus and a Victor portable

X-ray bedside unit. The hospital was getting crowded and the need for more beds was once again being expressed. Cancellations of surgery were not the order of the day, however, and there was some consternation that maternity beds were being used for surgery. This was seen to be counter to building up an active maternity service. Medical rooms in isolation were also being used for surgical cases.

The staff appointed for 1927-28 remains the same as for the preceding year with the addition of two new names: Dr. F.E. Boudreau and Dr. J.W. Dobson. Dr. Boudreau joined the staff as a junior specialist on the EENT service and Dr. Dobson as a senior physician.

Born in Arichat, Nova Scotia, on September 22, 1880, F.E. Boudreau received a BA from St. Anne's College in 1903 and his MD, CM from the Halifax Medical College in 1907. He interned at the Victoria General Hospital in Halifax in 1907, and then undertook postgraduate training in EENT. Surgery at l'Hôtel Dieu de Paris and St. Joseph's Hospital in Paris. He had a long association with the hospital and died in the spring of 1960.

J.W. Dobson was born in Hillsborough on September 18, 1899. He obtained a BA from Acadia in 1920 and graduated from McGill Medical School in 1925. He interned at the Royal Victoria Hospital in Montreal from 1924 to 1926 and established a general practice, including surgery, in Moncton, that was to last until his retirement in 1968. He was a heavy set man who enjoyed the outdoors and was renowned for his stamina and strength. Joe Dobson, being a "country boy" from Albert County, always thought that surgery should start at 6:30 am, rather than 8 am. This was before he had a serious heart attack. After that, he never booked surgery before 10 am. He was probably the first local person to quickly return to activity after a coronary. On being discharged from the hospital, he went to his cottage in Shediac and each day he would go for a long walk. At that time no one knew that he kept an axe hidden in a wood-lot area where he would go and use it to chop wood until he felt some chest distress. Apparently, he would do this every day until he fully recovered and returned to work. Dr. Dobson was instrumental in re-establishing the Moncton Gun Club from its original site on the McLaughlin Rd. to its present location on the Coverdale Road. Joe passed on his love of the outdoors to his son, Dr. Arthur Dobson, who has blazed a trail through the Albert County woods, and which has been named fittingly, "The Dobson Trail." Dr. Joseph Dobson died in 1973.

In the May 31, 1927, annual report, attention is again drawn to the increasing use of the hospital with 1,737 patients admitted, contrasted to 1,295 in 1922, and with an average daily census of 60 patients as against 42 in 1922. The cost of running the hospital for that year was $73,998.64.

On June 9, 1927, the sod was turned for the new l'Hôtel Dieu L'Assomption on Archibald Street, north of Mountain Road. Construction was begun that same year and the hospital opened in October 1928. It originally began as a 17-bed hospital on Church Street in 1922 and was operated by the Sisters of Charity of Providence.

The year 1927 saw the school, the VD and the chest clinics all running in a satisfactory manner. The Gyro Club of Moncton paid 50 percent of the cost of a chest X-ray for the chest clinic patients. Although the maternity service was gaining favour with the citizens of Moncton, it was still not large enough to provide adequate training for the student nurses. The three-month rotation period for obstetrical and infant feeding was transferred this year from St. Luke's Hospital in New Bedford, Massachusetts to the Royal Victoria Hospital in Montreal. There were 1,277 operations performed from May 31, 1926, to May 31, 1927, with 471 major and 806 minor operations. There were 1,643 outpatient treatments, an increase of 177 over the preceding year. There were 625 X-ray exams and 100 X-ray treatments carried out. The ambulance service made 463 calls.

The annual report for the year ending May 31, 1928, once again reports the need for expansion with the hospital operating at more than 100 percent of its rated capacity of 86 beds, which included 8 beds for contagious diseases and 10 nursery cots. The daily census averaged 65 patients. The average public patient was now being charged $5 a week if it were felt that he or she could pay but most did not contribute. In the fall of 1928, the hospital purchased a new Studebaker ambulance at a cost of $3,135.30. The rate for a call in the city was $2, with a mileage charge for calls outside the city.

The only new name appearing on the medical staff at this time is that of Dr. Leo Doiron. Dr. Doiron was born in Shediac on March 19, 1898, and obtained his BA from St. Joseph's in 1921 and his MD from Laval in 1926.

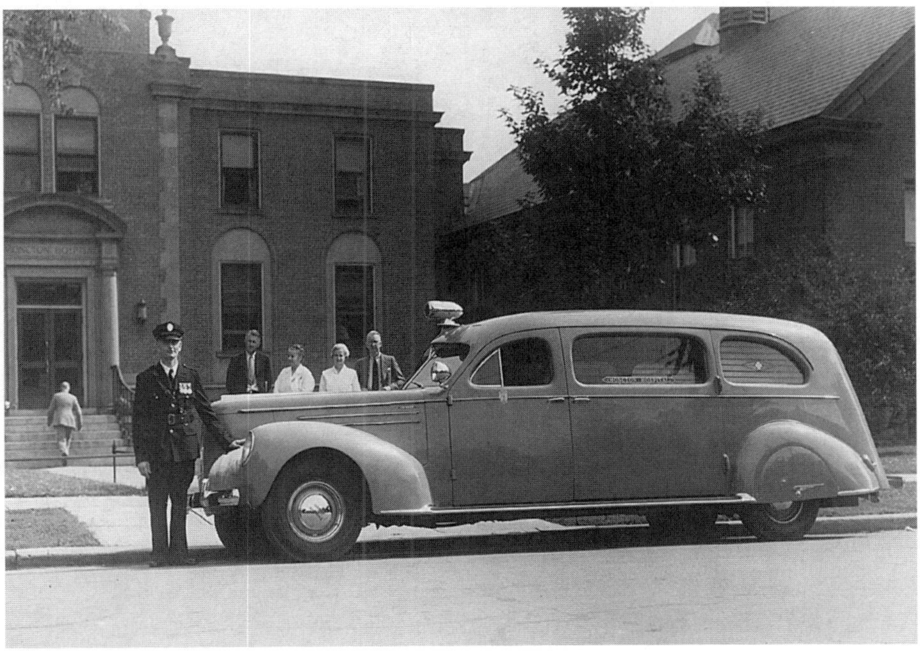

The new hospital ambulance in the 1930s. Standing (l to r): Sgt. William Walsh, Norman Dryden, Ruth C. Wilson, Miss A.J. MacMaster, and Dr. R.G. Girvan.

He then did postgraduate work in surgery at the Hôpitaux de Paris in 1926-27. Dr. Doiron must have prospered in his early years as he lived in the fine house which is now occupied by Cadman's Funeral Home. By the 1950s, however, alcohol had taken its toll on him and he was no longer licensed to practice.

The opening of the new l'Hôtel Dieu in 1928, did not relieve the bed shortage at The Moncton Hospital as admissions continued to climb with 2,060 admissions during the year ending May 31, 1929, with an average daily census of 70. There were 121 births, 1,408 operations, 2,136 outpatient visits, 801 X-ray exams and 145 X-ray treatments. No new physicians were added to the staff during the year and, in fact, the staff decreased by one with the death of Dr. H.A. Jones. The administration grew, however, with the addition of three new members bringing the total to ten. The new staff included an office secretary, a supervisor for the ward and an assistant housekeeper. Obtaining adequate case records remained a problem, according to the annual report, and would continue to be a problem until such time as a full-time record clerk and a suitable record room and equipment could be obtained. The staff were holding regular staff meetings once a month, in the board room of the hospital, with only an average attendance. Meetings of the local medical society were being held in the nurses' residence.

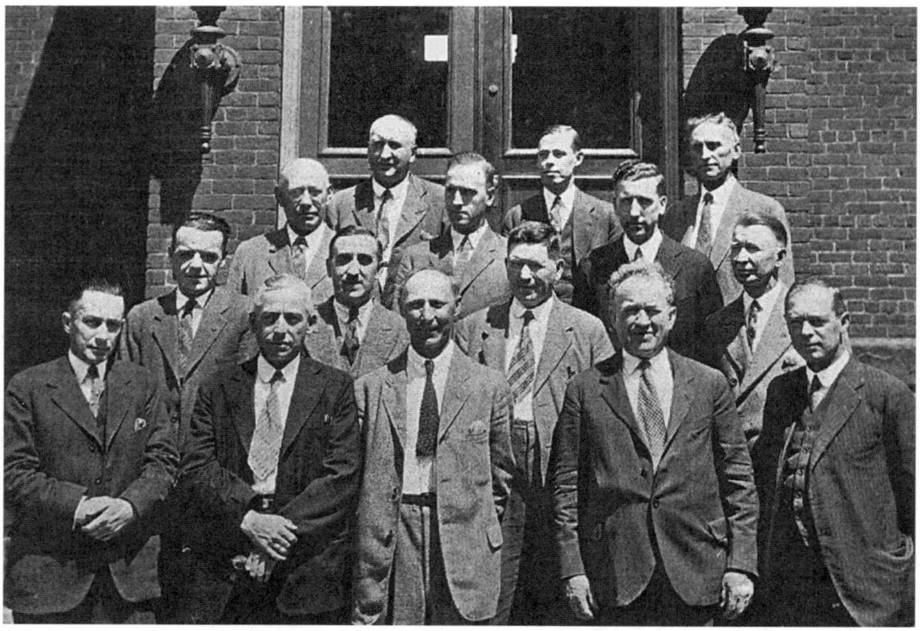

The medical staff of The Moncton Hospital in 1929. Front row: Dr. H.E. Britton, Dr. F.A. Richard, Dr. J.A. McNaughton, Dr. W.A. Ferguson, and Dr. W.P. Kirby; Second row: Dr. G. Lyons, Dr. Euclide Leger, Dr. Ambrose Myers, and Dr. R.G. Girvan; Third row: Dr. L.H. Price, Dr. J.A. Dobson, Dr. C.R. Baxter; Back row: Dr. A.E. Forbes, Dr. L.E. Goodridge, and Dr. S.W. Burgess.

In August 1929 a case record system was put into operation and in February 1930, a part-time health record person was appointed. In the annual report dated May 31, 1930, it was reported that 2,087 patients had been admitted during the year with 1,071 classed as private, 676 as semi-private and 340 as public ward. There were 1,397 operations performed of which 547 were major and 850 were minor. The school clinics continued to function and 34 T&A's were performed under the auspices of this public service. In the VD Clinic run by Dr. George Lyons, 553 treatments were carried out. The Public Health Gyro Chest Clinic was held every two weeks under Dr. Arthur Melanson, the Public Health Doctor, and assisted by Miss Findlay, the Public Health Nurse. There were 159 patients seen and 90 new cases of TB encountered. There were 153 live births with 4 stillbirths during the year and 4 of the births were by caesarean section. One point of particular note is that there were only 4 charity cases on the maternity service during the year, and it appears obvious that the poor were expected to have their babies at home.

As noted previously, the hospital was experiencing crowded conditions and the need for enlarged facilities was readily apparent. As early as November 1926 the hospital administration began a campaign to raise funds through public subscription for an addition and appointed a building committee consisting of A.C. Chapman, G.A. Robertson, Reid McManus, G.O. Spencer, Ambrose Wheeler, H.H. Grainger and Mrs. R.P. Dickson. As usual, the Ladies' Auxiliary pitched in and established a building fund. Mr. Chapman made a public plea for funds in a letter published in the *Moncton Times* on March 23, 1927. On the same date, the board applied to the provincial legislature in Fredericton for the authorization to issue bonds worth $150,000 for the construction of additional buildings and furnishings for The Moncton Hospital. The legislation passed in May, and the city council thereafter guaranteed $75,000 in hospital bonds. Efforts were also assisted by a $20,000 donation from the CNR. The architectural firm of Stevens and Lee was hired to draw up plans for the addition. The city council approved the plans in May 1929. After presentation of a second set of plans, tenders were subsequently called. The lowest tender submitted was from Ambrose Wheeler, vice-chairman of the board, in the amount of $323,639.24 and it was accepted at a board meeting on June 21, 1929. Construction was started shortly thereafter and the decade ended on a happy note.

CHAPTER FIVE

THE DIRTY THIRTIES— THE DEPRESSION YEARS

Although the stock market had crashed in November 1929, the Depression had not yet set in as the 1930s began, and the future of The Moncton Hospital looked bright. At this time a new wing was being built which was disrupting service, but the construction was nearing completion. It was opened on October 28, 1930, by the Lieutenant-Governor, Hugh Havelock McLean, before an audience that completely filled every foot of space in the reception room, the lobby, most of the rooms surrounding the central lobby, and spilled out onto the front steps. Also present and making speeches were Premier Baxter; Hon. C.H. Taylor, the minister of health; Dr. O.B. Price, MP; Senator Robinson, chairman of the Building Committee; Hon. A.A. Dysart; Col. S. Boyd Anderson, city clerk representing the city council; and the board chairman, Mr. Chapman. The reception area was decorated with flags, palms and chrysanthemums and an orchestra under the direction of Mrs. Ida Bremner Malcolm played musical selections throughout the event. The architects Stephens and Lee, who designed the new wing, sent their regrets at being unable to attend the opening. In his speech, Premier Baxter stated that while the rich and the poor were well looked after by the hospital, he felt there should be some scheme, such as that already in effect, whereby workers were covered by Workers' Compensation, to look after the hospital needs of those of modest means. Mr. Chapman, in his remarks, thanked the city for guaranteeing the bonds but announced that they were still short of money for the equipment and furnishings for the new wing and would soon be appealing to the citizens for more money to put the hospital out of debt. This would not be done before the board gave a full accounting of the expenditures to date.

The new wing contained 75 beds increasing the bed capacity of the hospital to 125. The building was of fireproof construction of reinforced concrete. The first floor contained seven wards of four beds each with a balcony off the wards. In addition, there was a solarium, an ambulance entrance, an admitting room, an outpatient department with surgical dressing rooms and clinic rooms as well as a board room, a doctors' room and offices for the superintendent and the training school. At a meeting of the medical staff on December 9, 1930, it was moved and seconded that the staff furnish the doctors' room, the members to be taxed $10 for this cause and the money to be given to the superintendent. The laboratory and X-ray department were also located on the first floor as well as a dining room for nurses that could seat 44. Private and semi-private rooms occupied the second floor. The third floor contained the operating rooms, which were equipped with an emergency lighting system, and there was a laboratory off the operating room. It was hoped that with this new building, a regular outpatient department could be developed. As a result of the enlarged facilities, a new cost-accounting system was deemed to be necessary.

The staff, with some changes, appointed for 1930-31 year, was as follows:

Senior Surgeons	Dr. W.A. Ferguson
	Dr. A.R. Myers
	Dr. W. Kirby
	Dr. H.E. Britton
Junior Surgeons	Dr. J.A. McNaughton
	Dr. G.A. Lyons
	Dr. P.McL. Atkinson
	Dr. C.R. Baxter
Senior Physicians	Dr. R.G. Girvan
	Dr. A.E. Forbes
Junior Physician	Dr. H.M. MacLean
Senior specialists EENT	Dr. S.W. Burgess
	Dr. L.A. Goodridge

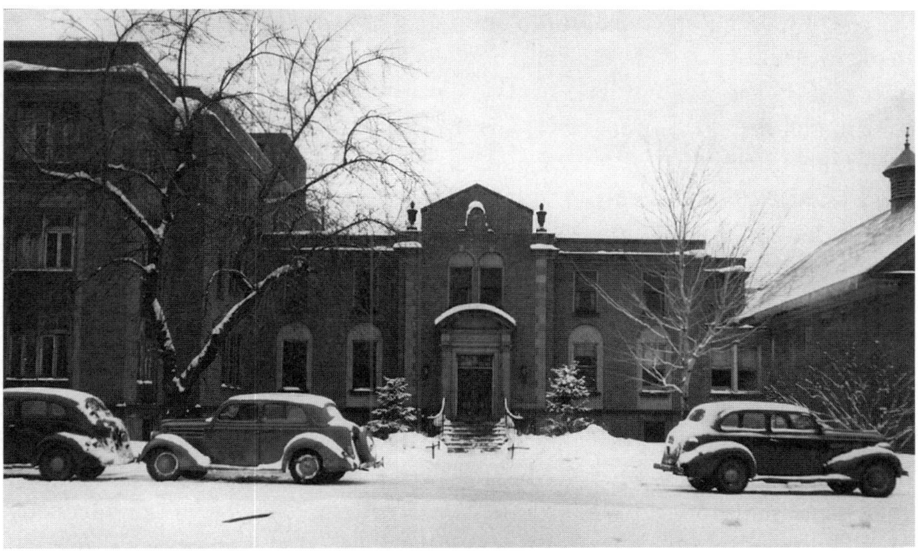

A new wing was added on to The Moncton Hospital in 1930.

Junior Specialist EENT	Dr. F.E. Boudreau
Anaesthetists	Dr. H.H. Coleman
	Dr. L.H. Price
Pediatricians	Dr. G.O. Taylor
	Dr. J.W. Dobson
Roentgenologist	Dr. F.A. Richard
Consulting Staff	Dr. L.H. Price—City of Moncton
	Dr. H.H. Coleman—City of Moncton
	Dr. H.L. Logan—Salisbury
	Dr. A. Sormany—Shediac
	Dr. R.D. Roach—Hillsborough

It is to be noted that four francophone members were no longer listed on the attending staff of The Moncton Hospital as of this year. They were: Dr. A.R. Landry, Dr. J.E. Leger, Dr. Leo Doiron, and Dr. J.A. Gaudet. These men figure prominently in the history of the new l'Hôtel Dieu and came to perform their public service in this venue. They were able, of course, to continue servicing private patients at The Moncton Hospital, but this period marks the beginning of a tradition whereby a member of the medical staff would serve on the active staff of one institution and the courtesy staff of the other institution.

A new addition to the medical staff was Dr. Hugh MacKay MacLean, known affectionately as "Kelly" MacLean. Kelly was born in Truro, Nova Scotia, on May 31, 1903. After taking one year of engineering at Acadia, he switched to medicine and graduated from Dalhousie University in 1928. While at university he was a star athlete and was captain of the Dalhousie rugby team. After graduation he interned at Charity Hospital in Cleveland and then came to Moncton, where his kind and gentle manner and professional competence allowed him to build up a large and successful practice. He became a fellow of the American College of Surgeons in 1938. He served overseas in the Second World War from 1940 to 1945, after which he remained overseas to undertake further postgraduate training in surgery at Hammersmith Hospital and became certified in surgery by the Royal College of Physicians and Surgeons. Although he didn't command a room like Charlie Baxter, he could tell some delightful stories. He used to say that his father would take the cow out to be serviced and, knowing what happened to the cow, he was always wary when someone was about to do him a "service." As was the tradition in Nova Scotia, families were always very partisan in their politics and his father was a staunch Liberal. Kelly used to tell the story that when he was a young boy during one election, he was paid 25 cents to sit on a wagon and blow a whistle and shout, "Vote Conservative." His father heard of this "sacrilege" and when Kelly returned home his father gave him a good whack and sent him off to his room. Apparently this had a lasting impression on Kelly because, as he would later relate, when he was overseas during the

Second World War, an election was being held and, the conscription issue being very much in the minds of the soldiers, they were against the Mackenzie King government of the day. Kelly went into the polling booth, intending to vote Conservative, but on entering the booth, he remembered the whack he had received from his father and ended up voting Liberal. He was a great outdoorsman, consummate bird watcher, fisherman and fly-tyer. He died on March 28, 1972.

Another new listing is that of Dr. R.D. Roach as a member of the consulting staff. Born in Tatamagouche, Nova Scotia, on November 26, 1898, Roach graduated from McGill in 1925. He undertook postgraduate training in internal medicine in England, receiving his membership in the Royal College of Physicians of London (MRCP). He practised first in Hillsborough and later moved to Moncton, appearing on the staff appointments as a paediatrician in 1933, and later as a senior physician. He was the first specialist in internal medicine in Moncton but it would take a few years before this was recognized as a separate department. He later received his Fellowship in the American College of Physicians and his Fellowship in the Royal College of Physicians and Surgeons of Canada and came to be recognized by his colleagues and the citizens of Moncton for his diagnostic ability. He served as president of the New Brunswick Medical Society in 1951-52 but died of cancer before his term expired.

In 1931, the year end for the hospital was changed from May 31 to December 31 so that reports for the year would now cover the calendar year. Restrictions on admission of certain cases continued: no one suffering from mental disease was admitted, nor was anyone with an incurable disease admitted or kept beyond the time that hospital treatment prove beneficial. Chronic diseases were to be admitted only for emergency treatment. The hospital would accept, however, all cases of a general medical and surgical nature for the public service, as well as for the private and semi-private service. It would now also accept for treatment certain contagious and infectious diseases, but not smallpox. Cases of tuberculosis and venereal diseases could only be admitted for emergency surgical intervention and the patients were to be removed to their homes at the conclusion of the emergency treatment.

Patients living in the City of Moncton admitted to the public ward were expected to pay $1.50 per day for their treatment. In applying for admission to the public ward, they were required to prove their inability to pay the cost of their hospital treatment and the services of an attending doctor. Patients applying for treatment in the public ward from any other locality were required to have the written order of their Overseer of the Poor, if they lived in the County of Westmorland, or a written order of their parish counsellor if they lived anywhere else in the Province of New Brunswick. Only bona-fide emergency patients were accepted from places outside the province. Although private patients could have visitors every day, visiting hours for ward patients were still restricted to 2-4 p.m. on Tuesdays, Fridays and

Sundays. Husbands who were working could visit from 7-8 p.m. on visiting days only, however. In the case of dangerously ill patients, relatives and friends would be admitted at any time.

As the new wing became occupied, it quickly became apparent that the hospital was burdened with buildings uneconomically planned, out-dated and inadequately adapted for modern hospital services. In response, the isolation building was moved from its former location on King Street to Carlyle Street, opposite the power house. It was then connected to the hospital with two passageways connecting the old annex through the isolation unit to the new wing. The maternity ward was transferred from the annex to the vacated old building with the annex then used to house members of the staff, and for sleeping quarters for the night nurses and for seven members of the domestic department.

The only purchases during the year were new laundry equipment and a new Zeigler obstetrical bed. In May 1931, the hospital instituted a system of purchasing staple provisions by tender. The pharmacy was contracted out to the private sector to Henry's Pharmacy, the objective being to lower the cost of medicines supplied to ward patients, and to increase service to hospital patients. In her annual report, the superintendent, Miss MacMaster, called attention to the deplorable method of conveying contagious patients (in the "contagious" wagon). She urgently recommended that some agency be approached to replace this method of conveyance, which was slow, cold, and, since a horse could not always be secured just when needed, extremely unreliable. She did not feel that The Moncton Hospital should be required to purchase a conveyance as the responsibility for this was clearly outlined in the Provincial Health Statutes. The VD clinic was a Department of Health responsibility as well, and the hospital only supplied the facilities. The Chief Medical Officer for the province had been approached on several occasions for an allowance to keep the facilities in good repair but no aid had ever been received since the clinic's inception.

With the increase in the bed capacity of the hospital, an increase in administrative staff was seen to be necessary, and so this was reformed and expanded to include the following fifteen positions:

Superintendent of Hospital and School of Nursing
Assistant Superintendent and Obstetrical Supervisor
Surgical Supervisor
Supervisor of Outpatient Department and Physiotherapist
Supervisor Day
Supervisor Night
Dietician
Laboratorian
Record Librarian
Bookkeeper
Stenographer

Matron and Housekeeper
Chief Engineer
2 Assistant Engineers (1, half-time)

There were two notable events at this time. Miss MacMaster attended a meeting of the American Hospital Association in Toronto in September, 1931, and at the formation of the Canadian Hospital Foundation, she was one of the representatives from New Brunswick.

There was only one new addition to the medical staff in 1931 in the person of Dr. W.A. Pullin. He was the first doctor on the EENT service who limited his practice solely to ophthalmology. Dr. Goodridge, on the other hand, limited his practice solely to ear, nose and throat. W.A. Pullin was born in Chanel, Newfoundland, on July 26, 1892. He started practice in Petitcodiac in 1926 and left in 1929 to specialize in diseases of the eye at the Marsfield Eye Hospital in 1929-30 and Debrien Eye Clinic, Hungary, in 1930. He then set up practice in Moncton and enjoyed a long association with the hospital. Dr. Pullin was a delightful man but somewhat absent minded. At one time, it is said, he examined Jerry Britton's eyes and gave him glasses. Jerry wasn't entirely happy with his glasses but thought he would get used to them. Then Dr. Pullin called to apologize. He had given Jerry his own glasses by mistake and wanted them back. Kelly MacLean used to tell the story that he had invited Dr. Pullin to a duck hunting expedition on an offshore location. Kelly, who never exerted himself unduly, retired to the back seat of the boat permitting Dr. Pullin to cast off and row. Dr. Pullin cast off and was holding his shotgun as he jumped on board. The shotgun went off and blasted a hole in the bottom of the boat. They never got to go duck hunting.

The Moncton Hospital continued to maintain its Grade A rating from the American College of Surgeons during this period. At a meeting in the summer of 1931, a motion was passed to adopt the by-laws as adopted by the General Public Hospital in Saint John, with necessary changes to apply to The Moncton Hospital.

In that August, a letter was sent to the chairman of the hospital board requesting an In-Out board for physicians. This request was obviously honoured as the old board now resides in the doctors' lounge of the present hospital. The names of those doctors who have died are now listed as "OUT." Those few who remain are listed as "IN." It has been suggested that a proper ceremony be held in the doctors' lounge when one of those remaining passes on with a proper toast in good wine as the name is moved to the "OUT" position.

A letter from Miss MacMaster to the staff in October 1931 stressed to the medical staff the necessity of having a consultation in all cases going to surgery for a D&C. In accordance with recommendations from the American College of Surgeons, two new staff positions were created at this time, as follows:

Supervisor of Pathological Department—Dr. J.W. Dobson
Supervisor of Fractures—Dr. W.A. Ferguson

In November, George O. Taylor resigned as pediatrician.

During the year 1931, there were 1,902 patients admitted with 69 deaths. Of these, 321 were ward patients. There were 876 major and 325 minor operations performed. The maternity service recorded 147 live births with eight stillbirths but no caesarean sections. There were only two charity patients admitted to the maternity service. The X-ray department carried out 731 exams and 87 treatments. There is a discrepancy in the percentage of private and public patients receiving X-ray treatments, as only four public patients received X-ray treatments. The new physiotherapy department appeared to be functioning well with 433 treatments given. The laboratory work was increasing with 4,258 examinations carried out. The ambulance made 424 calls. There were 47 student nurses in training with 15 senior, 17 intermediate and 15 junior students. The student nurses were now being given their course in dietetics by the recently hired hospital dietician.

The outpatient department was organized as a formal service in the new wing at this time but saw little use in its first year. The school clinic also saw a change in its operation. Due to poor hygienic conditions existing in many of the homes from where these children came, it was now felt that it would be better to hospitalize these children for several days following their tonsillectomies rather than treating them as day patients in the clinic. The children continued, however, to be referred to the hospital by the school nurse.

In 1932, the first effects of the depression began to make themselves felt at the hospital, although there were 203 more patients admitted in 1932 than in 1931. While there was this slight increase in the number of private patients, there was a decrease in the number of semi-private patients and an increase in the number of public patients. Moreover, the year's increase of 117 X-ray exams were practically all public ward exams. A reduction in X-ray fees, where practical, was adopted in November 1932. There was an increase of 16 births over 1931, but the increase was reflected in more semi-private than private accommodation. The lab showed an increase of 740 exams, of which more than 50 percent produced no income for the hospital. In his annual report, the hospital's accountant cautioned about the rapidly increasing total amount of accounts receivable.

The outpatient department which had been created with the opening of the new wing in October 1930 was now beginning to fulfil its mission and experienced an increase of 423 examinations. The outpatient department was provided for the benefit of the poor only. Patients who were able to pay ordinary fees for medical attendance were not entitled to treatment and would be refused. A flat charge of 25 cents per visit was made when the patient was able to pay. A pharmacy was conducted in the outpatient department of the hospital and ordinary prescriptions were dispensed at an average cost of 25 cents to outpatients. The previous arrangement for Henry's Pharmacy to operate a pharmacy in the hospital was cancelled but, as yet, the hospital did not have its own pharmacist.

New clinics were now held on an organized basis, with each clinic in charge of the public ward service as follows:

Surgery	Tuesday and Saturday—10-12 am
General Medicine	Monday and Friday—10-12 am
Gynaecology and Prenatal	Wednesday—10-12 am
EENT	Thursday—10-12 am

In addition to these new clinics, the previous special clinics continued to function as follows:

Venereal Disease	Wednesday—women, 2 pm; men, 6:30 pm
Gyro Chest Clinic	Alternative Sat.—10 am-3 pm

The Venereal Disease Clinic was operated as a Department of Health Service by Dr. George Lyons and statistics reported 2,600 cases treated during the year. There had been only 600 cases treated in 1931. I think these figures must represent the number of treatments and/or new and different treatments, as I don't think we could expect to see a 400 percent rise in promiscuity in one year! It may also reflect the times, however, with fewer patients going to their private practitioner for treatment.

Dr. W.S. Fitzpatrick was added to the staff in 1932. He was born on September 27, 1892, and, after taking premed at St. Thomas and one year of engineering at St. Francis Xavier, he entered Dalhousie University, graduating with his MD, CM in 1921. He interned at the Victoria General Hospital from 1920 to 1921 and the Nova Scotia Sanatorium in Kentville from 1921 to 1922. Between 1925 and 1932, he undertook residencies in surgery and urology at various hospitals in the New York area, including three years at the Jersey City Medical Centre. He is first listed on the staff appointments as a cystoscopist but carried on a general surgical practice as well as urology. He served as president of the New Brunswick Medical Society in 1945-46. He soon built up a loyal following of patients. In this point it is interesting to note that during the thirties and up until after the war, Moncton's citizens were divided not only on ethnic grounds, but also on religious grounds. Life in the community often revolved around the church, and although no hard and fast conclusions can be made, the Irish Catholic patients tended to go to Irish and English Catholic doctors, such as Dr. Fitzpatrick and Dr. Myers, while the Protestants went to the Protestant doctors and the French Catholics went to the French doctors.

Dr. R.J. Caldwell, who was also added to the staff this year, was born in Havelock on June 8, 1897. He took his premed at Dalhousie and graduated from McGill in 1928. He interned at the Royal Victoria Hospital from 1928 to 1932 and joined the staff as a senior physician. He only practised in Moncton for a short time, however, before continuing his practice in Petitcodiac. He died on October 18, 1975.

The 1933 staff appointments record the promotion of Dr. J.W. Dobson to the surgical staff as a junior surgeon.

One point of interest during the early years of the hospital is that individuals and organizations would often take it upon themselves to furnish and maintain rooms in the hospital as a project or a memorial. There were 13 such rooms designated in 1932 as follows:

New Wing—Endowed Rooms
Room 223—Mrs. Emma O'Neil
Room 220—Dr. R.C. Tait and Family
Room 212—Mrs. Hestor M. Boyd
New Wing—Furnished and Maintained
Room 224—Bonar Lodge Chapter, IODE
Room 226—Mr. and Mrs. A.J. Tingley
Room 227—Moncton Chapter, New Brunswick Association of RN's
Room 201—The children of Mr. and Mrs. Andrew Wheaton
Room 204—Fort Cumberland Chapter, IODE
Maternity Wing—Endowed Rooms
Room 14—In memory of Sir Albert James Smith
Room 16—In loving memory of son, George Roy Dobson
Maternity Wing—Rooms Furnished and Maintained
Room 15—Mrs. Victor Foster Dunlop
Room 16—Keith Lodge No.23 F & AM (Masonic Room)
Room 12—Marion White Room
Room 11—The Shediac Room

There were 2,105 admissions in 1932 of which 1,089 were private, 518 semi-private and 498 ward. There were 163 births with 15 stillbirths and 4 caesarean sections, 1,131 operations were performed on private patients and 353 on ward patients, in addition to 12 T&As on school clinic patients. There were 831 X-ray exams and 132 X-ray treatments and 471 physiotherapy treatments. In the outpatient department, 2,040 treatments were given with 25 reduction of fractures performed and 109 minor operations. The EENT clinic looked after 158 people and the medical clinic 62 persons but only 29 attended the surgical clinic.

The appointment of an anaesthetist for the public ward service was recommended to the board this year as an urgent need. It was stipulated that the person should be especially qualified to administer gas-oxygen and other methods of anaesthesia now being required for major surgery.

Since 1930, the medical staff had been complaining to city hall about the noise and traffic around the hospital, and in 1932, there was some response to their complaints. Removal of the street car tracks and the levelling of King Street in front of the hospital brought about a great improvement.

By 1933, the effects of the Depression were evident. The cost of running the hospital for the year was $109,062.94 with a net loss of $13,596.29. Fortunately, however, the hospital again enjoyed a surplus before depreciation, this being in the amount of $3,119.88. A sustained inability of paying patients to meet their obligations was occurring and deferred payments of funds due from municipalities were the major factors contributing to the deficit. Fifty fewer patients were admitted in 1933 with 132 fewer private patients, and 84 fewer semi-private patients, but an increase in the number of non paying ward patients again occurred, this time by 66. The only funds expended on the physical plant were to extend steam lines from the power plant to the old maternity building, for construction of a tunnel under King Street to the nurses' home, and for the transfer of main steam pipes from the new wing to the power plant proper. This not only produced increased comfort in the buildings but was cost effective, resulting in a savings of 24.6 percent over the heating costs for 1932. The replacement of equipment was kept to a minimum but a new ether suction pump with accessories was purchased for the specialist's operating room and it was also found to be necessary to replace the basal metabolism apparatus.

There were no new additions to the staff in 1933, but the death of Dr. L.H. Price did occur. Two of the junior surgeons on the staff, Dr. George Lyons and Dr. Charles Baxter, were made Fellows of the American College of Surgeons.

Admissions to the hospital in 1933 numbered 1955, of which 957 were private patients, 435 semi-private and 564 ward. There were 140 births including 3 sets of twins and 6 stillbirths. The caesarean section rate was increased this year with 6 performed. There were 992 private patients who underwent surgery as well as 372 ward patients. A total of 945 X-ray exams were carried out along with 71 X-ray treatments, 668 physiotherapy treatments and 4,776 laboratory exams were performed. Attendance at outpatient clinics doubled over the previous year with 121 attending the EENT clinic; 281, the medical clinic, and with the biggest increase, 121, in the surgical clinic. Attendance at the Gyro Clinic numbered 546 people and at the VD Clinic, 2,126. As a reflection of the economic times, the amount paid by the Gyro Club for X-rays in the Chest Clinic was reduced to $3 to from the previous $4 charge.

In 1933, The Moncton Hospital was the only one in Canada, and one of nine in Canada and the United States, to receive honourable mention in National Hospital Day awards. These award were under the jurisdiction of the American Hospital Association. During that year, Miss Ruth Wilson attended the Hospital Administrators Institute in Chicago and Miss King, the record librarian, attended the meeting of the Association of Registered Record Librarians in Chicago. At first glance this does not seem an unusual occurrence, but it is noteworthy in that both of these women attended these meetings during their vacations.

In her annual report for the year 1933, Miss MacMaster, much ahead of her time, reflected upon the possible development of insured hospitalization. I quote verbatim from her report:

> The conditions encountered during the past several years and brought to a focal point during the year just ended establish definitely the dependence upon the economic welfare of the community it serves. This dependence must continue until such time as some policy is evolved relieving the tension which must necessarily exist when such a hospital is called upon to sustain itself against overwhelming odds. These odds may be summed up in the matter of (a) finding itself in the hazardous position of having to rely upon the sustained inability of the public to pay for services rendered, and (b) facing the problem of supplying adequate hospitalization for municipalities finding themselves increasingly handicapped for funds to meet current obligations.
>
> The policy that I would suggest and which is meeting with varying degrees of success in many centres throughout Canada and the United States as well as Great Britain, is what might be termed "The Periodic Payment Plan for the Purchase of Hospital Care." In other words a system of hospital insurance carefully worked out whereby participants are able to avail themselves of mutually agreed upon hospital services through the payment of an annual premium.
>
> The machinery for its set-up and the particular type which might be best adapted to this community is a problem too complicated to be discussed in this report. There are many very excellent schemes each one acceptable to a particular communities needs, and I present this as a possible answer to mutual problems affecting both individuals and hospitals which serve them.
>
> It is almost needless to comment that such a scheme must first be endorsed by and have the full co-operation of our physicians.

No action was taken on this issue during the following year, but Miss MacMaster again raised the issue of group hospitalization in her annual report for 1934, stating that she had informally approached Sister DeBrescia, the administrator of l'Hôtel Dieu, on the matter and Sister DeBrescia had replied that l'Hôtel Dieu would be willing to be approached with a view to participating in such a community plan.

The effects of the Depression were beginning to diminish in 1934: 2,123 patients admitted, an increase of 168 over 1933, and with an average daily census of 71. There was an increase of 106 private admissions over 1933 and the hospital reported increased earnings of $10,000. The depression, however, was far from over as public ward hospital days made up 43.5 percent of the total of hospital days. The death rate showed an improvement with 74 deaths recorded versus 92 in 1933. Some monies were expended on new equipment this year and a new portable X-ray machine, together with other X-ray accessories, was purchased to replace one of obsolete design.

The hospital opened its own pharmacy for the first time on April 1, 1934, and besides insuring prompt delivery of drugs to the patients, it made a small profit for the hospital. In July 1934, the hospital was honoured by a visit from the Governor General of Canada, Lord Bessborough, and staff. That year Miss MacMaster attended the American Hospital Association conference held in Philadelphia and on the same trip attended the first convention of the American College of Hospital Administrators.

Two new physicians were added to the staff in 1934: Dr. Peter Dowd and Dr. H. Paul Melanson. Moncton could not have agreed with Dr. Dowd as his name vanishes from the annual report of 1935. Dr. H. Paul Melanson, on the other hand, built up a large practice and remained on staff for many years. He was born in Moncton on July 3, 1903, received his BA from St. Joseph's in 1920 and his MD, CM from McGill in 1929. He interned at the Royal Victoria Hospital from 1929 to 1932, undertook a residency at Alexandra Hospital from 1932 to 1934, and served overseas during the Second World War. He was known as a "doctor's doctor" and despite being, in effect, a general practitioner he was often called in as a consultant in several fields. He was president of the New Brunswick Medical Society in 1959-60. In 1966 he retired to Florida because of ill health and he died there on August 23, 1976. Dr. Melanson had been a prominent witness in the famous Bannister murder trial having performed the autopsy on Arthur Lake, discovering the bullet in the skull of Lake's burned body.

Another note of interest about the staff is that in October of this year Dr. J.W. Dobson received his fellowship in the American College of Surgeons.

During 1934, there were 2,123 admissions and 1,429 operations performed; 1,054 private and 375 ward. 960 of the operations were major and 358 minor. There were 166 births, 3 by caesarean section, and 10 stillbirths recorded. There were 1,083 X-ray exams, 271 X-ray treatments, 420 physiotherapy treatments, and 1,655 outpatient treatments, with 187 minor operations and 42 fractures reduced in the outpatient department. Outpatient clinics continued to flourish with 277 attending the EENT clinic, 178 the medical clinic, and 49 the surgical clinic, although there was only one visit to the gynaecological clinic.

Tragedy struck the medical staff in 1935 with the death of one its stalwarts, Dr. W.A. Ferguson. Although not one of the founding fathers, he was on the staff by the turn of the century. His wife Janet, a former superintendent and a long time member of the Ladies' Auxiliary, donated his library to the hospital. Appropriate bookcases were constructed in the old boardroom in the maternity wing and this room was thereafter to be known as the Medical Library, for the use of the attending staff. Since 1932, physicians had been assessed the sum of $5 yearly to purchase periodicals for a staff library but no separate room had previously been set aside for such a purpose.

In the annual report for the year ending December, 31, 1935, there were no new appointments made to the staff for 1936 as announced but there were some changes in the staff designations as follows:

Senior Surgeons	Dr. A.R. Myers
	Dr. H.E. Britton
	Dr. P.McL. Atkinson
	Dr. G.A. Lyons
Junior Surgeons	Dr. C.R. Baxter
	Dr. J.W. Dobson
	Dr. H.M. MacLean
	Dr. R.J. Caldwell
Senior Physicians	Dr. R.G. Girvan
	Dr. J.A. McNaughton
	Dr. A.E. Forbes
	Dr. R.D. Roach
Junior Physicians	Dr. H.P. Melanson
Special Senses:	
EENT	Dr. S.W. Burgess
	Dr. F.E. Boudreau
Ear, Nose & Throat	Dr. L.A. Goodridge
Ophthalmologist	Dr. W.A. Pullin
Pediatricians	Dr. R.D. Roach
	Dr. H.P. Melanson
Cystoscopist	Dr. W.S. Fitzpatrick
Roentgenologist	Dr. F.A. Richard
Anaesthetists	Dr. A.E. Forbes
	Dr. R.G. Girvan
	Dr. J.A. McNaughton
	Dr. H.H. Coleman (Emeritus)
Physician to Communicable Diseases Unit	Dr. H. P. Melanson
Consulting Staff	Dr. A.R. Landry—Moncton
	Dr. H.H. Coleman—Moncton
	Dr. A.S. Cowie—Salisbury
	Dr. A. Sormany—Shediac
	Dr. A.R. Richardson—Petitcodiac
	Dr. G.M. MacFarlane—Sackville

A net loss of $5,896.55 was recorded for the year 1935 on a budget of $118,178.66 which was 50 percent better than 1934. Omitting depreciation, however, a surplus was recorded so there was adequate cash flow. It is recorded that 175 more patients were treated in 1935 than 1934, 79 more private and 38 more semi-private patients. Forty percent of hospital days, however, were accounted for by public ward patients and 35 percent of all patients admitted from the City of Moncton were public ward patients. Urology received the only largesse from the budget with the purchase of a Sisk cystoscopic table at a cost of $903.80. In her annual report for this year Miss MacMaster continued to decry the lack of government support for renovations to the VD Clinic and to provide a suitable ambulance for transportation of infectious diseases patients. The regular ambulance, under its chauffeur, William Walsh, a long time member of the Moncton Police Department, made 662 calls that year travelling some 2,668 miles. Miss Marjorie Rodd took over the duties of pharmacist on November 1.

The Nursing School continued its affiliation with the Royal Victoria Hospital in Montreal for training in obstetrical nursing. Student nurses also underwent a three-month rotation at the Tuberculosis Hospital in East Saint John for training in tuberculosis nursing and public health.

There were 2,285 admissions to the hospital in 1935 with 91 deaths recorded; 1,142 were private patients, 503 were semi-private and 640 were ward patients. Seventy percent of all ward patients were from the City of Moncton. There were 158 births recorded, with 9 stillbirths and 3 caesarean sections. The first set of triplets born in The Moncton Hospital occurred this year. In operations performed, 1,099 were major and 358 were minor. The X-ray department performed 1,067 examinations with 781 on private and 286 on ward patients. A motion was passed this year that the X-ray exam for fractures include pre and post reduction X-rays for the one fee. The number of X-ray treatments show a much different story from that presented by statistics on X-ray examinations with 208 treatments on private patients but only 1 treatment on a public ward patient. Besides being used for malignancies, X-ray treatments were still being used for benign conditions which included in that year 37 cases of acne, 21 cases of tubercular glands, 14 cases of eczema, 7 of pruritus and 7 sycosis. In one sense the poor were perhaps fortunate not to be exposed to the radiation for these benign conditions but it would have been nice to see more equal treatment for their malignancies.

The outpatient clinics continued to function with 201 patients seen at the EENT Clinic, 199 at the Medical Clinic and 32 at the Surgical Clinic. In addition, 1,203 treatments were given in the outpatient department with 190 minor operations and 48 fracture reductions, and 568 physiotherapy treatments were also given.

There was a continued lessening of the effects of the Depression in 1936, with public hospital ward days dropping to 34 percent of the total from 40 percent the previous year and 43.6 percent in 1934. The hospital's financial reports show that the hospital was just about at the break-even point at this time. Good times had not entirely returned, however, as many people not eligible for admission to the ward service were barely scraping by. Although admitted to hospital as private or semi-private patients, they had trouble meeting their financial obligations and their accounts were carried on the books of the hospital.

The only new medical equipment purchased during the year was a "Victor Giant" Eye Magnet for the operating room.

There were no new additions to the medical staff in 1936 and the death of Dr. A.E. Forbes, a long-time senior physician on the staff occurred. At the annual meeting of January 7, 1936, the option of having 6 senior and 6 junior surgeons on staff was proposed by the staff but Miss MacMaster felt it was more efficient for the hospital to stay with 4 senior and 4 junior surgeons. Her option prevailed. It was adopted at this meeting that, from this time on the retirement age be set at 65 exclusive of those already on staff. Those who retired were to be automatically appointed as chief consultants to their respective services. At a meeting on April 14, 1936, a motion was passed that the attending ward staff be allowed to extend to any visiting doctor of specialist standing the courtesy of the hospital, if invited by an individual member of the staff in attendance and in accordance with the legal status as laid down by the New Brunswick Medical Society. The hospital again was inspected by the American College of Surgeons and, although approval was received, there was marked criticism of the state of the hospital records and the by-laws of the staff, suggesting that the latter needed immediate revision. Dr. Baxter was appointed to work with Miss Wilson, the assistant administrator, on revising the by-laws. Miss MacMaster declared that in the future, apart from emergencies, all case histories would require to be written up before any case would be accepted in the operating room.

Statistics for 1936 show an increase of about 10 percent in patient attendance and work for the year.

In 1937 there were two new appointments to the medical staff. Dr. Lea Allanach was appointed as dental surgeon, replacing Dr. Fred E. Burden who had served in this position for several years. Dr. Allanach had the distinction of being the first baby born by caesarean section at The Moncton Hospital.

Dr. K.W. MacKenzie was appointed a junior physician and was to enjoy a long association with the medical staff. He was a local boy born in Sunny Brae on June 20, 1908. He received his BA from Mount Allison in 1930 and his MD, CM from Dalhousie in 1935. He interned at the Victoria General Hospital in 1934-35 and then served as a resident in surgery at the Toronto Western Hospital (1935-1936). He was one of the few in the medical profession who planned for and looked forward to his retirement. Unfortunately, he died from a coronary attack in January 1973, in the first year of his retirement.

Dr. Henry Hicks Coleman, who was one of the founding fathers of the hospital and had served for many years as the staff representative on the hospital board, died in 1937. His death left Dr. A. R. Myers and Dr. L.N. Bourque as the only living founding fathers and Dr. Myers as the only remaining founding father on the active staff.

At a staff meeting on January 15, 1937, after some discussion as to the advisability of splitting up the surgical service into specialities, it was passed that Dr. Fitzpatrick be appointed as urologist. This met some resistance and the opposition was able to muster its forces and rescind the motion at a special meeting on January 20. However, the opposition did not prevail, as another meeting was held on February 2, 1937. At this meeting, it was again passed that there be a Department of Urology with Dr. Fitzpatrick as urologist but with the proviso that all junior surgeons would be appointed as assistant urologists.

On reviewing the 1937 annual report of Miss MacMaster to the board of Directors of The Moncton Hospital, one comes to appreciate how fortunate the hospital was to have such a dedicated and capable administrator. Fully forty-seven years before the hospital developed its mission statement, the preliminary part of her report expressed so succinctly the mission of a hospital that I quote it in full:

> We have emerged from the depression and with the improvement of the past year the hospital's economic pressure has become less intense. It seems time to take account of stock and consider the future in light of changed and changing conditions. Policies and standards must be reconsidered if hospitals are effectively to meet the demands which the future will impose; some indication of these developments will follow in this report.
>
> Since new methods, new procedures, and discoveries in medicine are developing faster than the profession itself is able to absorb, much less the public, it would appear that hospitals with their professional staffs might well act as a stabilizing influence to interpret these advances to the lay community. There is in every community and organization a laissez faire group who are content to leave things as they are. In scanning the history of hospitals and medicine an intelligent observer could scarcely concur in their opinion. We cannot remain silent and stationary among all the changes going on and progress. The education of the public for more healthful, abundant and happy living has been claimed as a legitimate responsibility of hospitals. The public health horizon has been expanded to include programs not only for environmental sanitation but control of communicable disease, pneumonia, diabetes, the degenerative diseases, mental health, etc. Such recognition focuses immediate attention upon the important part played by the hospital structure in dealing with the care of the sick and in the fostering of health, as well as the potentialities for better results which can come about from better co-ordination of effort among the health agencies. New conceptions of what constitutes an adequate health program and the services which must be included in the same, emphasize the gradual disappearance of the line of demarcation between the prevention and the treatment of disease. This changing point of view calls for greater unity of purpose and more intelligent co-planning and interrelationship by the agencies engaged in the various aspects of health services.
>
> If we divorce the hospital from its sentimental and scientific aspect, we may consider the management as a business, its plant in terms of shelter, work space and power and its budget from the angle that only what is left, after overhead and departmental costs have been met, is available for its essential function—the professional care of the patients. It has

> been said that it is strange that men can see sublime inspiration in the ruins of an old church and see none in the ruins of man. In presenting my report I would plead that the contents thereof be received not merely as a routine accounting of stewardship, but as a re-affirmation of our consciousness that we who are entrusted with the administration of the hospital are charged with a most solemn duty—that of helping to restore to their rightful place in society those inflicted in mind, body and spirit through physical sickness. That we may be granted the courage to look up and not down, to look forward and not back, to look out and not in, and to lend a hand.
>
> I submit, therefore, a picture of the year's activities not as a barren outline of statistics but as an index of ever growing service to a community which, judging from the facts presented, is paying greater heed to the essential benefits which may be obtained whenever needed in the standardized approved modern hospital of today.

Tired of waiting for the government to act, the hospital went ahead with the installation of the VD Clinic in new modern quarters, the only capital expense of the year. Three hundred dollars was donated that year by Mr. and Mrs. Henry Merkle of Anfield, Victoria County, New Brunswick, for the purchase of an up-to-date eye, ear, nose and throat operating table. One mark of increasing good times was the appointment of a committee to carry out a survey and to acquire data which would be of use should the board of Directors decide to complete the third floor of the new wing, which had been left unfinished when the wing was opened in 1930.

Representatives from all New Brunswick hospitals met with the Worker's Compensation Board in the fall of 1937, to discuss a proposed reduction of the fees paid to hospitals for Workers' Compensation cases. The discussions came to naught, however, as on January 1, 1938, the WCB put its revised and reduced fees into operation despite the protest of the Hospital Association.

A notable event of the year was the induction of Miss Ruth Wilson, the assistant administrator of the hospital, as a member of the American College of Hospital Administrators at the 1937 Hospital Conference. This meeting was also attended by Miss MacMaster, a charter fellow of the college.

Group hospitalization began operations in the city on September 1, 1937. Its administration was vested in an authoritative commission known as the Group Hospitalization Service Commission under the aegis of The Moncton Hospital Board and l'Hôtel Dieu. With the institution of the plan, the roentgenologist, went on a flat fee rate per month.

On April 27, 1937, a special meeting of the staff was called to study the question of forming a new set of by-laws. Eventually a new set was created, patterned after a set proposed by the American College of Surgeons. At another special meeting held on May 1, 1937, the new by-laws were passed with three amendments as follows:

1. Notice of vacancies or changes in the personnel be posted and discussed at a meeting one month before the changes are acted upon;
2. Regular monthly meetings to be held at 5 pm on the second Tuesday of each month instead of in the a.m.;
3. All members of the active staff shall be expected to attend all meetings. Absence for three consecutive meetings or six regular meetings of the year shall be dealt with at the regular meeting of the active staff on the advice of the executive.

Another rule passed this year, on November 9, was that every surgeon must provide himself with an assistant for all major surgical procedures, EENT being exempt, and that assistants for night work be called at the discretion of the operator. It was subsequently recommended to the board of Governors that the immediate engagement of two medical graduates as interns would lessen the financial burden incurred by the public as a result of this new rule. A resolution was also passed at this meeting in which the medical hospital staff recommended the appointment of a graduate nurse duly qualified in surgical technique to act as instrument nurse at all major operations.

In 1937, 2,527 patients were admitted to hospital with an average stay of 12 days and an average daily census of 83.8. Public ward hospital days were still high and accounted for 38 percent of the hospital days. There were 187 births with 5 stillbirths. There were 1,179 private and 452 ward patients who underwent surgery; 1,308 X-ray exams and 198 X-ray treatments took place. One point of note is that 34 public X-ray treatments were carried out this year. There were 6,589 laboratory exams carried out and 331 physiotherapy treatments. In the outpatient department, 881 patients were seen, 326 of which were private and 555 ward patients, who underwent 193 treatments, 126 minor operations, 30 fracture reductions and 533 dressings. In addition, 127 persons attended the EENT Clinic and 113 the Surgical Clinic. Only one person attended the Medical Clinic.

The only new additions to the staff in 1938 were those of Dr. L.J. Gaudet to the position of junior physician and Dr. Vincent Doucet as a junior EENT specialist. Vincent Doucet was born in Richibucto on June 11, 1902, and obtained his BA from St. Joseph's and his MD from Laval in 1927. He interned at l'Hôtel Dieu in Quebec City in 1926 and St. Luke's Hospital, New York, in 1927. He then did postgraduate work in EENT in Paris from 1928 to 1930 and at the New York Postgraduate Hospital during 1930-1931. He died in 1948.

June 1938 marked the first intern appointment to The Moncton Hospital. In August 1937 Dr. Philip Magmet from Glace Bay applied for an intern position but was turned down and it was recommended that only young recent graduates be considered for intern positions. The first intern committee was formed that same month and consisted of Dr. Atkinson, Dr.

Fitzpatrick and Dr. Dobson. Dr. Everett Crutchlow, a graduate of McGill University, was its first appointment.

On December 20, 1938, the medical staff recommended to the New Brunswick Medical Society that some method be arranged for procuring radium for cancer treatment.

By this time, the Depression's effect on the economy of the city had lessened and 1938 saw a slight increase in the admission of private and semi-private patients, with a drop of over 120 in the number of public ward patients treated. The pharmacy also experienced an increased workload and the pharmacist had her hours increased to a three-quarter time basis from her previous half-time basis.

There were 2,502 admissions in 1938 with 1,127 major and 460 minor operations performed. Among the operations were 8 caesarean sections. There were 222 births and 15 stillbirths recorded. The attendance at clinics, meanwhile, seemed to vary a lot from year to year during this period. Whereas there was only 1 visit to the Medical Clinic in 1937, there were 123 patients seen in 1938, while visits to the Surgical Clinic dropped to 18 from 113 the previous year.

By 1939, the depression years were definitely over but a new economic fact, inflation, comes into play. In September 1939, at the beginning of the Second World War, the cost of provisions began to rise. By the end of the year, the patient-day cost exceeded the previous year by 26 cents with every indication that prices would increase in 1940, although it was hoped this would be constrained somewhat by the Price Review Board. It was a happy year for those patients with contagious diseases, however, as a new Studebaker ambulance was purchased by the hospital on August 12, 1939. The old ambulance which it replaced was retained for use in conveying contagious diseases patients replacing the old horse-drawn wagon which had previously been used. In March 1939, the Knights of Columbus, Council No.1310, notified the hospital that it had developed a voluntary free blood donor service and offered the facilities of this service to the hospital in any emergency for the benefit of any needy patient. An application was made during the year to have the student nurses and staff trained in fire drills, under the instruction of the Chief of the Moncton Fire Department. The Fire Chief inspected the hospital and its fire extinguishers but no training program was implemented at this time.

The Group Hospital Service Commission became an incorporated body in April 1939. Although the reports for the year ending August 1939 were encouraging, Miss MacMaster pointed out that the plan was actuarially unsound and urged a policy of accepting subscribers in groups rather than on an individual basis.

Staff changes in 1939 saw the promotion of Dr. Baxter and Dr. Dobson to the status of senior surgeons and Dr. H.P. Melanson and Dr. H.M. MacLean to the positions of junior surgeons. Dr. H.L. McKeen and Dr. Ralph Myers were appointed as junior physicians.

Harry McKeen was born at Cumberland Bay, New Brunswick, on February 6, 1903, took his undergraduate BA degree in 1931 at the University of Alberta and graduated in medicine from McGill in 1936. After interning at the Montreal General Hospital in 1936-1937, he established a practice in Petitcodiac but then moved to Moncton where his general practice flourished until he retired in 1962. He was transferred to the honorary staff in 1976. He was very attentive to his patients and it would not be unusual for him to make house calls a couple of times a day to check in on his patients. He was a small man physically and quick of temper, often leaving many a nurse with tears in her eyes.

Dr. Ralph Myers was the son of Dr. Ambrose Myers and the first of the hospital's second generation physicians to join the staff. He underwent his medical training at Edinburgh, receiving his LRCP & S(Edin), and also received his Canadian qualifications with the LMCC. Ralph was always very active in the Saint John Ambulance Association and was invested as an Officer Brother by Governor General Alexander on November 12, 1951.

In other staff developments for the year, Dr. E. Crutchlow finished his term as intern in the summer of 1939 and was replaced by Dr. Vernon Dunfield, who left shortly after his appointment, however, to set up practice in New York State and so the hospital was left without an intern. As a result, the hospital applied to the medical school of Dalhousie University to be placed on its list of hospitals for rotating service of student interns.

When appointments were made for the coming year at the January 10, 1939, annual meeting it was moved and seconded that a Department of Orthopaedics be established (exclusive of fractures) and that Dr. E. W. Ewart be made orthopaedist. Dr. Ewart was born in 1894 in Bolton, Ontario, and served in the Navy in the First World War. After graduating in medicine from the University of Toronto, he interned at St. Michael's Hospital in Toronto in 1921-22 and then at the Vancouver General Hospital in 1922-23. After practising for six years in British Columbia, he embarked on a career in orthopaedics. He trained at several leading orthopaedic centres in the United States and these institutions are still renowned as excellent orthopaedic centres today. He was a resident under Steindler, a leading orthopaedist and kinesiologist at the University of Iowa and was an early fellow of the famous Campbell Clinic in Memphis. He also served as a resident at the Shriners

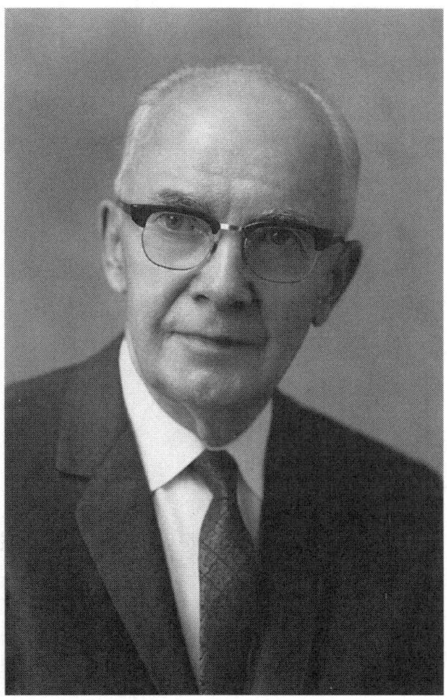

Dr. E.W. Ewart was the first orthopaedic surgeon at The Moncton Hospital.

Hospital in Shreveport, Louisiana. I once asked Dr. Ewart why he underwent such a long period of residency when at that time one or two years was the norm and he replied there were surgeons driving taxis in New York City and at least he was doing work he was enjoying and getting his room and board. He was on the attending staff of the New Jersey Orthopaedic Hospital when he was enticed to come to Moncton by his brother-in-law, Dr. R.D. Roach, whose wife was a sister to Edith Ewart. Dr. Ewart passed his certification exams of the American Board of Orthopaedic surgeons in 1937 and subsequently became a Fellow of the American Academy of Orthopaedic Surgeons in 1943. He thus arrived in the Maritimes as the first orthopaedic surgeon in New Brunswick and the first fully-trained orthopaedist in the Maritimes.

At the time of his appointment, most surgeons still considered that the treatment of trauma and fractures were the preserve of the general surgeon and this was why the department of orthopaedics was created with the exclusion of fractures. Mrs. Ewart told me that when Dr. Ewart arrived in town he went to see several of the surgeons and one surgeon remarked to him that there may be the odd fracture that he couldn't handle, but if so, he hadn't yet seen it. Dr. Ewart soon established a reputation for his excellent orthopaedic work, including the treatment of fractures, and it was not long before he was treating most of the fractures by popular demand. The treatment of bone tuberculosis for the province came under his care and all cases of bone tuberculosis were sent to Jordan Memorial Hospital for his treatment and then later to the Moncton Tuberculosis Hospital. The Moncton Tuberculosis Hospital was established in 1947 in the abandoned base of the Commonwealth Air Training Plan Hospital in Moncton. This was done because of a large backlog of bone tuberculosis in New Brunswick and because Dr. Ewart was the only qualified orthopaedic surgeon in New Brunswick at the time. Dr. Perry Knox, formerly superintendent of the Riverglade TB Hospital became CEO. In the ensuing six or seven years, with the advent of the anti-TB drugs and Dr. Ewart's surgical expertise, bone TB was eradicated in New Brunswick. Dr. Ewart was also responsible for the establishment of Crippled Children's Clinics in the province and was awarded the coveted Red Cross Service Medal for his work with these children. He was a founding member of the Canadian Orthopaedic Society in 1945 and became its president in 1961. As a prelude to the annual meeting of the Canadian Orthopaedic Society, to be held for the first time in New Brunswick in Saint Andrews, all the orthopaedists in the Atlantic provinces were enlisted to help in the organization of the meeting, resulting in the formation of the Atlantic Provinces Orthopaedic Society in 1960 with Dr. Ewart as its first president.

Dr. Ewart was a handsome, mild spoken and a very kind man. He was a superb operator and could not be hurried, making certain that any work was done to perfection. If things were not going well in the operating room, which was seldom, the only indication from Dr. Ewart that anything was amiss would be a soft-spoken "pshaw" and if things got really bad, a mild "damn." The only time Dr. Ewart ever appeared hurried was when he got behind the wheel of his car and was often stopped by the men in blue as he sped along Mountain Road on his way to the hospital. He had total devotion to his work and for a long time, being the only orthopaedic doctor in Moncton, the number of hours he worked were legendary. He would often make rounds at night and often after patients had gone to sleep. One amusing story concerns two young ladies in the same room who had had surgery but had not had a visit from Dr. Ewart in the daytime for some time. They sent him a telegram saying they were having a wonderful time and would be pleased to have a visit from him. He kept up well on current developments in orthopaedics and about the only vacations he ever took were to attend meetings of the American Academy of Orthopaedic Surgeons, the Canadian Orthopaedic Association and SICOT, an international orthopaedic society. He always thought of his patients first and would often fashion a brace for a crippled child. He had an OR table for use in hip pinnings constructed locally.

I can recall two cases when I was in general practice in which his generosity stood out. I saw an elderly lady who had fallen and sustained a Colles Fracture of the wrist. I gave her an anaesthetic and Dr. Ewart reduced the fracture. Sometime later, she came to my office and stated that she had gone to Dr. Ewart's office to get the bill but his office said there was no charge. I spoke to Dr. Ewart and he replied that, from the patient's address, he felt it would be a hardship for her to pay anything. I informed him that as she had fallen in the Bank of Montreal, their insurance covered her treatment and that he had better change his mind. On another occasion, he did an open reduction of a fracture dislocation of the spine on a young lad injured in a motor vehicle accident and did not send the family a bill as he felt they would have enough expense looking after this young man who had been rendered a paraplegic.

There were 2,619 admissions in 1939, an increase of 46 over 1938. The hospital days were less, however, indicating an improved length of stay per patient. There were 1,152 major and 354 minor operations; 428 of the operations were on public patients. The X-ray department carried out 1,599 examinations and 239 treatments; 704 persons were seen in the outpatient department with 137 treatments, 193 minor operations, 49 fractures reduced and 325 dressings. At the clinics, 174 people were seen at the EENT clinic, 266 at the medical clinic and 43 at the surgical clinic. 24 Gyro chest clinics were held during the year with 551 examinations by Dr. J.A. Melanson, the public health doctor, and there were 1,755 treatments in the VD clinic.

With the thirties ending, and Canada "at war," there arose the challenge of providing increased services with fewer personnel and rationed resources.

Chapter Six

The Forties—The War Years and After

With the beginning of the fifth decade of the twentieth century, Canada was at war and three members of The Moncton Hospital's medical staff took leave of absence to join the army. The 14th Field Ambulance Corps was recruited in July 1940, and among those on staff accepting the call to duty was Dr. George Lyons, who became a lieutenant colonel and was the corps' commanding officer at its mobilization. The other doctors from the medical staff who went to war were Dr. H.P. Melanson and Dr. H.M. MacLean. Dr. Arthur Melanson, the public health doctor and Dr. Raoul Landry, who later became a public health doctor in Moncton, also joined the war effort by joining the corps. Also among the original officers of the corps were Dr. F.J. Desmond and Dr. R.B. Eaton, who would become staff members after the war. Dr. Andy Richardson from Petitcodiac was another officer with the corps. As well, several of the orderlies from the hospital were included among the enlisted men. Training began in Sussex where the unit was brought to its full strength of 250 officers and other enlisted men. On July 31, 1941, the unit sailed for England with "A" Company under Dr. MacLeod, and "B" Company under Capt. A.R. Richardson from Petitcodiac. Major Paul Melanson was appointed second in command of the unit in July 1942. On June 6, 1944, the 14th Field Ambulance Corps was in the thick of battle as it landed on the Normandy beaches with the third Canadian Division. Dr. Lyons was awarded the Canadian Efficiency Decoration in February 1942, the first Moncton native to win a decoration in the Second World War. Dr. Lyons returned to Canada in 1944 and rejoined the medical staff. Dr. Joseph Tanzman of Saint John was the last commanding officer of the corps.

Dr. Eaton had gone overseas with the 14th Field Ambulance but later he served with the Canadian Number 1 Neurological Division and was in charge of a surgical team during the Normandy invasion. His work as a surgeon in the field during the European campaign was noted in the British Journal of Surgery War Supplement No.3, in an article about chest and abdominal injuries, and in Ian Aird's Companion of Surgical Studies. After the war, Dr. Eaton joined the Sackville Clinic as a surgeon but then moved to Moncton in 1950, where he enjoyed a long and distinguished surgical career.

Many of the doctors who joined the staff after the war had also served in the armed services during the war. Many, such as Dr. C.E. Doyle, Dr. J.S. Wright and Dr. C. Leighton, had graduated from medical school during the war years, joined the army, and then took postgraduate work after the war. Others, such as Dr. Brent Stewart, served in the army during the war and only took their medical education after the war.

In 1940 there was a marked increase in the use of the hospital facilities, with 500 more admissions than in 1939. In her annual report for 1940, Miss MacMaster stressed the need of finishing the third floor of the new wing as provided for in the original architect's plans of 1930. City of Moncton ward cases accounted for 35 percent of all Moncton patients and 18 percent of total hospital services. Only $242 was collected directly from these patients but the city of Moncton did contribute $25,030.99 or about 16.6 percent of the total hospital revenues for the year. The board of directors increased the rate for public ward patients of Westmorland and Albert counties from $2 to $3 per hospital day plus the cost of X-ray examinations in order to cope with the increased cost of providing hospitalization to these patients.

To comply with Department of National Defence regulations, all build-

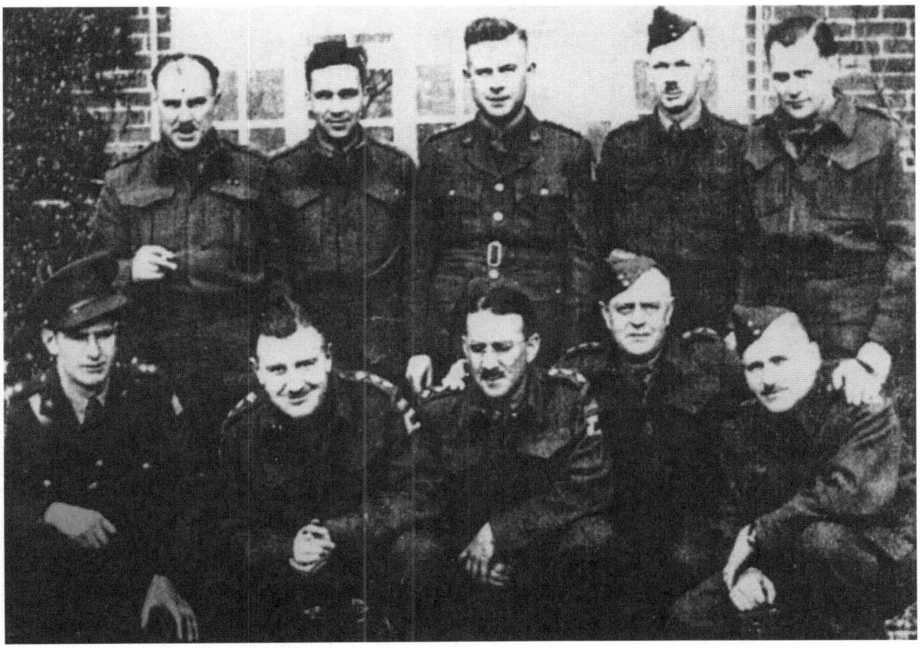

Doctors gone to war in 1940—the 14th field ambulance. Back row, L-R: Dr. Art Melanson, Dr. Bud Desmond, Dr. Esmond Stiles, Dr. A.R. Richardson, Dr. R.B. Eaton. Bottom row: unidentified, Dr. Kelly MacLean, Dr. Paul Melanson, Dr. Len Reid, Dr. Raoul Landry.

ings were prepared in June 1940, for emergency and blackouts in case of air raids. As a result of recommendations from the Fire Marshall, the basement floor in the old wing and service departments occupying this space were demolished and replaced with fireproof materials. This resulted in a new stores department and receiving room, linen and sewing rooms, an eye clinic and several offices and other service rooms. Another result of the fire inspection was that the Fire Marshall of the province ordered the destruction of all charts of patients dating back before 1930.

An electrocardiographic service was arranged under the direction of Dr. R.D. Roach, as well as a cardiac clinic in the outpatient department. Very little medical equipment was bought during the year, but a new surgical treatment and examination table was purchased for the isolation building and a new steam table was purchased for maternity. The most expensive purchase was a Hess Infant Incubator with oxygen attachment at a cost of $400. An Iron Lung was presented to the hospital by Lord Nuffield.

There were 3,140 patients admitted in 1940 with 1,673 operations performed and 340 births, including 17 stillbirths and two sets of twins. Four caesarean sections were performed, 3,749 X-rays were taken and 265 X-ray treatments given; 207 physiotherapy treatments were done; 817 treatments including minor surgery, fracture reductions and dressings were performed in the outpatient department with 291 patients seen at the EENT, Medical and Surgical clinics.

The slack in the staff created by the departure of three staff members to the army in 1940 was taken up in 1941 when three new doctors were appointed: Dr. A.W. Ross, Dr. John Stewart and Dr. Robert Cox. The attending staff for 1941 was as follows:

Senior Surgeons	H.E. Britton, MD, CM, FACS
	P.McL. Atkinson, MD, CM, FACS
	G.A. Lyons, MC, MD, CM, FACS (On leave of absence in RCAMC)
	J.W. Dobson BA(Acadia) MD, CM, FACS
	C.R. Baxter, MD, CM, FACS
Junior Surgeons	John Stewart, BA, MD, CM
	H.M. MacLean, MD, CM, LMCC, FACS (On leave of absence in RCAMC)
	H.P. Melanson, BA, MD, CM (On leave of absence in RCAMC)
	K.W. MacKenzie, BA, MD, CM
	R.P. Myers, BSc, RCP&S(Edin), LMCC
Senior Physicians	J.A. McNaughton, MD, CM
	R.G. Girvan, MD, CM
	R.D. Roach, MD, MRCP(London),FACP
Junior Physician	H.L. McKeen, MD, CM, LMCC

Department of Orthopaedics	E.W. Ewart, MD, Dip. ABOS
Eye, Ear, Nose and ThroatSpecialists	S.W. Burgess, MD, CM, FACS
	F.E. Boudreau, MD, CM
Junior Eye, Ear, Nose and Throat Specialists	Vincent P. Doucet, MD, CM
	A.W. Ross, BSc, MD, CM
Ear, Nose and Throat	L.A. Goodridge, MD, CM, FACS
Ophthalmologist	W.A. Pullin, MD, CM
Senior Pediatrician	R.D. Roach, MD,MRCP (London), FACP
Junior Pediatricians	Junior physicians on service
Urologist	W.S. Fitzpatrick, MD, CM, FACS
Assistant Urologists	Junior surgeons on service
Roenthenologist	F.A. Richard, BA, MD, CM
Anaesthetists	R.G. Girvan, MD
	J.A. McNaughton, MD, CM
Communicable Disease Unit	Senior and junior physicians on service
Dental Surgeon	John A. Folkins, DDS
Consulting Staff	A.R. Myers, MA, MD, CM, FACS, Moncton, New Brunswick
	A.R. Landry, MD, CM, FRCS(Canada), Moncton, New Brunswick
	A. Sormany, MD, CM, Shediac, New Brunswick
	A.R. Richardson, MD, CM, Petitcodiac, New Brunswick (On leave of absence in RCAMC)
	R.J. Caldwell, BSc, MD, CM, Petitcodiac, New Brunswick
	Dr. C.A. Gass, Sackville, New Brunswick
	Dr. P.L. Oxley, Hillsborough, New Brunswick
	Dr. R.P. MacDonald, Shediac, New Brunswick

In contrast to 1995, at which time there were twenty-seven committees of the medical staff, in 1941 there were only five committees as follows:

Executive Committee:	Dr. Britton, Dr. Goodridge, Dr. Girvan
Records Committee:	Dr. Girvan, Dr. MacKenzie, Dr. Atkinson
Program Committee:	Dr. Roach, Dr. Goodridge, Dr. R. Myers
Credentials Committee:	Dr. Britton, Dr. Fitzpatrick, Dr. McNaughton
Intern Committee:	Dr. Atkinson, Dr. Fitzpatrick, Dr. Dobson

Although it was the custom to appoint new members to the staff at the beginning of the year, the appointments of Dr. A.W. Ross to the eye, ear, nose and throat staff was recorded in the minutes of a July 9, 1940, meeting. No mention of the appointments of Dr. John Stewart and Dr. Robert Cox is made until the presentation of the medical staff for 1941.

Dr. Arthur Ross was born in Pictou County, Nova Scotia, on January 10, 1905, but as his family moved shortly thereafter to Cape Breton he always considered this his native land. After graduating from Dalhousie in 1929, he practised in Saint John for a short period of time and then several years in Souris, Prince Edward Island, before undertaking postgraduate work in EENT in Montreal. Arthur Ross was a man of many talents and, besides being a competent surgeon, he was an excellent storyteller and poet. He could tell many amusing stories of his practice on the Island and could easily have compiled them into a book but did not feel it would be ethical to do so while the characters he described were still alive. He did publish one children's book called *Percival Pup*. He wrote scripts for pieces of entertainment for the medical society and for the Gyro Club in Moncton. He was an amateur photographer, notably taking 16 mm films when 8 mm would keep most amateur photographers happy. A lot of the films he took in Moncton during the war years now rest in the archives of the National Film Board. He was an avid salmon fishermen and on his death on December 19, 1969, was laid to rest in a churchyard on the banks of his favourite fishing spot, the Margaree, in Cape Breton.

Dr. Robert Cox was born in Aroostook Junction on October 10, 1912. He took his premed at Mount Allison University and graduated in medicine from McGill in 1940. He interned at the Royal Victoria Hospital from 1939 to 1940 and then served as a resident in surgery at the Homeopathic Hospital in Montreal before coming to Moncton. He practised in Moncton for about 25 years. After developing angina, he left Moncton to spend the rest of his career in the upper Saint John River valley.

Dr. John Stewart was born in Campbellton on January 21, 1907. He received his BA from Mount Allison in 1928 and his MD,CM from Dalhousie in 1934. He interned at the Halifax Infirmary and served as a resident at the Saint John General Hospital from 1934 to 1935. He then undertook a surgical residency at the Royal Victoria Hospital in Montreal. After practising in Corner Brook, Newfoundland, for two years, he arrived in Moncton and established a general practice with surgery, although his training allowed him to be recognized as especially knowledgeable in obstetrics and gynaecology. He was a tall, gaunt-looking man who soon had a large obstetrical practice and, seemingly, never went to bed. In the middle of the night he could be seen drinking coffee at the Blue Circle Restaurant which, during the forties and fifties, was the only place open in Moncton in the wee hours of the morning and which was usually the hangout for some of Moncton's more unsavoury characters. The busy life took its toll on John Stewart, however, and after recovering from one heart attack, he took another fatal attack in the Montreal airport at the age of 46.

The year 1941 recorded an increase of 508 patients over the number admitted in 1940. With an average daily occupancy of 86 percent, including bassinets and cribs, which increased at times to 116 percent the facilities were overcrowded. With this increased use, however, the hospital ended the year with a surplus. On a positive note for the hospital's future finances, beginning January 1, 1942, the Workmen's Compensation Board increased their hospital rates from $2 to $2.50 per day. A special committee was also formed to investigate the possibility of engaging the interest of federal defence authorities in obtaining additional hospital bed space but Ottawa showed no interest in its proposals. During the year, the hospitals were placed under the provisions of the Wartime Price and Trade Board and room charges were fixed by government control.

In 1941, there were 3,648 admissions with an average length of stay of 10.6 days and an average daily census of 108.5 patients. There were 2,029 operations performed and 5,628 X-rays were taken with 308 X-ray treatments. An upsurge in the use of the maternity service took place with 422 births recorded, including 13 by caesarean section. There were 1,113 visits to the outpatient department mostly for dressings, but there were 170 fractures reduced and 314 minor operations carried out. The use of the free clinics was significantly down probably as a result of increased prosperity and reduced unemployment resulting from the war. In the Medical Clinic 41 patients were seen, 4 in gynaecology, 24 in EENT, 2 in surgery, 2 in ophthalmology and 1 in orthopaedics. The VD Clinic was active with 1,300 treatments carried out on 134 patients. Tuberculosis was also still active with 377 patients seen at the 12 clinics held during the year. During the latter part of the year, Moncton had a poliomyelitis epidemic and 21 patients were admitted to the isolation unit. Four iron lungs were pressed into service, including the one donated the previous year by Lord Nuffield. The Department of Health for the province engaged the services of a trained physiotherapist to supervise therapy for polio victims and this service was made available to The Moncton Hospital, financed in part by the government.

Blue was the predominant colour in Moncton in 1942. On a Friday or Saturday night, Main Street was awash with airmen dressed in their blue uniforms. During the war years, Moncton became an important Air Force Centre. No. 8 Service Flying Training School was opened up in December, 1940, at Lakeburn, now the site of the Moncton Airport. No. 5 Supply Depot began operations on November 11, 1940, and after November, 1941, handled all equipment required in the Maritimes for the air force. Another air base was constructed at Scoudouc and became the home of No. 4 Repair Depot. The largest concentration of airmen, by far, was at No. 31 Personnel Depot which was opened up in Moncton to serve as a manning depot for airmen coming to Canada for training under the Commonwealth Training plan for aircrews. This was a stopping-off point for the airmen on their way to and from the British Isles. Although the air force bases had their own hospitals, the increased activity and construction in Moncton during this period led to a growth in the population and this naturally had an impact on The Moncton Hospital. In the four years from 1939 to 1942, the number of patients treated each year increased 65.5 percent. The only encouraging point was the reduction of public ward hospital days to 15.47 percent due to the improved economic and employment conditions. The hospital facility built by the air force at No. 31 would play a future role in Moncton, becoming the Moncton Tuberculosis Hospital after the war, and then later being converted into the Moncton Hospital Annex.

Around this time, the efforts of the Special Building Committee and the hospital board to build an addition to relieve the acute congestion were stymied by government regulations. The committee was informed by the Hon. Mr. Howe, Minister of Munitions and Supply, that the hospital would not be given a permit to purchase essential plumbing and electrical supplies or allowed to build a fireproof structure. Nevertheless, a special building fund was established to assist a possible building program when circumstances permitted. To help ease the congestion in the meantime the superintendent made two recommendations in her annual report. Firstly, discretion be exercised in the admission of patients to the hospital and that admission be limited to those unable to remain at home, particularly the "rest-cure" and chronic ailment type of cases. Secondly, that control of admission of maternity cases be set up and that, during the current period of congestion, normal multipara cases be cared for at home. Maternity cases admitted to hospital were recommended to be discharged and removed to their homes at the end of a week. To ease the congestion in the maternity ward it was also suggested that a student nursing classroom in one wing of maternity be converted to maternity use and a new student classroom be constructed in the basement. Because of recruitment in the armed services, staff turnovers were common and it was especially difficult to obtain and keep orderlies and housekeeping staff. Supplies were also hard to come by and a Scanlan-Morris high pressure autoclave ordered in August 1942, had still not been obtained by the end of the year. A Wapply shortwave diathermy machine was obtained and added to the equipment of the physiotherapy department. At long last, the Sub-District of Health took over the task of providing a conveyance for the transportation of communicable diseases patients. The hospital was now able to use the old ambulance, previously used for infectious diseases, as a backup.

There were no new additions to the staff in 1942. The hospital was inspected by the American College of Surgeons and received only provisional approval. A special meeting was called to discuss this with Dr. DuBois, the visiting examiner from the American College of Surgeons. The loss of approval was based on: (1) poor case histories, (2) poor progress notes, (3) incomplete minutes and (4) poor attendance at staff meetings. The hospital board was unhappy with this turn of events and a special meeting was held on December 8, 1942, between a committee of the board and the medical staff. The chairman, Mr. Chapman, was quick to point out that the blame for the loss of standardization rested solely with the medical staff. Suggestions for improvements included obtaining the services of one or more interns as well as a stenographer and dictation equipment. Mr. Chapman pointed out, however, that it was impossible to get interns at this time with the war raging. During the meeting Dr. Roach expressed his belief that the hospital should obtain a trained pathologist if it really wanted to raise the standard of the hospital. Some improvements must have occurred over the next year, because in 1943, the hospital was restored to its previous rating.

There were 4,140 admissions to the hospital in 1942, an increase of 527 over 1941, with an average daily census of 120.4 and an average length of stay of 10.65 days. There were 2,040 operations performed with only 174 of them on ward patients. The number of births increased to 580 with 17 stillbirths, 4 sets of twins and 13 caesarian sections. Only 114 patients attended the free outpatient clinics. The VD clinic was still quite active with 482 patients receiving 1,480 treatments; 276 examinations were carried out at the Tuberculosis Clinic with 161 new patients seen; 5,992 X-rays were taken and 294 X-ray treatments were given; 633 physiotherapy treatments were also given.

The facilities of the hospital continued to be taxed into 1943 with over 400 more admissions than in 1942, and with the hospital consistently working at over 100 percent occupancy of its rated capacity of 125 beds. Equipment purchased during the year included an electrocardiographic machine at a cost of $340. A special fluoroscopic tube with complete shockproofing of the electrically driven table in the X-ray department was among the other medical items purchased this year. It was a great year for the surgeons. Up until then the surgeons supplied their own instruments for use in the operating room but, at this time, they agreed to pool these. In addition, the hospital agreed to buy $1,000 worth of surgical instruments and to take on the responsibility of obtaining and maintaining a supply of instruments in the future. The pharmacist, Marjorie Rodd, left during the year to join the Canadian Army Women's Corps and until a new pharmacist could be obtained, the firms of G.O. Spencer and F.W. Patterson carried on the work of the pharmacy.

During 1943, the Maritime Hospital Association organized the Maritime Hospital Service Association and The Moncton Hospital became a participant. Ruth C. Wilson, a long-time assistant administrator of the hospital and secretary to the board of Directors, resigned to assume a leadership role in the association.

A new constitution and set of by-laws was adopted by the board at its November meeting that year. The new constitution and by-laws were drafted by a committee under the chairmanship of Alderman J. Edward Murphy in consultation with the hospital solicitor, T.T. Goodwin, KC. The hospital community was saddened that year by the death of the chairman of the hospital board, A. Cavour Chapman, who had served in this position for the past twenty-five years. He was succeeded by Ambrose Wheeler.

Dr. F.J. (Bud) Desmond and Dr. R.I. McKenna were added to the courtesy staff in 1943, and became part of the attending staff in 1944, when Dr. Desmond was appointed to the senior eye, ear, nose and throat staff and Dr. McKenna to the position of junior physician. During the year, the deaths occurred of Dr. S.W. Burgess, who had served on the senior EENT staff for many years, and of Dr. J.A. Gaudet, who had been on the courtesy staff for many years.

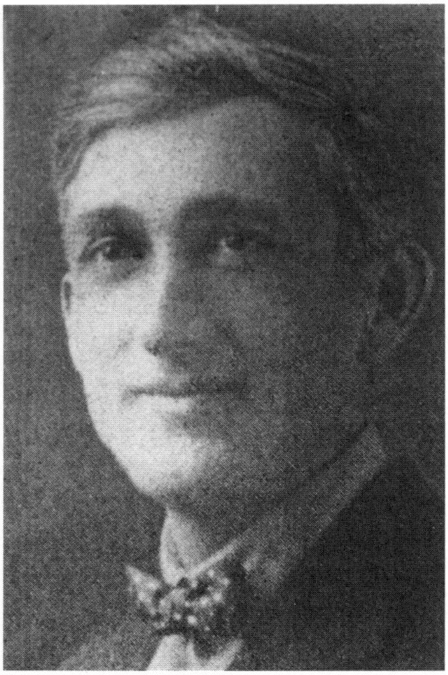

Ambrose Wheeler was Chairman of the Board from 1943 until 1947.

Dr. Desmond was born in Newcastle on October 19, 1915. He took his premed at Saint Francis Xavier and graduated from McGill in 1938 after interning at the Royal Victoria Hospital from 1938 to 1939. He then underwent a residency in EENT at the Royal Victoria Hospital from 1939 to 1943, although he interrupted his residency in 1940-41 while he served overseas with the Third Canadian Division of the Army. He served for many years on the staff and his life ended tragically in a car accident in 1969.

Reg McKenna carried on a general practice, including surgery, for many years. A Prince Edward Island native, he had in his blood the Islanders' love of horse racing and always owned some race horses. He could be found on the phone at noon talking to his stockbroker, and rumour has it that he did very well in the stock market over the years.

After serving as the radiologist at The Moncton Hospital for 40 years, Dr. F.A. Richard retired in 1944, and was replaced by Dr. Howard Ripley, who had just finished his training as a radiologist at the Royal Victoria Hospital in Montreal. Dr. Ripley would remain a mainstay of the radiology department for the next 30 years. Howard Ripley was born in Amherst, Nova Scotia on September 18, 1907. He received a BA from Mount Allison in 1928 and his MD,CM from Dalhousie in 1940. His medical education was interrupted in his second year of study when he contracted pulmonary tuberculosis. After five years of treatment, he was fortunately able to resume his medical studies. After graduation he served on the medical staff of the Nova Scotia Sanatorium (1940-1941), then from 1941 to 1943 he did a residency in radiology at the Royal Victoria Hospital in Montreal and finally, in 1943-44 he did a residency in radiation therapy at the Toronto General Hospital. He was certified by the Royal College of Physicians and Surgeons of Canada in diagnostic and therapeutic radiology in 1945 and was made a Fellow of the American College of Radiology in 1959. With his appointment, came the acquisition of some modern X-ray equipment. He organized a training school for radiology technicians in 1945 which continues to produce well trained technicians to this day. He retired in 1968 and died on May 31, 1970.

The year 1944 also saw the return of Dr. George Lyons and Dr. Paul Melanson to again take an active part in the staff of the hospital. An addition to the staff was Dr. R.A. Auffrey as a junior physician. A few years later, Dr. Auffrey, like Dr. Desmond, would die tragically in a car accident.

The hospital's resources were again strained to the limit with overcrowding this year, as well as with staff shortages. Three front sun porches and two rear sun porches were converted into wards to increase the bed capacity to 150. There were 4,926 patients admitted in 1944, an increase of 360 over 1943. The number of operations performed was 2,582, an increase of only 24 over 1943. Despite efforts to limit the growth of the obstetrical department, there was an increase of 114 in the number of births over 1943 for a total of 766, including 6 sets of twins and 11 caesarean sections. There were 1,027 patients seen in the outpatient department but only 54 seen in the free clinics. There were 692 patients seen in the tuberculosis clinic and 158 patients made a visit to the VD clinic. Use of the electrocardiographic service was increasing with 80 ECG's done on inpatients and another 18 on outpatients. There were 773 physiotherapy treatments carried out.

An important event halfway through 1944 was the introduction of penicillin, of which the hospital received a monthly quota. It was expected that this quota would be increased in 1945 and that the cost would be reduced as well.

The strain on the resources of the institution continued through 1945. Average daily occupancy increased by 13.15 percent with 508 more patients admitted in 1945 over 1944 and 468 more operations performed, including 20 more caesarean sections. Births increased in number by 73 and 697 more X-rays were taken. There was an increase in the per diem cost of care to $4.16 from $3.95 in 1944 but earnings and collections increased and the hospital ended the year without a deficit. An increased use of Group Hospital Service Association and Blue Cross Plans is also observed through the year. Miss MacMaster recommended to the board at that time that a retirement and pension plan be considered for the benefit of the employees of The Moncton Hospital. She stressed, however, that the major need of the hospital was additional accommodation and modern facilities for both patients and staff.

At this time, Dr. George V. Parsons joined the staff as the first fully-trained anaesthetist at the hospital. He was born in Carbonear, Newfoundland, and graduated from Dalhousie in 1940 after interning at Camp Hill Hospital, the Nova Scotia Sanatorium and the Victoria General Hospital. He then spent one year in an anaesthetic residency at the Victoria General Hospital in Halifax, taking further training at the Royal Victoria Hospital, Montreal, from 1941 to 1942 and then at St. Anne's Hospital, St. Anne-de-Bellevue, Quebec. He received his certification in anaesthesia in 1946, as well as his fellowship in the American College of Anaesthesiology. George was an excellent anaesthetist and later obtained his FRCP in 1955 when this fellowship was usually only obtained by those working in academic centres. On his arrival at the hospital, George also took over the job of organizing and expanding the blood and plasma bank. The Department of Health began supplying a quantity of dried human serum at this time. George had an inordinate amount of testosterone flowing in his veins and this tended to make the nurses keep their distance from the head of the operating room table.

With the war over, the No. 31 Personnel Depot became No. 10 Release Centre for processing air force veterans returning from overseas. During the fall of 1946 several doctors stationed at No. 10, worked as part time interns at The Moncton Hospital to gain experience in surgery and obstetrics.

Strain on the hospital resources continued in the post war period in 1946, and an additional 842 patients were treated with 307 more operations performed. Births showed an increase of 224 over the previous year with 1,063 recorded. The workload of the X-ray, laboratory, physiotherapy and pharmacy departments all increased. The pharmacy dispensed 5,725 vials of the new wonder drug penicillin at a cost of $5,371. The largest expense for the year was the installation of new X-ray equipment, with structural changes to accommodate the equipment costing $22,180.26. Hospital expenditures for the year were $271,822.22 with an income of $290,854.41, resulting in an operating profit of $19,032.19. Public ward patients now accounted for only 7.5 percent of patient days.

The biggest event of 1946 was the establishment of a Department of Pathology with the appointment of Dr. Ian MacLennan as pathologist. Dr. MacLennan was born in Campbellton on February 18, 1912, and after attending the University of New Brunswick for premed, he attended McGill, obtaining his MD in 1937. From 1937 to 1941 he served as intern and then resident in pathology at the Montreal General Hospital. He then served in the Royal Canadian Air Force until October, 1945. He was certified as a pathologist by the Royal College of Physicians and Surgeons of Canada and was a charter member of the Canadian Association of Pathologists. He resigned from the staff in June 1963 to become Director of New Brunswick Laboratories in Saint John. In another staff change, Dr. H.M. MacLean resumed his practice after finishing his war service and spending extra time in England doing postgraduate work in surgery. Finally, Dr. Lea Allanach was appointed as the dental surgeon. With his wartime experience he became the main surgeon for the treatment of fractured mandibles with the use of interdental wiring. This procedure was often combined with open reductions performed by Dr. Ewart and, in later years, by other members of the Department of Orthopaedics.

With the closing of No. 31 air base, the base hospital was given to the province and it was used to establish the Moncton Tuberculosis Hospital with Dr. P.M. Knox as superintendent. As a result, the chest clinic was transferred to the Tuberculosis Hospital late in the year. Besides serving as a facility for the treatment of pulmonary TB, this hospital became the main centre in the province for treating bone tuberculosis, as a result of the recognition of Dr. E.W. Ewart's experience.

A special hospital building committee, charged with planning a new addition to the hospital facilities, was appointed in 1945, and consisted of G.O. Spencer, Ambrose Wheeler, Ruth Wilson, Miss A.J. MacMaster, Reid McManus, Dr. J.W. Dobson, Dr. R.D. Roach, B.A. Taylor, Hon. C.H. Blakeny, H.J. Crudge, A.W. Jamieson, M.J. Elsliger, J.E. Murphy, Ald. F.M. Brown, Ald. A.E. Stone and Ald. W.D. Hoar. The building committee hired A.J. Swanson from the Toronto Western Hospital as a consultant, and it was his opinion that it would be too expensive to build on a new site and he, therefore, recommended an expansion of the present plant at a cost of about $800,000. In August 1946 the city council, under Mayor G.F.G. Bridges, agreed to guarantee the bonds the hospital might issue to finance the project. This would be done if the Act of Incorporation of 1917 was changed by the provincial legislature so as to transfer ownership of the hospital to the City of Moncton rather than the board of Trustees. The city council also proposed a board of Trustees consisting of eleven members, with two from the city council, and the other nine appointed by city council. In the meantime the architectural firm of Govan, Ferguson and Lindsay was employed to draw up plans for the expansion. They submitted plans for a new wing of five stories and another wing of four stories with a capacity of 153 adult beds, 32 children's beds and 71 bassinets. The board of trustees and city council gave its tentative approval to the plans on October 28, 1946, but the latter indicated it would withhold final approval until the new board was appointed.

In the meantime, there was a groundswell of opinion in the community that the board was making a mistake with its expansion plans, and that an entirely new hospital should be built on a new site. This opinion was also shared by the medical staff and their spokesman on the board, Dr. J.W. Dobson, made their opinion well known. An active Taxpayers Association was formed, which held a meeting at the King George School on February 17, 1947, and proposed as an alternative to the present board's plans that a new hospital be built on a new site. Much discussion followed in the radio and newspapers and the issue came to a head when the revised Act of Incorporation was enacted by the provincial legislature and at a city council meeting of the whole on May 13, 1947, a new slate of trustees was named to replace the present 25 -member board. Rather than single out several and let others go, the mayor, J.E. Murphy, stated that the council would appoint an entirely new board as follows: Leonard W. Lockhart, chairman, W.V. Creaghan, W.J. Kirby, G.W.R. Myles, J.E. Surette, R. Eric Raworth, A.O. Fownes, Dr. E.W. Ewart, Mrs. H.F. Radcliffe plus Mayor J.E. Murphy and Ald. E.G. Gaskin representing the city council. The next day, the chairman of the board, Ambrose Wheeler, angrily denounced the mayor and city council, indicating that he had not been informed or asked for any input into the changing of the Act nor informed of the new appointments to the board and had to read it in the newspapers. He and the board consequently resigned *en masse*. Ruth Wilson described the appointment of the new board as "tricky, dirty, petty politics." She was probably not far from stating the truth as the new board consisted of many young businessmen in the community known to be in favour of a new hospital on a new site, some of whom had attended the Taxpayers Association meeting on February 18, 1947.

With the resignations of the old board and having served as superintendent for 36 years, Miss MacMaster submitted her resignation. Her assistant, Miss MacLaren, submitted hers at the same time on May 14, 1947. Both resignations were to take effect on June 10. Miss MacMaster left big shoes to fill, and it eventually took two people to do so. The reality was that the job had become too big for one person to handle effectively in any event. On December 5, 1947, Miss B.A. Beattie became Superintendent of Nurses and on December 21, George Filliter was hired as Administrator, assuming his duties on January 2, 1948.

Significant changes in the administration and in the direction of the hospital were soon apparent. Significantly, the question of ancient and inadequate facilities was to be addressed at last. On June 3, 1947, Dr. J.C. MacKenzie, a hospital consultant from Montreal, was employed to make a survey. One of his recommendations that was put into effect was the purchase of dictating equipment which the doctors had wanted for years. Other recommendations mostly concerned administrative matters, such as the purchase of large refrigerators so that meat could be purchased in bulk, the rewiring of the maternity facilities, a redecoration program and employment of a maintenance man to take care of all building repairs and small remodelling jobs. He recommended the purchase of a large amount of equipment from the War Assets Corporation. This recommendation was carried out. Another significant recommendation which was implemented, was the employment of staff to take over the operation of the ambulance service by the hospital from the police department, which had operated this service in the past. Dr. MacKenzie further recommended that the large Studebaker ambulance be reconditioned and a second ambulance purchased from War Assets and a garage constructed to house both vehicles. The hospital has continued to run the ambulance service for the city since October 4, 1947.

At this time a complete audit of the books was made by the accounting firm of Hudson, McMackin and Company. Their recommendation was that a new system of hospital accounting be installed. This was done with the necessary work being completed in the month of September.

An advisory committee, consisting of three members of the medical staff, was also appointed to work with the executive committee of the board to help them in their task of providing hospital services. On September 10, 1947, the following resolution was passed by the board:

> WHEREAS the Trustees of The Moncton Hospital are satisfied after giving careful consideration of the matter that the present hospital building is wholly inadequate to meet the demands and requirements of the

City of Moncton and surrounding territory, and that the construction of additions or annexes to the present hospital building are inadvisable, and would in the long run prove most costly to the City of Moncton. THEREFORE BE IT RESOLVED that the Trustees of The Moncton Hospital place themselves on record as follows:

1. That they are in favour of and strongly recommend to the City Council of the City of Moncton the construction of a new hospital building with 200 beds and nurses home on a new site in the City of Moncton or adjacent to the City of Moncton at a cost of approximately $2,500,000.00.
2. That subject to the approval of the City Council of the City of Moncton a competent firm of architects be engaged at once to prepare plans and specifications for such a hospital building and nurses' home.
3. That the City Council of the City of Moncton be requested to approve of the construction of a new hospital building with 200 beds and nurses' home on a new site in the City of Moncton costing approximately $2,500,000.00 and to apply for legislative authority to guarantee bonds for a sufficient amount to cover the construction of such a hospital and nurses' home.
4. That the City Council be requested to assure the Trustees of The Moncton Hospital it will, when required, grant such monies to the Trustees of The Moncton Hospital as may be required for the architects' fees for plans and specifications in connection with such new hospital building and nurses' home.

A short time after passing the above resolution, the members of the board attended a meeting of the Committee of the Whole of the city council to discuss the details of this proposal and in September, the city council approved the recommendations of the Hospital board.

With new houses, new cars, and new brides, the Allanach twins, Gerald and Ralph, returned to their native city around this time to join the staff as junior physicians. They were born in Moncton on September 7, 1916, and graduated from Mount Allison with BSc degrees in 1938 and from the University of Toronto with their MD degrees in 1943. They both interned at St. Joseph's Hospital in Toronto. General practice did not suit them, however, and Ralph departed in 1948 to pursue a career in public health. Gerald took a leave of absence in 1950 to take postgraduate work in urology at Roosevelt Hospital in New York and, after passing his certification exams in urology, he rejoined the staff in 1953 and served many years on the urology staff until his retirement in 1990. Gerald could have a heart of gold at times. When any of his colleagues or friends were sick they could expect to see Gerald appearing at their hospital room with lobster or a steak. On the other hand, Gerald could have been a role model for Archie Bunker with his not so subtle opinions on any subject. Once Gerald purchased an article there was never any doubt but it was the best on the market. There was never any car built, for instance, that could compete with an Oldsmobile 98!

Another addition to the staff was Dr. S.A. Hopper, who was appointed to the staff as a senior pediatrician. Alan Hopper was born in Moncton on June 12, 1907. He received his BA from Mount Allison in 1934 and then served as principal of the Sackville High School from 1934 to 1937. The teaching profession's loss was the medical profession's gain as Alan moved on to enter Dalhousie University where he obtained his MD,CM in 1942, after interning at the Jordan Memorial Sanatorium and the Victoria General Hospital. He then joined the Royal Canadian Air Force and in 1946 was in postgraduate work at the Montreal Military Hospital. Although never certified, he confined his practice to internal medicine and pediatrics and, in particular, he had a large geriatric practice. During a 'flu' epidemic when I was in general practice, I remarked that I had a busy weekend making over twenty house calls and Alan remarked that this was just a usual weekend for him. What I found out later was that Alan would often spend his weekends going around and making calls on all his geriatric patients, spending his time having tea and conversation. A lifelong bachelor, he devoted his spare time to the Boy Scout movement. From 1946 to 1965, he was Assistant Provincial Commissioner and from 1965 to 1971, Provincial Commissioner of Boy Scouts. Among the honours received from the Boy Scout movement were the Medal of Merit in 1937, the Silver Acorn in 1950 and scouting's highest award, the Silver Wolf, in 1966. He received the fifty year pin for service to scouting in 1977. Other honours bestowed upon him were the Centennial Medal in 1967, and the Queen Elizabeth Jubilee Medal in 1977. He was made a senior member of the New Brunswick Medical Society and the Canadian Medical Association in 1980. His alma mater, Mount Allison, awarded him an honorary degree at the fall convocation in 1983. Alan was a large man and loved food. He lived with his mother and two unmarried sisters and every now and then, they would place him on a diet and so Alan would go to a restaurant and have a meal before proceeding home for his "diet" dinner.

Dr. Patrick Murphy joined the staff in May 1947 and began an association that was to last for over 40 years. The Murphy clan had long been a prominent family in Moncton in the legal profession and community affairs and Pat marked the beginning of the clan's spreading its wings to become dominant forces in the medical profession as well. His brother, J. Edward Murphy, was mayor in 1947 and 1948 and served on the hospital board. His brother, Henry, was also a lawyer and a prominent judge and former MP for Moncton. His younger brother, Fred, followed him into the medical profession and later would play a major role in the story of The Moncton Hospital. Pat was born in Moncton on May 18, 1917, and obtained his BSc from the University of New Brunswick in 1940 and his MD from the University of Toronto in 1944. He interned at the Saint John General Hospital and then worked at the Sussex Military Hospital from 1945 to 1946 and the DVA Hospital in Saint John (1946-47). As an apprentice surgeon he was caught up in the hospital's change of by-laws, however, and his application for appointment to the surgical staff in 1952 was denied. He retired on August 1, 1989. Dr. Pat was always soft-spoken and dedicated to his practice. He lived and worked in the east end of the city and before the introduction of Medicare likely had a large number of uncollectible bills on his books—if he had even bothered to enter them. No down-and-out alcoholic was ever refused treatment by Pat Murphy.

Another addition to the staff in 1947 was Dr. Ralph Fitch, the first doctor in Moncton to devote his practice solely to pediatrics. Ralph was born in Sydney, Nova Scotia, on May 26, 1915. He received his BSc from Acadia in 1939, his MD,CM from Dalhousie in 1945 and served as a resident in pediatrics at the Halifax Children's Hospital from 1946-1947. Taking a leave of absence in 1954, he completed his training and obtained certification in pediatrics from the Royal College of Physicians and Surgeons of Canada. He retired in 1987, becoming a member of the honorary staff, and died only three years later. Besides being dedicated to his pediatric practice, Ralph was very active in the Rotary Club. He loved music, and could always be found at noon on Mondays, leading the Rotarians in a singsong. He had also been a very active member of the First Baptist Church and initiated and directed a handbell choir there. The choir gained widespread renown in the city, and, although the membership has changed, continues to perform to this day.

A slight reduction in the number of patients treated took place in 1947, with 6,241 discharges versus 6,277 in 1946. This was not because of lack of demand for beds but rather because of efforts to control admissions at times when the hospital was badly overcrowded. There was less ward work throughout 1947 with only 63 operations performed on ward patients out of a total of 3,209 operations and exams carried out in the operating room. Ward patients were no longer treated as second class citizens and were now allowed the same visiting hours as the other patients, except for evening visiting hours which were 7-8 pm compared to 7-8.30 pm for private and semi-private patients. There were 1,113 births in 1947 with 45 caesarean sections. There were 1,712 patients seen in the outpatient department but only 63 patients in the free public clinics. Venereal disease was still prevalent with 130 patients making 1,714 visits to the VD clinic. The number of visits and treatments given, however, showed a slight decline, probably indicating more use of penicillin. X-rays were performed on 4,295 patients and the number of X-ray treatments given had soared to 2,156. In his annual report of the X-ray department, Dr. Ripley stressed the need for another therapy machine to be used exclusively for superficial and moderate voltage Roentgen treatments if the hospital was to keep abreast of modern procedures which required small flexible equipment and easily manoeuvred tubes. Such a machine would also relieve the present "Max'mar 250" and fulfil increasing demands for higher voltage service. The request of the Department of Health, through Dr. Porter, Director of Hospital Services, for space in The Moncton Hospital to open a Cancer Diagnostic Clinic was granted in September.

In 1948, the County of Westmorland approved a resolution to build, and provide financial support for a new hospital. This enabled planning to proceed. The offer by D.A. MacBeath to donate ten acres of land on West Lane was accepted, thus establishing the site for the new hospital. At this time, West Lane really was just a lane, and I recall that my friends and I, as children, would look upon going to West Lane on our bicycles as quite an excursion. Indeed, a number of the citizens at the time thought that this was quite a remote site. One must remember, however, that for the ordinary working man at that time, a car was a luxury, and travel about the city, was for the most part, done on foot or via the Grey Bus Line. There was certainly input from the medical staff concerning the new facility, as the advisory committee of the medical staff consisting of Dr. R. Myers, Dr. J.W. Dobson and Dr. R.D. Roach met twelve times during the year with a committee of the board of Trustees with many common problems being worked out. It was estimated that the cost of the new hospital would be $2 million. On December 3, 1948, the hospital was represented by Leonard W. Lockhart, W.J. Kirby and Dr. J.W. Dobson at a meeting in Fredericton. The meeting was held to discuss distribution of hospital grants of $5 million available from the federal and provincial governments on a 50-50 split. As a result of this meeting, it was expected that The Moncton Hospital would obtain $400,000 in grants and that two-thirds of the remainder of the cost would be financed by the City of Moncton. The city would guarantee bonds to be issued by the hospital and the County of Westmorland would guarantee bonds issued for the other one-third. The Director of Planning of Health Services for the Province of New Brunswick at that time was Dr. A.M. Clarke, who would later become an administrator of The Moncton Hospital.

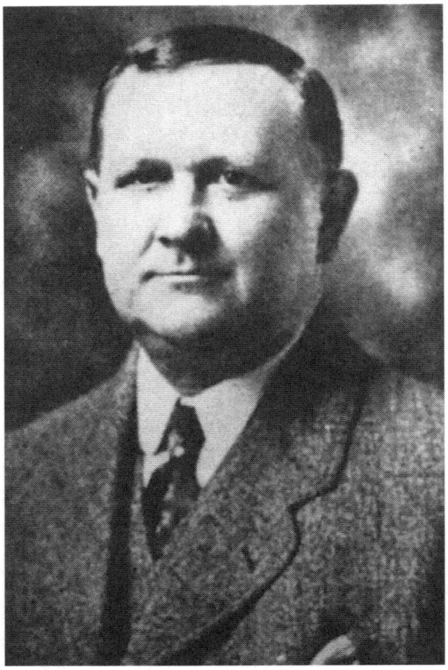

Mr. D.A. MacBeath

During the year, Miss Beattie, the new superintendent of Nurses and the Nursing School, began to make her presence known about the school and the hospital and made several changes. Firstly, a School of Nursing Committee was established to act in an advisory capacity on educational matters. It included in its membership: (a) a member of the medical staff; (b) a member of the board of Directors; (c) a representative of the City Educational Department; (d) an alumnae of the School of Nursing, as well as the Director of Nursing, Assistant Director of Nursing, Instructors and the Hospital Administrator.

Secondly, a pediatric service with a teaching program was arranged. Twenty-two beds and cribs were segregated on the first floor and this included an infant ward with cubicles. Thirdly, with over 1,000 births a year, it was now felt appropriate to establish an obstetrical teaching department, the affiliation at the Montreal Maternity Pavilion, Royal Victoria Hospital, being discontinued. Fourthly, arrangements were made for student nurses for short observation periods in Community Health Services such as the VON, school nursing and various clinics. Finally, the nurses' residence was rearranged to provide a study room and a reference library for the students.

Among the graduates of the Nursing School that year was Katherine Richardson whose name appears among the prize winners at the graduation ceremonies. She also led the province in the spring Registered Nurses' examinations. Better known by her married name, Katherine Wright, she later had a distinguished career as the Superintendent of Nurses at The Moncton Hospital. Also among the graduates that year was Ailene Alexander. Also better known by her married name, Ailene Forsythe, she served for many years as supervisor in the operating room.

Miss Beattie recognized that the days of slave labour were coming to an end, especially for nurses, and recommended the establishment of an 8-hour day or 44-hour week for student nurses, graduate nurses and nurses' aides. She championed the organization of a students' council as a form of self-government in the School of Nursing, and, as a mean of improving morale, she initiated a recreational programme for the students and for the hospital staff as a whole.

Anyone working in the hospital, as well as patients and visitors is familiar with the volunteers who bring their carts around to the wards with reading material. This service was first started in June 1948 and was provided twice weekly by members of the staff of the city library. A short time later, the service was taken over by a committee of the Dr. John Clarence Webster Chapter of the IODE.

In February 1948 Dr. Ian MacLennan, the hospital's pathologist, was selected by the Scholarship Committee of the New Brunswick Branch of the Canadian Cancer Society to attend Cornell University Medical Branch in New York to study the most recent technique in cancer diagnosis, the Papanicolaou Cancer Smear Test.

In 1948, the provincial Department of Health began giving grants to hospitals based on a certain amount per patient day, with the amount to be expended as far as possible on additional equipment and improvement to techniques and services. This money was used to provide a diathermy machine, stretchers, an incubator, to equip the new pediatric floor and to obtain surgical instruments for the OR, as well as for some non-medical purchases such as steam irons for the laundry, a tubular fire escape for the second floor of maternity, and for the overhaul of the elevator and dumb-waiter. This money was also used to introduce the use of disposable equipment for intravenous therapy and the use of radiopacque sponges in the operating room.

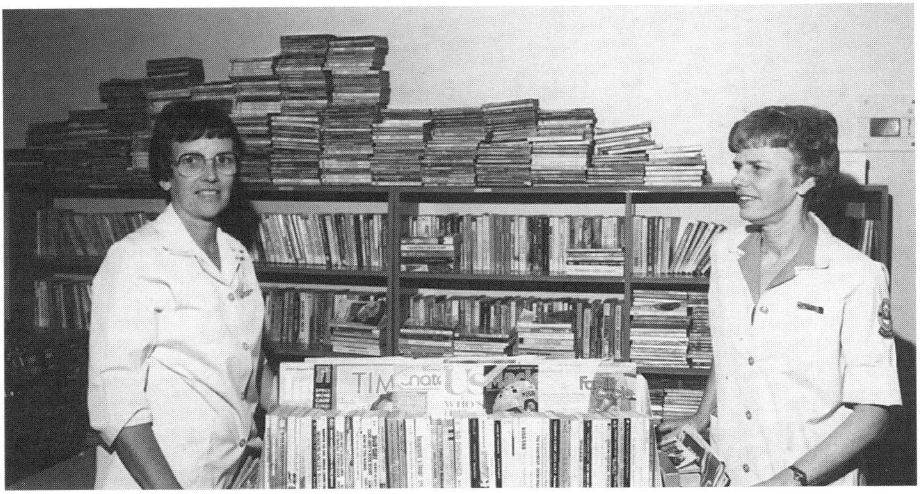

Volunteers Alma Stewart (left) and Hughena Sommerville (right) bring a cart of reading material to patients.

Several new doctors were added to the medical staff in 1948. At that time Dr. O.J. White joined the Department of Orthopaedics. Jack White was born in Winnipeg on March 26, 1922, and after graduating from medical school at the University of Manitoba in 1945, he interned at the Winnipeg General Hospital. He was a resident in orthopaedics there from 1946 to 1947 and then served a fellowship at the Winnipeg Clinic before coming to Moncton at the request of Dr. Ewart. He took a two-year leave of absence beginning in 1950, to pursue further postgraduate work at the Royal National Orthopaedic Hospital in London, England, returning to Moncton in 1952 and obtaining his certification in orthopaedics from the Royal College of Physicians and Surgeons of Canada. In 1989 he received the Award of Merit, a distinction awarded to senior members of the Canadian Orthopaedic Association. Dr. White pursued an active orthopaedic practice until his recent retirement and was made a member of the honorary staff in 1994.

Dr. Normand J. Belliveau, Dr. Philip d'Entremont, Dr. Peter Lyons, Dr. J.Chipman McCrea and Dr. H.C.J. LeBlanc were all appointed to the staff as junior physicians.

Normand Belliveau, born at Belliveau Cove, Nova Scotia, on April 9, 1922, received a BA from St. Ann's College in 1942 and, after serving an internship in university hospitals in Quebec City, he received his MD from Laval in 1946. He did an advanced rotating internship from 1946 to 1947 and then served as chief resident house surgeon in Jersey City. In 1951, he took a leave of absence for further surgical training and was appointed to the active surgical staff in 1955. He practised in Moncton for a few years and then moved to Montreal where he has had a distinguished career. He became very active in the Canadian Medical Association and served a term as its president.

Like Dr. Belliveau, Dr. Phil d'Entremont was also a Nova Scotian

Acadian, being born in Yarmouth on April 8, 1920. He attended St. Ann's College obtaining a BA in 1940, and graduating from Laval with his MD in 1944. He served as a medical officer in the RCAF from 1944 to 1946 and then did a rotating internship at the Ottawa Civic Hospital from October 1946 to April 1948. Beginning in 1951 he took a leave of absence from the staff to do a residency in general surgery at the Montreal General and Queen Mary's Veterans Hospital in Montreal from 1951 to 1954. He obtained his certification in general surgery and rejoined the staff in the Department of General Surgery in 1954. He subsequently served on the staff for many years, although the majority of his work was carried out at the Dr. Georges-L. Dumont Hospital (formerly l'Hôtel Dieu).

Henry LeBlanc also carried on most of his work at the l'Hôtel Dieu. He was born in St. Anselem on January 17, 1905 and received his BA from St. Joseph's University in 1927 and his MD from Laval in 1932. He interned at the Jeffrey Hale Hospital in Quebec City (1931-32) and at St. Luke's Hospital in Montreal (1932-34). Henry was a lifelong bachelor and would always appear at medical dances and functions with a young woman whom he would always introduce as his cousin. He must have had many cousins, however, as he always seemed to have a different one for each occasion. He was appointed to the honorary staff in 1978.

Peter Lyons, the son of Dr. George Lyons, was born in Moncton on July 9, 1923. He took his premedical education at St. Francis Xavier University and in 1947 graduated from McGill with his MD,CM. He interned at the Montreal General Hospital from 1947 to 1948. In 1951, he began a three-year leave of absence to pursue postgraduate training in surgery at the Henry Ford Hospital in Detroit. Peter enjoyed a lengthy general and surgical practice in Moncton until his untimely death from a coronary on December 7, 1987, while out walking. He served as chief of the Department of Surgery in 1960, 1981 and 1982 and he was president of the medical staff in 1972 and 1973. He was an avid sportsman and will be long remembered by the golfing and curling fraternities of the hospital and the city. Dr. Phil d'Entremont, Dr. Dollard Cormier and his brother-in-law, Dr. Bob Dysart, were often his curling teammates.

J.C. (Chip) McCrea was born in Moncton on October 18, 1920, received a BA from the University of New Brunswick in 1940 and graduated from McGill in 1943 with his MD. He interned at the Royal Victoria Hospital in 1943-1944. He was a resident physician at the Moncton Tuberculosis Hospital in 1947 and then did a residency in general surgery at the Queen Mary's Veteran Hospital in Montreal from 1947 to 1948. In 1951 he was appointed to the anaesthetic staff. He was still engaged in active practice in 1995.

There were 6,033 patients treated in hospital during 1948 and that year 2,888 operations were performed, 4,516 X-rays were taken and 2,305 X-ray treatments given. There were 225 electrocardiograms done and 663 physiotherapy treatments given, 15,543 tests were performed in the laboratory on 5,317 patients and the number of births recorded was 1,021.

As the decade ended, the light began to appear at the end of the tunnel after ten tough years. All the arguments and rancour of the past two years were over and the building of a new hospital on a new site is an established fact. In July 1949, architects, with input from the staff, began working on the plans. Dr. D.F.W. Porter took over the position of executive director on September 1, 1949, replacing Mr. Filliter, and most of his time was taken up in working with the architects in preparing plans and specifications for the new hospital with the expectation that they would be complete by June 1950. The executive committee of the board, consisting of Leonard W. Lockhart (chairman), W.J. Kirby, W.V. Creaghan, R.E. Raworth and D.S. Smith, together with A.O. Fownes and H.H. Trimble, formed the Building Committee. With a commitment of funds by the County of Westmorland in February, four members from the county were appointed to the hospital board, which had consisted of only citizens of Moncton up until that time. During the year the board also established a Personnel Relations Committee which was given full authority to deal with difficulties arising out of staff employment.

From the newly established federal and provincial health grants, funds were allotted for training of personnel and for the purchase of new surgical, laboratory and X-ray equipment. The Department of Pathology and Bacteriology continued to increase its volume of work, providing an ever-broadening service to the hospital and to the area, albeit with some difficulty, because of the lack of space. There was no increase in the volume of work in the X-ray department, but this service received the largest of the grants from the Department of Health. A general diagnostic and fluoroscopic radiographic machine, a complete urographic unit and two new therapy units were evidence of this largesse. In addition, wiring was completed for the accommodation of a photo-flurographic unit for the admitting department of the hospital.

The decade closed with 3,098 operations performed, showing an increase of 210 over 1948. The number of births was down, however, with only 854 recorded. In the outpatient department 1,336 minor operations were performed with 283 dressings done and 353 treatments given. The new cancer clinic saw only 15 patients and the other free clinics showed a falling attendance, with only 20 patients seen at each of the medical and E.E.N.T. clinics. No one attended the surgical clinics. No report is given for the VD clinic for the year, apparently having been disbanded.

Chapter Seven

The Fifties—New Horizons

The plans for a new 225-bed hospital were completed by the architects Messrs. Govan, Ferguson, Lindsay, Kaminker, Maw, Langley, Keenleyside in the summer of 1950. Tenders were called that September and the lowest bid, submitted by a Toronto firm of contractors, George Hardy Limited, was accepted by the board and then approved by the Moncton City Council and the Westmorland County Council. Construction was started on November 30, 1950. The hospital board accepted a proposal from the Department of Health in Fredericton to provide a new building adjacent to the new hospital to accommodate a provincial zone laboratory, regional offices for local health authorities and space for clinics on a non-profit basis. The provincial government agreed to pay sufficient rent to cover the cost of heat and other services and to retire the bonds required to finance the Health Unit over a 30-year period. Dr. J.W. Dobson, along with the executive director, Dr. Porter, and superintendent of nurses, Miss Beattie, made an exhaustive tour of many American and Canadian hospitals during the year, in order to become better acquainted with recent developments in hospital equipment and hospital administration and this proved most helpful in completing effective plans for the new building.

In 1950 Dr. R. Burnell Eaton was appointed to the surgical staff of the hospital. He was born in Canning, Nova Scotia, and graduated from Acadia with a BSc in 1927 and from Dalhousie with a MD, CM in 1932. After a general practice in River Hebert and Joggins, Nova Scotia, he went to England in 1936 and took postgraduate work in surgery at Hammersmith Hospital in London and then in Edinburgh and received his FRCS(Edin) in 1938. He started to practise surgery in Amherst but joined the army in 1940 and went overseas with the 14th Field Ambulance Corps. After the war, he started a surgical practice at the Sackville Hospital and Clinic but moved to Moncton in 1950. He obtained his FRCS(C) in 1947 and his FACS in 1949. He was a governor of the American College of Surgeons from 1960-1963 and served as president of the New Brunswick Medical Society in 1973. He received an

Honorary DSc from his alma mater, Acadia University, in 1972 and was made a member of the Order of Canada in 1982. He was the first member of the staff to devote his practice solely to general surgery and it did not take long for his fame as a surgeon to spread. He had an incredible skill. Although extremely fast he never seemed hurried and his diagnostic skills and pre- and post-op management were equal to his technical skills.

Dr. George Lyons and Dr. McNaughton both retired from the active staff this year with Dr. d'Entremont replacing Dr. McNaughton on the anaesthetic staff. The nursing staff of the hospital now numbered 114 but included in this number were 65 student nurses. April 3, 1950, marked the commencement of the eight-hour day for the nursing staff. Miss Beattie resigned as superintendent of nurses and was replaced by Florence Breau.

Admittance figures for 1950 show 5,730 patients with an average length of stay of 9.2 days. The number of operations was 2,856 operations, and X-rays, 4,190, with 225 patients undergoing 2,017 X-ray treatments. There were 174 ECGs and 339 physiotherapy treatments performed. The hospital birth rate showed a drop with 858 recorded. The laboratory carried out 18,039 tests on 4,190 patients. An important innovation in the laboratory service this year was the commencement of the Red Cross Blood Transfusion Service on March 13, 1950.

As planning for the new facilities continued to proceed in 1951, it became evident that the plans for a Medical Health Centre in connection with the new laboratory were too costly and the plans were scaled back so that only a Regional Laboratory would be built and attached to the hospital. A new set of medical staff by-laws was approved this year, and one of the major changes was the limitation of surgical privileges to those who were qualified to write the certification examinations of the Royal College of Physicians and Surgeons of Canada. It was stipulated that, after appointment to the staff, it was necessary to pass the examinations within 28 months, thus giving the surgeon three chances at writing the examinations.

On April 1, 1951, The Moncton Hospital was one of four hospitals in the province selected to partake in the Cancer Control Programme financed by the Department of Health.

In 1951 four new doctors were added to the surgical staff: Dr. F.J. Hogg, Dr. J.S. Wright, Dr. C.E. Doyle and Dr. W.D. MacDonald. There were also two internal medicine specialists added to the medical staff: Dr. E.D. Levittan and Dr. J.A. Fownes, as well as four physicians appointed to the staff as junior physicians: Dr. D.C. Cormier, Dr. Eugene Leger, Dr. R.D. Landry, and Dr. J.H. West. The death of Dr. W.S. Fitzpatrick occurred this year leaving the surgical staff without a trained urologist.

F.J. Hogg was born in Sherbrooke, Quebec, on August 8, 1914. After obtaining a BA from Bishops, in 1934, he received his MD, CM from McGill in 1939. He interned at the Hamilton General Hospital in 1939-41 and then did a surgical fellowship at the McGregor Clinic from 1941 to 1942. After serving in the army, he became a resident in surgery at the Queen Mary's

Veterans Hospital in 1946-47 and obtained his FRCS(C) in 1947. He then practised at St. Martha's Hospital in Antigonish from 1947 to 1951. He came to Moncton with the intention of devoting his practice solely to surgery but this proved to be unsuccessful and he left Moncton after a year.

On the other hand, Dr. J.S. Wright and Dr. C.E. Doyle, although certified in surgery, were willing to abide by the custom of the time and combine a general practice with surgery and remained on the staff for years to come. Syd Wright was born in Prince Edward Island on June 14, 1919, and attended Dalhousie University, obtaining his BSc and MD, CM in 1940 and 1943 respectively. He interned at the Saint John General Hospital. After serving in the army, he carried out a general practice in North Sydney from 1946 to 1948 and a residency in general surgery at the Victoria General Hospital from 1948 to 1951 and then passed his certification exams in general surgery. Since his retirement from active practice, he has continued to serve in the Pain Clinic at the hospital.

Charles Doyle was born in Moncton on July 13, 1920, and likewise, received his education at Dalhousie, receiving his BSc in 1941 and his MD, CM in 1945 after interning at the Victoria General Hospital. He then undertook a residency at the Saint John TB Hospital (1946-1947) and a surgical residency at the New York Polyclinic Hospital and obtained his certification in general surgery. He served as the second chief of staff and retired to the honorary staff in 1992.

W.D. MacDonald (aka "Blind Bill") was also a Moncton native, born on March 2, 1921. He took the premed course at Dalhousie and received his MD, CM in 1944 after interning at the Halifax Infirmary and St. Martha's in Antigonish. He did a residency in surgery at the Montreal General Hospital in 1944-1946 and then undertook further postgraduate work in EENT at London Post-Graduate School, Hammersmith, and completed his training with another term at the Montreal General Hospital from 1949-1951. He then joined the hospital's EENT staff but failed to obtain his certification in surgery so that his practice was subsequently restricted to a non-surgical one. Bill took great pride in his Mercedes car and the story goes that, when he would park his car in the parking lot at the hospital he took down the license plate numbers of those parked on either side of him and then later, on leaving the building, checked the car for any scratches.

Dr. E.D. Levittan and Dr. J.A. Fownes were fully trained in internal medicine but as yet there was no separate department for this speciality, so Dr. Levittan was appointed as a senior physician and Dr. Fownes as a junior physician to the medical staff. Dr. Ed. Levittan was born in Brooklyn, New York, on May 29, 1913. He obtained a BSc from Columbia University in 1935 and then came to Canada and received his MD, CM from Dalhousie in 1940. He fell in love with Canada and never returned to the United States. He first carried out a general practice in Guysborough County, Nova Scotia, and then from 1948 to 1950 he did postgraduate work at the National Hospital for Nervous Diseases, the famous Queens Square and Hammersmith Hospital in

England, receiving his MRCP(Edin). He was a brilliant diagnostician but was not a man to be hurried. When asked for a neurology consult, he might do the history one day, the physical exam the next day, a lumbar puncture on the third day and then on the fourth day finally present his diagnosis, which was usually right on the mark. He was very meticulous in his habits. Each tool in his workshop was always carefully slotted in the right place and never left lying around after use. On taking a European holiday he had his itinerary made up so that he would be at a certain museum at a certain hour with no wasted time in his schedule. He was an amateur astronomer and electronics buff. He retired from the active staff in 1972 and died on August 21, 1980.

J.A. Fownes was born in Portland, Maine, on January 4, 1915, took his premed at St. Francis Xavier and graduated from Dalhousie with his MD, CM degree in 1942 after interning at the Saint John General Hospital from 1941 to 1942. After serving in the RCAF during the war, he took postgraduate work in internal medicine at the Royal Victoria Hospital in Montreal from 1946 to 1949 and then served as a clinical assistant in the cardiac department at the London Hospital, London, England, and at the National Heart Hospital, London, in 1950. He obtained his FRCS(C) and began the practice of internal medicine in association with Dr. R.D. Roach. Like Dr. Levittan, he was a brilliant diagnostician and if, at death rounds, it was stated that the patient had been seen by Dr. Fownes that usually would suffice to allay any criticism as to treatment the patient may have received, and would provide assurances that everything possible had been done for the patient. Al is a great story teller with the stories often told in colourful language.

Dollard Cormier was born at Cormier's Cove, New Brunswick, on February 9, 1915. He obtained a BSc from St. Joseph's University in 1945 and an MD from Laval in 1950. He then interned at l'Hôtel Dieu and St. Sacrement Hospital in Quebec City (1949-50) and at Christ Hospital, Jersey City, New Jersey, from 1950 to 1951, after which he entered general practice. He took a leave of absence to specialize in obstetrics and gynaecology, first, for a year at the Victoria General Hospital and then he completed his training at the Montreal General and Royal Victoria Hospital, obtaining his certification in 1963. He was made a Fellow of the American College of Obstetricians and Gynaecologists in 1967. He carried out the bulk of his practice at l'Hôtel Dieu and changed from active staff to consulting staff in 1968. An active curler, he served a term as president of the Beausejour Curling Club. He was also active in Acadian affairs and in 1954 was president of the Richelieu Club and in 1970, president of the Acadian Club. He was also president of the medical staff of l'Hôtel Dieu in 1957-58. He died in September 1977.

J.H. West was born in Moncton on July 8, 1886, and graduated from McGill in 1915. He interned at the Homeopathic Hospital in Montreal in 1915 and then worked at the Grenfell Mission from 1915 to 1918. He interned again at the Saint John General Hospital in 1918 and then spent 25 years as a Baptist medical missionary at Serango Mission Hospital in India from 1924 to 1949. After joining the staff, he served for a while as an assistant to Dr. Clarke who had become the administrator. He died in 1960.

Eugene Leger was born in Memramcook West on September 3, 1923, graduated from St. Joseph's College with a BA in 1945 and from Laval with an MD in 1950. He did an internship at Chest Hospital, Jersey City, from 1950 to 1951. He carried out his practice almost exclusively at the Dr. Georges-L. Dumont Hospital and was not reappointed to the staff in 1972 because of delinquent records.

Raoul D. Landry was born in Bouctouche on March 25, 1910, obtained his BA from St. Joseph's College in 1930 and his MD from Laval in 1936. After joining the army, he trained in army radiology at the Toronto General Hospital in 1944-45 and studied tropical medicine in London, England, in 1945. After the war, he took the diploma course in public health in Toronto in 1946-47. He became the District Medical Health Officer in Moncton and in this capacity, joined the medical staff in February 1951. He was appointed to the honorary staff in 1976 and died on February 28, 1981.

There were also two appointments to the nursing staff in 1951 of people whose names became legend. Both were graduates of The Moncton Hospital School of Nursing. Shirley MacLeod took postgraduate training in obstetrics at the Margaret Hague Maternity Hospital in Jersey City and became the Head Nurse in Obstetrics, a position she occupied for many years until she undertook further studies and was lured away to academic centres. Ailene Alexander (Forsythe) was appointed to the position of OR Supervisor where she ruled both doctors and nurses with an iron hand for the next 25 years.

There were 5,728 patients discharged from hospital in 1951 with 2,796 operations performed and 863 births recorded. The number of operations on the public ward service had dropped to 95 and no surgical patients were seen in the public outpatient clinic although 35 were seen at the EENT clinic. The new Red Cross Transfusion Service was proving to be valuable but Dr. MacLennan pointed out that it was not entirely a free service as the hospital had to supply all the required pre-transfusion examinations free-of-charge.

In his annual report for 1952 Dr. Porter was slightly off the mark in his assessment of future needs of the hospital. He stated, "Abnormally high occupancy rates have benefited us financially in recent years but I hope sincerely that you do not expect these rates to continue indefinitely. The day is fast approaching when the efficiency of a general hospital will be judged in a broad sense by a continued surplus of unoccupied beds. This will be accomplished by expanding outpatient diagnostic and treatment facilities, by higher standards of community health due to closer working with the Department of Health in preventive measures and by an expansion of the availability of hospital services for home care, probably best accomplished by a rapid expansion of VON services in our community." It is certainly true that most of these predictions came about. However, one major question must be asked, "Where are the unoccupied beds?"

In 1952, there was a severe epidemic of poliomyelitis with a total of 50 such patients being treated at the hospital with their hospital bills being paid by the New Brunswick Department of Health.

In 1952 the opening of the Department of Psychiatry was a doubly eventful occasion as it marked the first appointment of a female doctor to the medical staff. Dr. Phyllis Bursey was born in Moncton on October 21, 1921, and studied pre-med at Acadia, and received her MD, CM from Dalhousie in 1950 after interning at the Saint John General and the Victoria Public hospitals. She then did a residency in psychiatry at the Victoria General, Camp Hill and the Nova Scotia Hospitals. Dr. Bursey left Moncton in 1953 to go into institutional work as she found the volume of work at The Moncton Hospital too much for one psychiatrist to handle. Dr. Porter had appealed to Dr. J.A. Melanson, Chief Medical Health Officer, Department of Health, for assistance to Dr. Bursey, but to no avail. Meanwhile, planned for the new hospital, was an eleven-bed psychiatric service, along with outpatient service in that field.

Another appointment to the medical staff in 1952 was Dr. C.M. Leighton and, with his calming and kindly demeanour, it was only fitting that pediatrics was his chosen field. Claude was born in Moncton on May 3, 1919, the son of Dr. G.T. Leighton, a dentist who served on the staff of the hospital in its early years. He received his BSc and his MD, CM in 1943 from Dalhousie after interning at the Halifax Infirmary. He then served in the army where he contracted TB of the spine. After undergoing treatment for this, he began his medical career again with a general practice in Shediac. He did a residency at the Children's Memorial Hospital in Montreal in 1948-50 with further training at the Children's Medical Centre in Boston in 1952. He ceased his pediatric practice in 1988, but remained on the consulting staff until 1991, joining the honorary staff in 1992.

Also admitted to the staff in 1952 was Dr. J. Arthur Dobson, the son of Dr. Joseph Dobson. He was born in Montreal on June 8, 1925, received his BA from Acadia in 1946 and his MD, CM from McGill in 1949. He interned at St. Mary's Hospital in Montreal (1949-1950) and then did a residency in anaesthesia at the Vancouver General Hospital (1951-1952). He returned to Moncton when his father became ill, and joined the anaesthetic staff. He took a leave of absence from the staff from 1954 to 1955 to take further anaesthetic training at McGill University teaching hospitals and was certified in anaesthesia in 1956. He has remained on the anaesthetic staff ever since. Arthur has always been very physically active and is in better physical shape than most men 20 or 30 years younger than himself. As mentioned before, most notable among his activities has been the creation of a hiking trail through Albert County, which has been very appropriately named the Dobson Trail. He has always had a keen interest in aviation and was also a private pilot and a glider pilot. Every April, for years, Arthur also would take a week off to tap sugar trees on his woodlot and make maple syrup. He has always been a keen gardener and is also active in his church, singing in the church choir and taking an active role in a Boy Scout troop.

Another addition to the staff in 1952 was Dr. R.C.E. Bourgeois, a native of Tracadie, born on September 20, 1913. He attended St. Francis Xavier University obtaining his BA in 1933, and then went to McGill from 1934 to 1936. After an interruption in his medical education, he attended Laval from 1939 to 1942 and received his MD from that institution in 1942. He then did residencies in EENT at l'Hôtel Dieu du Précieux-Sang, Quebec (1946-48), the New York Polyclinic and Hospital (1948-50) and the Toronto General Hospital (1950-51). After practising in Moncton for five years, he was appointed to the consulting staff, because of illness. He died in 1967.

There were 5,988 admissions during 1952 with 2,741 operations performed and 1,003 births recorded with 13 stillbirths. The pediatric service was flourishing with 1,184 admissions to the service, although it is noted that T&A was still a pretty common operation accounting for 533 of the admissions. Records show that 5,303 patients underwent X-ray examination and another 1,696 had X-ray treatments.

The following year was a banner year for The Moncton Hospital and August 21, in particular, was a banner day when all the patients were transferred from the old hospital to the vastly improved facilities of a brand new building on MacBeath Avenue. There were increased costs as a result of the move, however, and the hospital ended the year with a deficit of $100,703, compared to a deficit in the previous year of $7,899.99. The nursing staff now totalled 172, although this number included 72 student nurses and 5 nurses on the faculty of the School of Nursing. There were 11 head nurses and 47 general duty nurses, 11 nurses aides, and 7 medical orderlies. Senior positions consisted of one maternity supervisor, two maternity night supervisors, two

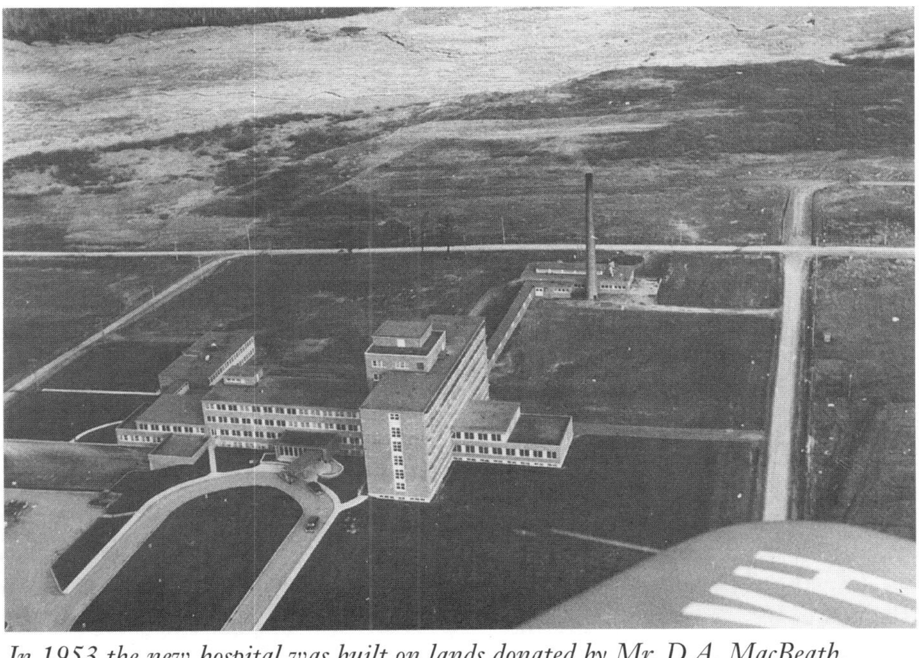

In 1953 the new hospital was built on lands donated by Mr. D.A. MacBeath.

general night supervisors, one operating room supervisor and one central supply supervisor. One feature of the new hospital was the new central supply rooms with twelve central supply workers. The eight-hour work day was now in effect and a new method of teaching student nurses was instituted. Instead of having to attend classes before or after working an eight-hour shift, the nurses were taken off the wards and attended classes in a block system. While the student nurses were attending classes, their places were taken by nurses obtained from the Private Duty Nurses' Registry. Members of the medical staff continued to play a prominent role in the School of Nursing, continuing their teaching assignments for the student nurses.

During the year, Miss Breau, the superintendent of nurses, died. Katherine Richardson (Mrs. Katherine Wright) took over her duties, a post she continued to occupy for many years. Although a nurse of the new generation with fresh ideas, she maintained the traditional reputation of superintendent of nurses as an all-powerful boss. Her trademark was a box of Kleenex. Any time a nurse was summoned to her office, either for good news or a reprimand, the box of Kleenex was immediately pushed across the table, quickly establishing who held the upper hand in any discussion that was to ensue.

Dr. Leonard J. Gaudet was appointed to the active staff in 1953 as a junior surgeon. He was born in Memramcook West on June 3, 1909, obtained a BA from St Joseph's University in 1931 and an MD from Laval in 1936. He interned at St. Michael and St. Sacrement Hospitals in Quebec from 1936 to 1937 and then undertook a one-year surgical residency. He was appointed to the courtesy staff in 1943, but in 1953 he applied for admission to the active staff in order to continue to receive surgical privileges under the grandfather clause. He resigned from the staff in 1967 because of ill health.

Another member of the courtesy staff who applied and was appointed to the active surgical staff in 1953 as a junior surgeon under the grandfather clause, was Dr. F.E. Leger. Emery Leger was born in Moncton on March 31, 1917, and after obtaining a BA from St. Joseph's University in 1937, he proceeded to Quebec where he obtained his MD from Laval in 1942. He interned at Misericorde Crèche, St. Sacrement Hospital and l'Hôtel Dieu in Quebec City in 1942-43 and underwent a residency in surgery at St. Joseph's Hospital, Saint John (1943-1944). He had an additional year of residency at the Lahey Clinic in 1947-48. He had been on the active surgical staff at l'Hôtel Dieu since 1944 and the courtesy staff of The Moncton Hospital since 1948. He was granted a leave of absence from both hospitals in May 1966 because of illness. He reapplied for admission to the staff in 1973, but his application was not approved by the Medical Advisory Committee on the recommendation of the credentials committee.

A notable addition to the medical staff in 1953 was Dr. Arthur Oatway. Arthur was born in Smiths Falls, Ontario, graduated from Queen's University in 1943 with his MD, CM and interned at the Ottawa Civic Hospital from 1943 to 1944. He then did a residency in anaesthesia at the Montreal General Hospital and Queen Mary's Veteran Hospital. From 1947 to 1953 he served as assistant medical superintendent at the Moncton TB Hospital. He was appointed to the staff in June 1953 and immediately took a leave of absence to pursue further studies in anaesthesia at the Montreal General Hospital and the McGill Diploma Course in Anaesthesia, obtaining his certification in 1955. Since operating rooms at that time only did elective cases until one o'clock with the surgeons going to their offices at two o'clock, Arthur took on another job as assistant administrator to Dr. Austin Clarke in February 1960. He continued to occupy this post until December 31, 1971, at which time the operating room hours expanded, leaving him little time for administration. It was a job that he did admirably as he was always able to see both sides of an argument and had the diplomatic skills to resolve contentious issues and yet still make the difficult decisions. Now retired, his advice is still often sought in helping to resolve disputes between opposing factions. Arthur has a great sense of humour and can calm down any tense moment with an appropriate story or joke. Besides serving as president of the medical staff and on numerous committees, he was the medical representative on the hospital board from 1983 to 1986. In addition to his medical duties, he has always been quite active in community affairs. He served on the Moncton Family and Children's Services Board before welfare was taken over by the Province and he has been active in the Boy Scout movement, the Moncton Art Society and on the board of the Friends of the Moncton Hospital Foundation.

An addition to the EENT staff this year was Dr. Nadgar Nadeau who was born at Baker Brook, New Brunswick, on March 2, 1918. He was awarded a BA from Sainte-Anne-de-la-Pocatière, Quebec, in 1940 and an MD from Laval in 1944. From 1946 to 1948 he practised in Tracadie but then decided to specialize. He took a basic science course in Otolaryngology at Harvard Medical School in 1948-49 and an ENT residency at Brooklyn Eye and Ear Hospital in 1949-51. He then took a basic science course in ophthalmology at New York University (1951-52) and another year of residency at Grasslands Hospital, Westchester, New York, from 1952 to 1953, receiving his certification in EENT in 1953. He stayed in Moncton for only a very short time.

Another addition to the staff as a junior physician was Dr. R.B. Abel who, like Dr. Nadeau, departed for greener fields within a short time.

One new addition to the medical staff who did stay and who eventually ended his career in Moncton was Dr. R.S. Wadup. Rex was born on June 11, 1913, and attended St. Dunstan's University from 1931 to 1933. He became a registered pharmacist in 1938 and from 1940 to 1945 he served as a pharmacist in the army in Canada, Italy and northwest Europe. After the war, he obtained his BSc in 1948 and his MD, CM from Dalhousie in 1952. He practised in Bath and Fredericton Junction after graduation but moved to Moncton in 1953. Having been first a pharmacist Dr. Wadup was naturally always appointed to the pharmacy committee. It would seem that his experience as a pharmacist must have made a great impression on him since he never learned to write like the stereotypical doctor. He wrote prescriptions in a printing style, which never needed verification. He retired from the active staff in December 1977 and was appointed to the honorary staff in 1988. He died in 1992.

During 1953, 6,466 patients were admitted to hospital with an average length of stay of 9.2 days. 3,179 operations were performed, an increase of 438 over the previous year. There were 5,405 patients X-rayed and 1,892 X-ray treatments given; 2,540 physiotherapy treatments were given to 303 patients and 960 births were recorded for the maternity department. The laboratory carried out 20,431 tests on 6,542 patients. In the special clinics in the outpatient department, 71 patients were seen at the EENT clinic and 302 at the cancer clinic. A new clinic was opened this year with 45 shock treatments administered by the new Department of Psychiatry.

A milestone was reached in 1954 when the hospital budget went over one million dollars for the first time with the net operating expenses for the year being $1,097,678.25. Due to the increased complexities of hospital cost accounting, a new position was created with the appointment of R.R. Rice as comptroller. There were 6,746 patients admitted and 3,648 operations performed; 6,122 patients underwent X-ray examination and 1,368 X-ray treatments were given, 1,128 deep and 240 superficial. By the end of the year, there was a waiting list for elective cases.

The salaried staff of the hospital now consisted of 308 persons: administration (32), dietary (44), housekeeping (36), laundry (15), plant operations (7), maintenance and repairs (8), central sterile supply (12), nurses (82), nurses' aids (14), orderlies (11), relief nurses (11), nursing education staff (5), medical records (5), X-ray (8), pharmacy (2), operating and delivery room (10), physiotherapy (1), outpatient department (1), ambulance (2) and professional services (1). There were 77 unpaid student nurses.

During the year the hospital accepted the very generous gift of a summer cottage property at Shediac Cape from Mr. and Mrs. Leonard W. Lockhart. Although primarily used by the nursing staff, the medical staff chose it for the location of its annual lobster party until it was destroyed by a fire.

There had been no separate urology department following the death of Dr. W.S. Fitzpatrick in 1951 but in 1954 Gerald Allanach returned from New York, certified in urology and the Department of Urology was re-established. Times had changed, however, and Gerald, unlike Dr. Fitzpatrick, was able to devote his practice entirely to urology. Another department was created in 1954 with the establishment of the Department of Thoracic Surgery as a multidisciplinary department with Dr. R.B. Eaton as coordinator. Other members of the department included: Dr. C.E. Doyle, Dr. G.V. Parsons, Dr. H.R. Ripley, Dr. J.A. Fownes, Dr. I.A. MacLennan and Dr. A.W. Ross.

The X-ray department became a two-man department for the first time in 1954 with the addition of Dr. Colin Ibbotson to the staff. Born in Liverpool, England, on August 3, 1915, Ibbotson took premedical education at the University of Pennsylvania in 1933-34, and then attended the University of Liverpool from 1934 to 1940, obtaining his MB, ChB degree

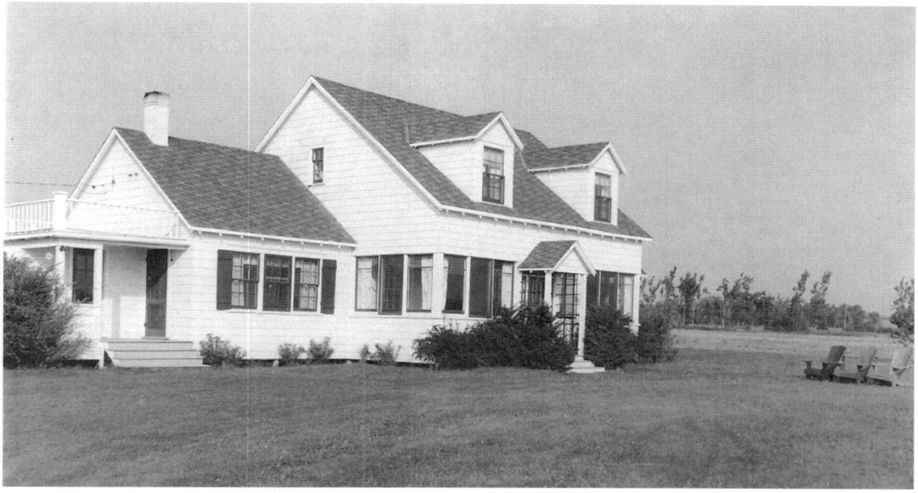

A nurses' cottage was donated by Mr. and Mrs. Leonard Lockhart in 1954.

in 1940. He interned at the Royal Infirmary in Liverpool (1940-41) and then served as a medical officer in the Indian Army from 1941 to 1946. After the war, he served an internship at the Chester County Hospital, West Chester, Pennsylvania (1947-48). He began a residency in radiology at the Chester County Hospital and the General Hospital, Wilmington, Delaware (1948-49) and then came to Canada, completing his residency at the Royal Victoria Hospital in Montreal from 1949 to 1951. He became certified in both diagnostic and therapeutic radiology by the Royal College of Physicians and Surgeons of Canada. Dr. Ibbotson worked as an associate radiologist at the Royal Jubilee Hospital in Victoria, British Columbia, but preferring to live in the east, came to Moncton when the position of associate radiologist became available. With the addition of a second radiologist, the hospital began offering consulting radiology services to the Miramichi Hospital in Newcastle and l'Hôtel Dieu in Chatham. Colin Has a good knowledge of his field but had one defect. Abraham Lincoln used to complain that General George McClellan had the "slows." Well, unfortunately, Colin Ibbotson also had the "slows." He was a slow talker and any doctor who went into the department to review a film with him would find himself engaged for the next fifteen minutes, at least. He was also slow getting to work in the morning, as well as returning from lunch breaks, and this did not sit well with the well-organized Howard Ripley. On October 8, 1963, he resigned to take a position at Albert Einstein Medical Centre in Philadelphia. He only lasted a year as the Americans apparently piled on more work than Colin was used to handling. He had a ramrod straight posture, undoubtedly developed during his army years, and at a party could miraculously hold a tray of canapés while leaning forward at a 15 to 20 degree angle, seemingly defying all the laws of gravity, as though his feet were nailed to the floor.

Although the departure of Dr. Phyllis Bursey had been a loss, the Mental Health Clinic and hence, the hospital were fortunately able to obtain the services of another very capable psychiatrist, Dr. John Stanley. Dr. Stanley was born in Ireland on August 19, 1921, and received his MB, BCh from the National University of Ireland in 1947. He came to Canada and interned at the Saint John's General Hospital, Newfoundland, in 1948-49, and then did residencies in psychiatry at the Wilshire County Mental Hospital in 1950-51, the Montreal General Hospital in 1951-53 and the Children's Memorial Hospital in 1953-54. He received a Diploma in Psychiatry from McGill in 1954. His stay in Moncton was short, however, leaving in 1956 to become superintendent of the William F. Roberts School in Saint John.

Another new addition to the staff in 1954 was Dr. D.I. MacLellan. Donald MacLellan was born in Moncton on May 30, 1929, received his BSc from Dalhousie in 1950 and his MD, CM from Dalhousie in 1954 after interning at the Saint John General Hospital from 1953 to 1954. Although enjoying a very successful general practice, he found the ever increasing changes in the medical field to be exasperating, so joined those who were abandoning general practice to go into specialization. During his general practice he came under the influence of Dr. E.W. Ewart and embarked on a training program in orthopaedics long before this was to become one of the most coveted specialities. He did a year of general surgical residency at the Boston City Hospital from 1961 to 1962 and then a three-year residency in orthopaedics at the New York Orthopaedic Hospital at the Columbia Presbyterian Medical Centre in New York from 1962 to 1965. He obtained his FRCS(C) in Orthopaedics in 1966 and his American Boards in Orthopaedic Surgery in 1968. He served as president of the Moncton and District Medical Society in 1960 and of the Atlantic Provinces Orthopaedic Society in 1970. He has served as Chief of Orthopaedics and was president of the medical staff in 1969, 1985 and 1986. He served as a volunteer for Care-Medico in Indonesia in 1974 and Tunisia in 1976, teaching orthopaedics in these countries. He retired in 1994, and has been busily engaged in developing this history of The Moncton Hospital as his contribution to mark the centennial year of the hospital.

Dr. D.F.W. Porter, the executive director of the hospital since 1949, resigned in 1955. He was replaced by Dr. Austin Clarke who had been assistant chief medical officer and director of Health Planning Services with the New Brunswick Department of Health and Social Services. His experience in government was to stand him and the hospital in good stead in the ensuing years, as government was becoming more and more involved in the regulation and funding of hospitals.

Plans were proceeding at this time for the construction of a new nurses' residence. This became imperative when an agreement of sale for the old hospital, now used as a nurses' residence, was signed during the year by representatives of the board of Trustees of The Moncton Hospital and Les Religieuses de Notre Dame du Sacré Coeur. One wing of the building was to be made available to the purchaser in July 1956, with the remainder of the building to be available in the late summer of 1957.

The American College of Surgeons inspected the hospital for accreditation of the Cancer Clinic in 1955, and gave provisional approval. The Cancer Clinic operating at The Moncton Hospital had served the district, and had not been confined to The Moncton Hospital patients. In order to get full approval, it was necessary to provide an additional register for The Moncton Hospital patients, to appoint a special cancer committee of the medical staff and to arrange for medical staff conferences on cancer. Plans for these changes were completed in 1955 to become effective January 1, 1956.

During 1955, ident-a-bands were first introduced into the hospital for use on newborns replacing the old system of using beads. The system would later be adopted for all patients in the hospital. This year also saw the publication of the first yearbook by the student nurses.

In 1955, Dr. J.A. Delaney appeared on the scene as the first fully-trained obstetrician and gynaecologist on the staff, confining his practice solely to that specialty. Austin Delaney was born in Bouctouche on October 18, 1918, received his BSc from the University of Montreal in 1938, an MD, CM degree from the same institution in 1943 and interned in 1943 at Notre Dame Hospital and St. Justine's Children's Hospital. He then practised in Summerside, Prince Edward Island. In 1949 he attended the Cook County Post Graduate School for surgical training and in 1953-54, he was a resident in obstetrics and gynaecology at the Victoria General Hospital. He had a similar residency at the Saint John General Hospital in 1954-55 and became

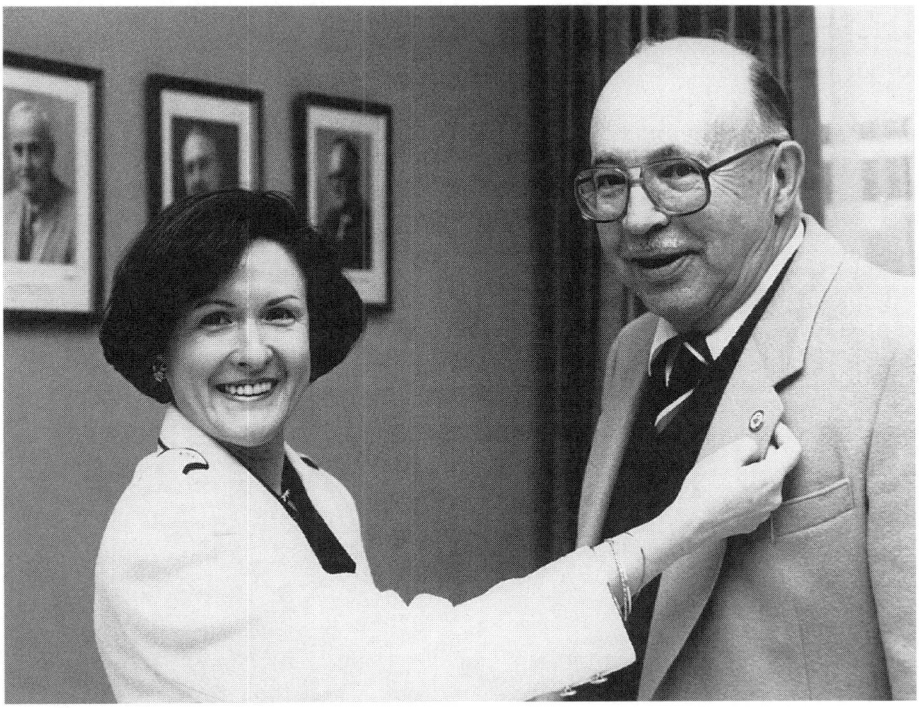

Dr. Ginette Gagné-Koch (left) presents a service pin to Dr. J.A. Delaney, the first obstetrician on staff.

certified in obstetrics and gynaecology in 1955. During the time he lived on Prince Edward Island, he developed a love of horse racing and after moving to Moncton kept his own stable of race horses at the track. He was an early riser and would go to the racetrack to exercise his horses and then go to the hospital and make rounds in his race barn attire before going home and preparing for the day's medical tasks. He very seldom had to listen to any complaints from his patients as they were usually asleep or pretty drowsy at the time of his rounds. On one occasion, as a number of us were sitting in the doctor's lounge, Austin got on the phone to Al Fownes and asked him if he would go to the Island with him to do a cardiogram on a friend of his suspected of having angina. What Austin neglected to tell Al, however, was that the "friend" was a race horse. Austin enjoyed a long association with the staff until ill health forced him to restrict his activities and he transferred from the active staff to the consulting staff in 1973 but he kept practising until 1990 when he was appointed to the honorary staff. He died in 1997. For many years he also served as coroner. One story he liked to tell of his experience as a coroner, concerned a fatal stabbing. On arrival at the scene of the crime, Austin found one of the policeman holding a knife. On being asked where he had found it, the policeman replied that it had been in the corpse. Austin told him he should not have removed it; whereupon, the policeman immediately put the knife back in the corpse.

A new name appears on the surgical roster in 1955 with the appearance of Dr. Edgar Girouard's name as a junior surgeon. Edgar "Jigger" Girouard was born in Moncton on August 26, 1923. He obtained a BA from St. Joseph's University in 1951 and a BM, MD from Laval in 1951. He interned in Quebec City from 1950 to 1951 and at Christ Hospital, Jersey City, from 1951 to 1952. He then did a residency in general surgery at Doctor's Hospital, Washington, D.C., from 1952 to 1953 and at the Rochester General Hospital (1953-55). Having practised mostly at the Dr. Georges-L. Dumont Hospital, he was not reappointed to The Moncton Hospital staff upon his resignation from practice at the Dr. Georges-L Dumont in 1983.

Four new doctors made their appearance on the scene as general practitioners in 1955. Drs. Hazel and Raymond Murphy were appointed as the first husband and wife team on the medical staff and Hazel was the second female doctor appointed to the staff. Hazel was born in England on July 12, 1920, and, after serving in the services during the war, took her premed at Acadia and received her MD, CM from Dalhousie in 1954 after interning at the Victoria General Hospital, the Halifax Children's Hospital and the Prince Edward Island Hospital. Her classmate at Dalhousie, Raymond Murphy, was born in Placentia, Newfoundland, on May 2, 1915, and, following Hazel on the same internship rotations, graduated from Dalhousie in 1954. After graduation, the Murphys set up practice at Riverside, Albert County, and then a year later opened an office in Gunningsville, at which time they became members of the staff of The Moncton Hospital, an association which continued until their retirement in 1996.

Paul Auffrey was born in Moncton on March 11, 1927, and attended St. Francis Xavier and the University of Montreal, obtaining his BSc from the former in 1950 and his MD from the latter in 1955. From 1954 to 1955 he interned at Hôpital de la Misericorde and Hôpital Sacré-Coeur. He practised mainly at the Dr. Georges-L. Dumont Hospital and was suspended from the medical staff in January 1976 for incomplete charts.

Dr. Bernard Kanter was born in Saint John, New Brunswick, on March 4, 1929, and received his BSc from University of New Brunswick in 1950, and after interning at the Victoria General Hospital and the Saint John's General Hospital in Newfoundland, he received his MD, CM from Dalhousie in 1955. He was a competent general practitioner but resigned from the staff in 1962 to specialize in psychiatry.

During 1955 there were 8,055 admissions which included 1,177 births. The number of operations was 3,584 and 7,232 patients were seen in the X-ray department, 284 of them for X-ray therapy. The laboratory carried out 61,422 examinations and 1,984 transfusions were given. 837 electrocardiograms were done and 4,822 physiotherapy treatments carried out on 350 patients. There were 4,062 visits to the outpatient department, including 1,637 minor operations and fracture reductions.

A fire occurred in the medical library on May 14, 1956. When it burned through to the door to the corridor, a fireball developed resulting in much damage to the corridor and front lobby although no damage was done to the patient areas. The medical library, including its furnishings, was completely destroyed. The library, which had books largely of historical interest, was

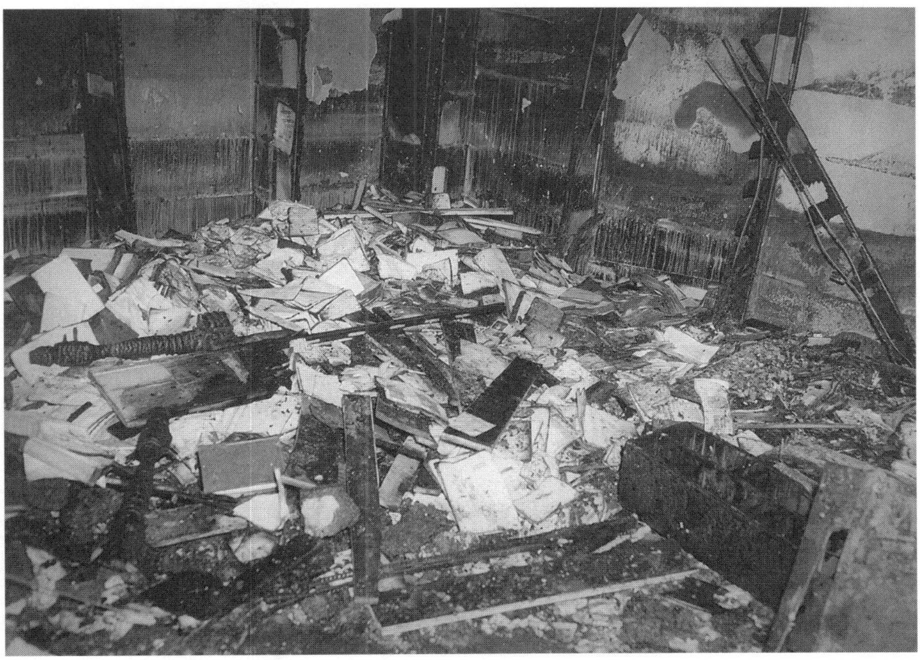

The medical library at The Moncton Hospital was destroyed by fire in 1956.

replaced eventually with some $6,000 of insurance money and became the foundation of the present-day superb medical library. The entire administration section of the first floor required renovations. As a result of the fire, a number of changes were adopted to provide for better safety in the future. Firstly, long corridors were divided by partitions with fire doors to provide relatively small compartments. The wooden doors on the cafeteria were replaced by steel ones. Secondly, fire detector heads were installed in rooms of the first and ground floors, where such protection had not been provided previously. Thirdly, a night watchman was put on duty from midnight to 8:00 a.m. daily to visit regularly the parts of the hospital where personnel were not on duty at night. Fourthly, fire regulations for the hospital were revised. Finally, fire lectures and drills were scheduled, with instructions being given to the hospital staff by City Fire Chief Murray McKie.

On June 1, 1956, plans providing for pensions and life insurance went into effect. The hospital would thereafter pay, on behalf of the employees, the entire cost of past service pensions, the entire cost of life insurance benefits and the difference between the cost of future service pensions and the contributions of the employees. The employees were to contribute approximately five percent of their salary. The plans were made voluntary for members of the permanent staff, but all employees engaged after June 1, 1956, were required to join the plan when they became eligible.

A sod-turning ceremony was held on August 29, 1956, for the new nurses' residence with the first sod turned by Margery MacManus, president of the Students' Council.

The only new additions to the staff in 1956 were Dr. P. Leger, who was admitted as a junior surgeon, and Dr. Leigh Ramsay to the EENT staff. Dr. Paul V.J. Leger was born in Moncton on June 10, 1925, and obtained a BA from St. Joseph's College and an MD from Laval in 1951. He interned at St. Joseph's Hospital in Saint John from 1951 to 1952 and did residencies in surgery at the Royal Victoria Hospital from 1952 to 1954, the Montreal General Hospital and the Montreal Children's Hospital from 1954 to 1955 and at University Hospital in Baltimore (1955-56). His medical career was cut short by his sudden death on December 14, 1962.

Dr. Leigh Ramsay was born on Prince Edward Island on June 14, 1915. After taking premed at Prince of Wales College, he obtained his MD, CM from Dalhousie in 1942, interning at the Victoria General Hospital from 1941-1942. He did residencies in EENT at Camp Hill Hospital, Halifax (1948-49), Beth Israel Hospital, Boston (1949-50), and Arkansas Baptist Hospital, Little Rock, Arkansas (1952-53) and an assistantship to Dr. C.K. Fuller in Yarmouth, Nova Scotia (1950-52). He became certified by the Royal College in ophthalmology in 1953 and the American Board of Ophthalmology in 1955. Before coming to Moncton in 1956, he practised at the St. John General and Lancaster Veterans Hospital from 1954 to 1956. He soon established himself as a hard working doctor who always obliged his colleagues by seeing requests for consults in the shortest possible time. A request for a consultation was often met with the reply to send the patient to the office at 5 pm. The patient, however, would usually arrive at the office to find it packed and would wish he had brought a snack. Leigh would never rush a patient through the office, and the person with the 5 o'clock appointment might only be seen by 11 pm. At his own request, Leigh was not reappointed to the staff in 1985, when the long hours had finally taken their toll on his health. He retired to Prince Edward Island where he died in 1994.

During 1956, 7,954 patients were admitted including 1,122 newborns; 3,591 operations were performed; 1,020 electrocardiograms were done and 7,884 physiotherapy treatments were given to 588 patients. The X-ray department looked after 7,217 patients for radiography and another 269 for radiotherapy. The laboratory did 74,636 examinations and 1,643 blood transfusions were given; 5,051 patients made 5,734 visits to the outpatient department.

The most significant event for the hospital in 1957 was the opening of the new residence for nurses on December 11, 1957, by His Worship Michael Baig, the mayor of Moncton, and Percy J. Eagles, Warden of the County of Westmorland. The building was built by Modern Construction of Moncton with Mott and Myles of Saint John serving as architects. The nurses moved to their new residence on December 13, 1957, and on December 17, 1957, the old hospital buildings on King Street were transferred by deed to Les Religieuses de Notre Dame du Sacré Coeur at a sale price of $160,000. To preserve part of the old hospital's heritage, the beautiful crystal chandelier from the lobby of the old hospital building was installed in the corridor at the entrance to the auditorium of the new residence. On its first and second

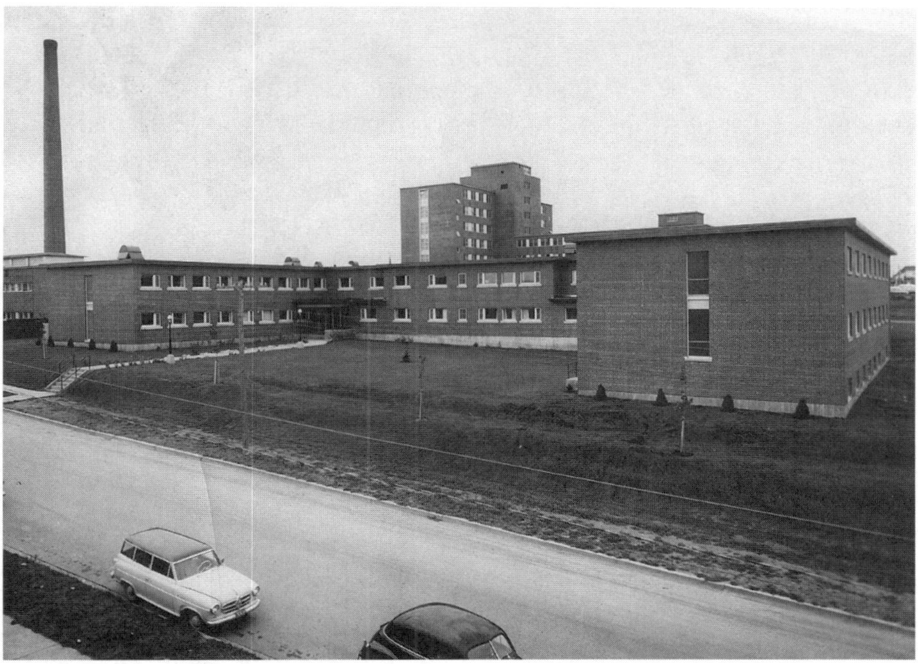

A new nurses' residence was opened in 1957.

floors, the new residence provided living quarters for the superintendent of nurses, a house mother, a female intern and 120 nurses. There were also lounges and reception rooms. Teaching space on the ground floor included two large classrooms with a sound-proof folding door between, a large demonstration room for teaching nursing arts, a library and an office for teaching staff. A large room on the ground floor was designed so that it could be used as an auditorium, a gymnasium or a recreation room. A two-storey passageway connected the nurses' home to the other hospital buildings. The completed construction project provided for an extension to the laundry, with extra space being provided for the workshop of the maintenance and repair department.

Dalhousie had been sending six interns a year to the hospital on a pediatric rotation but at this time the hospital began its own intern program, accepting three interns with rotations through medicine, surgery and obstetrics.

In the nursing field, three nurses who would continue to play prominent roles in the nursing staff were off for the year on postgraduate study leave. Shirley MacLeod went to McGill University School for Graduate Nurses to pursue studies in maternal and child care. Lois Good spent a year at the University of Toronto School for Graduate Nurses taking a course in the teaching of medical and surgical nursing. Harriett Hayes also took a course in teaching of medical and surgical nursing but at McGill University School for Graduate Nurses.

In 1957, the Department of Obstetrics and Gynaecology suddenly expanded from a one-man department to a three-man department with the arrival of two newly-trained specialists. The first, Dr. Victor D. McLaughlin, was born in St. Boniface, Manitoba, on February 25, 1928, but grew up in Nova Scotia. He attended Acadia University from which he graduated with a BSc in 1948, attended McGill obtaining an MD, CM degree in 1952 and then interned at the Montreal General Hospital in 1952-53. He remained at that institution as a junior assistant resident in surgery in 1953-54, an assistant resident in obstetrics and gynaecology in 1954-55 and then resident in 1956-57. During 1955-56 he served as a resident at the Margaret Hague Maternity Hospital in Jersey City. He was certified by the Royal College of Physicians and Surgeons of Canada in obstetrics and gynaecology in 1958. His decision to come to Moncton was no doubt, influenced by the fact that he had married Peggy Dobson, the daughter of Dr. Joseph Dobson. In addition to his skills in the surgical field, his organizational ability was soon apparent and, besides serving as co-ordinator of obstetrics and gynaecology the year after his arrival, he was elected president of the medical staff in 1963. In 1971 he served on a committee with Dr. Carl Brown and Dr. Bill Turner to revise the medical staff by-laws. One of the features of the new by-laws was to create the position of Chief of Staff. When elections were held in 1972 for this position, Victor was chosen to be the first Chief of Staff at the hospital. He held this position until 1975. On November 25, 1974, he addressed the Moncton Rotary Club with his address entitled: "A Tale of Two Hats." In it, he explained that since he was a member of the medical staff his work could be evaluated by the chief of his service. As Chief of Staff, however, he was required to oversee the work of the entire medical staff so that quality care was always provided to the community it served. In 1981, when the administration felt the time was ripe for the appointment of a Medical Director to Assist the Executive Director, Victor assumed this position on August 1, 1981, but resigned from this position on June 30, 1982, because he thought that it was apparent that some members of the medical staff felt that he now had only one hat, the administrative hat, and no longer the hat of a member of the medical staff. He resumed his practice, but still had the administrative bug and in August 1986 he became Registrar of the College of Physicians and Surgeons of New Brunswick. He resigned from the medical staff in 1986, and was appointed to the honorary staff in 1988. After retiring from the position as registrar of the college, he was appointed to the position of chairman of the new Peer Review Committee. When the hospital began preparations for centennial celebrations, it was fortunate that Victor was available to take on the task of chairman of the Centennial Celebrations Committee. In his spare time, he indulges in his hobbies of woodworking and weaving.

The second addition to the obstetrics and gynaecology staff that year, was Dr. Paul Pugh, who continues on the senior active staff to this time. Paul was born in Burtt's Corner, New Brunswick, on November 1, 1925. He received his BSc degree from University of New Brunswick in 1947 and his MD, CM from Dalhousie in 1953 after interning at the Victoria General Hospital from 1952-1953. He then took a residency in obstetrics and gynaecology at the Victoria General, Camp Hill and Grace Maternity Hospitals in Halifax from 1953-1957 and obtained his certification in obstetrics and gynaecology from the Royal College. In his quiet unassuming manner he has remained a mainstay of his department throughout the years and still carries on a busy practice at this time. In his spare time he skies, golfs and enjoys poker, a game in which he possesses some skill.

Although he would practise principally at the Dr. Georges-L. Dumont Hospital, Dr. Eugère Cormier was admitted to the active staff in internal medicine in 1957 and so would participate in caring for those patients admitted to the public service. He was born in St. Paul, New Brunswick, in 1920, and attended St. Joseph's University, from which he obtained a BA in 1942. He then attended Laval and received a BM, MD in 1946 and following this, interned in Quebec City Hospitals. He did general practice in Shediac for a few years and this was followed by an internship at Christ Hospital, Jersey City, from 1951 to 1952, a medical residency at the New England Deaconess Hospital in Boston (1952-53) and then residencies at St. Alexis Hospital, Cleveland (1953-54) and at St. Vincent's Charity Hospital, Cleveland (1954-55). He was awarded a Fellowship in the American College of Cardiology in 1956. He did not apply for reappointment in 1981 after he underwent open heart surgery. Eugère had suffered his first coronary around the same time in 1971 as I had suffered my own. Both of us lost weight but some time later I met Eugère in the record room one night and remarked that he seemed to have put all his weight back on. Eugère's comment was that he was a cardiologist and all his thin patients seemed to die just as quickly as the fat ones so he was going to continue to enjoy his French cuisine.

An addition to the Department of General Practice was Dr. Joyce Boillat. She was born in Toronto on November 20, 1927, and took both her premed and her medical education at the University of Toronto receiving her MD degree in 1954. She interned at the Toronto East General and Orthopaedic Hospital from 1954 to 1955 and practised at a clinic in Toronto (1955-57). She came to Moncton when her husband was appointed as minister of the French Baptist Church, La Bonne Nouvelle. While she was in practice in Moncton, Joyce's husband had a coronary and was hospitalized. Joyce obeyed visiting rules quite strictly, usually, but one evening she was particularly busy in her office and decided to ignore the rules for once and visited her husband after the usual visiting hours. As she was sitting with him, he had a sudden cardiac arrest and Joyce sprang into action and brought him around. She was quite certain thereafter, that divine providence had arranged her day. On July 1, 1958, she took a year's leave of absence while her husband was on study leave in Montreal. At the end of the year, her husband received an appointment in Montreal and so Joyce submitted her resignation and began work at a geriatric hospital there.

The Department of Psychiatry continued on a course of musical chairs with Dr. John Stanley departing for Saint John. Dr. J.R. Beesley, who was born in Saint John on February 27, 1924, came to take Dr. Stanley's place in Moncton. He obtained his BSc from University of New Brunswick in 1947 and his MD, CM from McGill in 1951. He interned at the Queen Elizabeth Hospital in Montreal 1951-52. He then studied psychiatry at the Psychiatric Ontario Hospital, Toronto (1952-53), the Toronto Psychiatric Hospital and Toronto General (1953-55) and at the Ontario Hospital, London (1955-57). He received his diploma in psychiatry from the University of Toronto in 1955 and was certified in psychiatry by the Royal College. He resigned from the staff in 1961.

During 1957, 7,297 adults and children were admitted to hospital, as well as 1,281 newborns. There were 1,620 major and 1,982 minor operations performed. The physiotherapy department carried out 6,794 treatments on 440 outpatients and 119 inpatients; 1,194 electrocardiograms were done. The laboratory did 93,120 tests, broken down as follows: 2,243 tissue pathology; 7,631 bacteriology; 48,089 chemistry; and 35,157 haematology. 1,666 blood transfusions were given. X-rays were taken on 3,574 inpatients and 3,594 outpatients. Radiotherapy treatments were given to 43 inpatients and 188 outpatients. The outpatient department showed a steady increase in the number of visits with 5,558 patients treated including 922 fracture cases, 2,814 medical patients, 1,563 surgical patients, 170 dental patients, 34 patients for electroconvulsive treatments and 45 patients for ENT clinic and 10 for prenatal clinic. The outpatient department saw 768 patents classified as emergencies and 590 general anaesthetics were given.

The demand for beds at the hospital in 1958 exceeded the supply with the result that no cases other than emergencies could be admitted for considerable periods of time. Preliminary plans were drawn up for the addition of a 170-bed wing but this would have to wait for the approval of the Hospital Services Commission of New Brunswick, the City Council of Moncton and the County Council of Westmorland.

The year 1958 is remarkable only by a scarcity of exciting events but it is notable, however, that for the first time in years the medical staff was empowered to appoint a representative to the board of Trustees of the hospital and Dr. George Parsons was chosen for this post.

New additions to the staff in 1958 included two surgeons. The first of them, Georges Grondin, was born in Grand Falls, New Brunswick, on January 13, 1928, received a BA from St. Joseph's University in 1948 and an MD from Laval in 1953 after interning at Quebec university hospitals in 1952-53. He then did a residency in general surgery at Memorial Hospital, Worcester, Massachusetts (1953-55), a surgical basic science course at the University of Pennsylvania in Philadelphia (1955-56) and completed his surgical residency at St. Mary's Hospital, Rochester, New York (1956-58). He was first appointed to the staff as a junior physician until such time as he provided evidence of eligibility to write the Royal College Exams. In 1960, he was appointed to the consulting staff. He did very little work at The Moncton Hospital but played a very prominent part in the history of l'Hôtel Dieu and Dr. Georges-L. Dumont Hospital where he became "Lord of the Manor."

The second addition to the staff, Dr. Robert M. Dysart, the son of Premier Allison Dysart, was born in Bouctouche on May 22, 1924. After taking premed at St. Francis Xavier he received his MD, CM degree from McGill in 1947, interned at the Montreal General Hospital from 1947 to 1948 and stayed on at the Montreal General until 1949 studying pathology. He then embarked on a career in internal medicine with a residency at Charity Hospital in New Orleans (1949-52) and he obtained his FRCP(C) in 1954. Not satisfied with a career in internal medicine, he took a surgical residency at the New York University-Bellevue Medical Centre from 1953 to 1958 and obtained his FRCS(C), thereby becoming one of very few in Canada and the only member on the staff to ever hold specialist qualifications in both medicine and surgery. Surgery, however, was his first love and it was to this that he confined his practice. He is fluently bilingual and until his recent retirement divided his practice between both The Moncton Hospital and the Dr. Georges-L. Dumont serving, on the active staff of both institutions. His sister was married to Dr. Peter Lyons and he and his brother-in-law became constant companions in the operating room, assisting each other, as well as being companions in the curling rink.

On January 1, 1958 the pathology department became a two-man department with the appointment of Dr. Alfred Bastarache to the staff. Born in Bouctouche on January 11, 1921, he obtained a BA from seminary of Rimouski in 1942 and an MD from Laval in 1946. He interned at St. Sacrement Hospital, Quebec City, from 1946 to 1947 and then did general practice in St. Anthony, New Brunswick, from 1947 to 1951 and in Shediac from 1951 to 1954. He proceeded to do postgraduate work in pathology at the Saint John General Hospital (1954-55) and at the Montreal General and St. Mary's Hospital, Montreal (1955-57). He became certified in pathology by the Royal College in 1959 and became a Fellow of the American Society of Clinical Pathologists in 1964. He served as associate pathologist at the Moncton Regional Laboratory from 1957 to 1963 and, on the resignation of Dr. Ian MacLennan in 1963, he was appointed its director, a position he held until 1973. He remained on the staff and accepted the position of acting director in 1976 on the departure of the director, Dr. Aubrey Hudson, and again resumed the position of director in 1977. He retained this position until 1980 when he resigned to accept a position as Director of the Laboratory at the Dr. Georges-L. Dumont Hospital. Unfortunately, the ever present cigarette which could be found in his mouth resulted in his untimely death from cancer of the lung on August 8, 1984. Besides being an excellent pathologist, Alfred soon became known as one of the most gifted after-dinner speakers in the community. He had a perfect sense of timing and could make any topic humorous and entertaining in both English and French. He was quite active in the National Society of Acadians and the Acadian Education Association. He served as president of the New Brunswick Cancer Society and also as president of the Richelieu Club.

In 1958 there were 8,545 admissions to hospital including 1,235 newborns; 3,791 operations were performed; 279 patients received X-ray treatments and there were 7,848 visits to the X-ray department. The laboratory carried out 96,883 examinations. 1,304 electrocardiograms were done and 5,510 physiotherapy treatments were given to 787 patients.

As the 1950s drew to a close, socialized medicine made its appearance on the medical scene when the Hospital Insurance Program under the Hospital Insurance Commission was inaugurated on July 1, 1959. Ever since, the destiny of the hospital has depended on government largesse. With "free hospitalization", the occupancy rate took a jump. In June 1959, the waiting list for both medicine and surgery stood at 242 patients and by December, this had jumped to 577. Considerable time was spent by the board of Trustees and the Administration on plans for a 160-bed expansion and the architectural firm which had been responsible for the new hospital in 1953 was engaged to draw up plans. The City of Moncton and the counties of Westmorland and Albert agreed to participate in guaranteeing the bonds that would be issued to finance the project, so it would appear that the board still had a lot of input when it came to financial matters. It was hoped to have legislation approved in the provincial legislature in the spring of 1960 with construction to commence in June 1960. On January 1, 1960, the Moncton Hospital Annex, formerly the Moncton Tuberculosis Hospital, was to open, to serve as a chronic care facility. It was understood that patients from both The Moncton Hospital and l'Hôtel Dieu could be transferred there.

New additions to the staff in 1959 included Dr. D.K. Senn, and Dr. W.A. Turner. Dr. Senn was born in Chittagong, East Pakistan, on March 21, 1921. He attended Calcutta University and received an M.B. degree from Carmichael Medical College, Calcutta, in 1944. After serving in the Indian Army Medical Corps from 1945 to 1949, he went to England where he did a residency in anaesthesia at Culsa Hospital, Coventry, England, from 1951 to 1952 and at St. Catherine Hospital, Birkenhead, England, from 1953 to 1954. He received a diploma in anaesthesia from the Royal College of Surgeons of England in 1954. He was appointed both to the staff as a general practitioner and to the anaesthetic staff but his anaesthetic privileges were withdrawn on February 28, 1961.

Dr. W.A. Turner established a general practice in Salisbury in 1957 and was appointed to the courtesy staff at that time, later joining the active staff in the Department of General Practice in 1959. He took a leave of absence from the staff in 1964 to take postgraduate work in internal medicine. More will be said of him when he rejoins the staff in 1968.

Drawing the decade to a close, 1959 saw 8,506 patients admitted to hospital and 3,442 operations performed. The radiology department performed X-rays on 9,490 patients with 35,656 films read. In addition, 1,720 X-ray treatments were given to 239 patients; 7,491 physiotherapy treatments were given to 1,061 patients; 1,572 electrocardiograms were taken and 309 basal metabolism tests performed.

Chapter Eight

The Sixties— Specialization and Departmentalization

The beginning of the 1960s heralds a decade long period of change in the medical profession and in the history of the hospital with a movement towards greater specialization. New doctors begin to arrive with special skills and other doctors on staff leave to pursue specialization, returning to use their added skills for the benefit of the citizens of Moncton. As will be apparent, this specialization and growth resulted in changes in the structure of the hospital and also growth in the administrative complexity of the hospital.

In 1959, Harold Tait replaced Leonard W. Lockhart as chairman of the Board. He was, however, transferred by his company, the T. Eaton Company Ltd., to the head office in Toronto and on February 1, 1960, Mr. Lockhart again resumed the chairman's duties. That February also marked the appointment of Dr. W.A. Oatway as Assistant Executive Director or Medical Director on a part-time basis, with supervisory duties over the professional aspects of administration, and over the phases of work dealing directly with patient care. The demand for beds kept increasing and extra beds were set up bringing the capacity to 225 whereas the rated capacity was 215 beds. Despite this, the waiting list for medical and surgical cases continued to grow so that there were 590 cases on the waiting list in December 1960, compared to 577 in December 1959. Architectural plans were completed for an extension to the hospital to provide for an additional 160 beds. While the Toronto architects were responsible for the design, the local architectural firm of LeBlanc, Gaudet and Associates was retained as associate or resident architects. The general contract for the building was awarded to Abbey Landry Limited, with the main sub-contracts being W.S. McKnight for mechanical and Acadia Electric Limited for electrical. Extensions and alterations were also planned for the outpatient department, physiotherapy department, administration wing, X-ray department, delivery room, operating room, nursery, kitchen, boiler room and laundry. Provision was also made for a 19-bed psychiatric section and an intensive care unit. There were also to be improved facilities for the isolation of patients with communicable diseases. At a special ceremony on July 4, 1960, Jeanne Odgen, president of the Student Nurses' Council, had the honour of turning the first sod for the new addition. For the first time, the total operating expenses of the hospital exceeded $2 million.

The Moncton Hospital Annex opened its doors on January 1, 1960, and was operated as a separate financial unit with Jean Lyons serving as administrator but with ultimate control resting in the hands of the executive director and the board of The Moncton Hospital. The psychiatric service was transferred to the Annex, where it remained until new facilities were provided with the opening of the Joyce Wing in 1962.

When the nursing school was opened in 1906, it had been called the Moncton Hospital Training School. In 1960, an amendment to the Hospital Act changed the name to the Moncton Hospital School of Nursing. This reflected a change in thinking to the effect that the purpose of the school was not to train the students, but rather to educate them. University trained nurses' programs were also begun at this time and during the summer 14 students from the University of New Brunswick School of Nursing were at the hospital to gain experience in medical and surgical nursing.

For the first time in many years, and for the only time in years to come, there were no additions to the medical staff.

During 1960, 9,692 patients were admitted and 4,044 operations were performed. 12,277 patients underwent X-ray examination and 1,697 X-ray treatments were given. 2,188 electrocardiograms were done and 359 basal metabolism tests performed. 13,493 physiotherapy treatments were given to 1,804 patients. Increased use of laboratory services was experienced with 87,450 hematology, 55,079 biochemistry, 25,131 pathology, 34,903 bacteriology and 1,064 cytology examinations. There was also increasing use of the outpatient department, with a total of 9,126 visits.

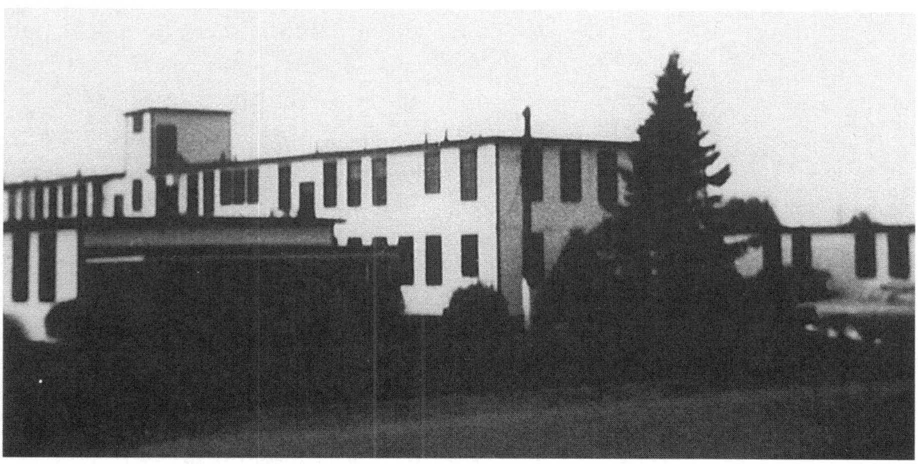

The Moncton Hospital Annex was opened in 1960.

Work progressed on the new wing throughout 1961, as the hospital continued to increase its waiting lists which grew from 656 at the end of 1960 to 934 at the end of 1961. In changes to the administration, John Dingle was appointed Assistant Administrator-Non Medical. He served as Personnel Officer and also had supervision over some of the non-professional and non-technical departments.

Up until 1961, the medical staff had been organized into several departments but all business was conducted at a monthly meeting of all members of the medical staff. This was to change with a revision of the by-laws completed and approved by the medical staff in May 1961. The staff was now to be organized into ten clinical departments: anaesthesia, general practice, internal medicine, obstetrics and gynaecology, ophthalmology and otorhinolaryngology, pediatrics, pathology, psychiatry, radiology and surgery. Each department would have a chief appointed and the departments were to meet monthly. The chiefs of each department, along with the executive of the medical staff, would then meet monthly as the Medical Advisory Committee (MAC). A meeting of the whole staff would be held each quarter, which would receive reports from the committee and provide a forum for discussion on the business carried out by the MAC. The president of the medical staff served as chairman of the MAC and this form of government has continued to the present day except for the addition of more clinical departments. The meetings have been chaired by the Chief of Staff since this position was created in 1972. Prior to 1957, the Department of Medicine was divided into junior and senior physicians. A Department of General Practice was formed in 1957 but this was created for administrative purposes rather than to act as a separate clinical department. In 1959, the Canadian Council on Hospital Accreditation, which was now carrying out the task of hospital certification in place of the American College of Surgeons, demanded that hospitals of certain size have departmentalization so that the category of junior physicians was dropped and junior physicians were listed only in the Department of General Practice. When the by-laws changed in 1961, the members of the Department of General Practice voted to hold their monthly meetings with the Department of Medicine. In 1963, the department would, however, become an active department separate from the Department of Medicine.

In addition to attendance at departmental and quarterly staff meetings, members of the staff could be appointed to any one of eleven standing committees: the Executive Committee, Medical Advisory Committee, Credentials Committee, Medical Records Committee, Hospital Practice and Tissue Committee, Infection Committee, Intern Committee, Infant Mortality Committee, Cancer Committee, and Library Committee. These committees would meet monthly to deal with the specific problems which fell within their terms of reference. In addition, another standing committee was formed, the Joint Conference Committee, and this consisted of the executive of the medical staff and the executive of the hospital board and it would meet on a quarterly basis. It serves as a forum for expressions of opinions between the medical staff and the board of trustees apart from the medical staff representation on the board. In addition to the standing committees, four special committees of the medical staff were also created:

1. The Disaster Plan Committee;
2. The Pharmacy and Therapeutics Committee;
3. The Admission and Bed Occupancy Committee; and
4. The In-Hospital Education Committee.

The student nurses still continued to provide 50 percent of the nursing services at the hospital and class size was now increased with 58 students accepted in September 1961. Student enrolment on December 31, 1961, was 131. With increased enrolment, however, the students no longer could all be accommodated at the nurses residence and a second building located near the Hospital Annex was opened to accommodate twelve students. By this time, most of the faculty members had completed post graduate courses in their clinical fields and in nursing education and several served as full time teaching staff. Gwendolyn Herman, who received her Bachelor of Nursing Degree at McGill School for Graduate Nurses, became the first degree nurse to be appointed to the Nursing School Faculty. In 1961, the Faculty of the School of Nursing consisted of fourteen members:

Katherine Wright, RN	Director of Nursing
Gwendolyn Herman, BN, RN	Assistant Director of Nursing
Flora Moroney, RN	Science Instructor
Kathleen Estabrooks, RN	Nursing Arts instructor
Myrna Sherrard, RN	Nursing Arts instructor
Heather MacLean, PDt	Dietetic Instructor
Harriett Hayes, RN	Medical-Surgical Clinical Instructor
Edith Warman, RN	Medical-Surgical Clinical Instructor
Shirley MacLeod, RN	Obstetrical Clinical Instructor
Margaret MacCallum, RN	Paediatric Clinical Instructor
Ailene Forsythe, RN	Operating Room Clinical Instructor
Joy Lewis, RN	Psychiatric Clinical Instructor
Marion Wilbur, RN	Assistant Director of Nursing Service, Charge of Student Rotation
Hilda Welling, RN	Student Health Service Nurse

An innovation introduced by the School of Nursing this year was the supplying of clinical practice for student nursing assistants from the New Brunswick Technical Institute after they had completed their theory at the school. Catherine Bannister, RN was Chairman of the Advisory Committee of the Nursing Assistants Course at the New Brunswick Technical Institute and Katherine Wright also served as a member of this committee.

The psychiatric department became a two man department in 1961 with the addition of Dr. Fred Houston to the department joining Dr. J.R. Beesley. Dr. Beesley would soon depart, however, again making it a one man department. Fred Houston was born in London, England, on May 24, 1917. He graduated from the University of Leeds (MRCS, LRCP) in 1942 and interned at Whiston Hospital and Chatterbridge Hospital, England, from 1942 to 1943. He then did a residency in psychiatry at the Kingsway Mental Hospital, Derby, England, from 1943 to 1946 and served in the Royal Army Medical Corps from 1946 to 1948. Prior to immigrating to Canada in 1957, he served at various hospitals in England. In Canada, he worked at the Provincial Hospital in Lancaster from 1957 to 1960 before coming to Moncton. He obtained his certification in psychiatry from the Royal College of Physicians and Surgeons of Canada in 1958. His stay in Moncton was short as he resigned on June 30, 1963, to accept a position at the Ontario Hospital in Hamilton.

With the increased bed capacity naturally there would be increased need for auxiliary services and the X-ray department was fortunate to obtain the services of Dr. W. Brenton Stewart as a third radiologist. He was born on April 1, 1920, in Norboro, Prince Edward Island. After serving in the army's Tank Corps in Italy during the Second World War, he embarked on a medical education and took his premed and his medical degree at Dalhousie, graduating in 1952, after interning at the Victoria General Hospital in Halifax. He was a member of the courtesy staff of The Moncton Hospital from 1952 to 1957 while he was engaged in a general practice in Salisbury. He left general practice and served as a resident in radiology at the Victoria General Hospital from 1957 to 1960. He then became a postgraduate student at the Harvard Medical School in Boston, serving as a resident at the Peter Bent Brigham Hospital and the Children's Hospital Medical Centre in Boston from 1960 to 1961. In 1967, he became director of the School of Radiological Technology and in 1968, he became the chief of radiology and remained in these positions until 1974. On March 7, 1969, he was selected by the Executive of the New Brunswick Medical Society to write a history of medicine in New Brunswick, a task which resulted in the publication of a book in 1974. In 1976, he retired from the active staff but remained on the courtesy staff and has worked at locums at various locations in the Atlantic provinces since, including The Moncton Hospital. Brent enjoys golf and loves telling jokes. The punch line, however, is often rendered inaudible as a result of his own chuckling laughter. He is also seemingly indestructible making a marvellous comeback after being at death's door following coronary artery surgery in 1994.

Dr. Leon Richard joined the active staff in ophthalmology in 1961. Leon was born in Richibucto Village on June 16, 1923. He obtained his BA from Saint Joseph's in 1946 and his MD from Laval in 1951 after interning at hospitals affiliated with Laval from 1950 to 1951. After a basic science course at Harvard Medical School from 1956 to 1957, he did a residency in ophthalmology at the Boston City Hospital from 1957 to 1959 and at the Mass. General Eye and Ear Infirmary from 1959 to 1960. He remained on the active staff at both The Moncton Hospital and the Dr. Georges-L. Dumont

Hospital until January, 1978, when he elected to change to courtesy staff. Subsequently, on his retirement from active practice, he became the medical director of the Dr. Georges-L. Dumont Hospital. His success in recruiting staff and raising the standards and reputation of the Dr. Georges-L. Dumont Hospital is attested to by the naming of the new oncology centre in his honour in 1994. Leon was also active in local, provincial and national medical politics and served a term as the President of the Canadian Medical Association, the only Moncton doctor to be so honoured. He died in December 1997.

Another addition to the medical staff in 1961, and one whose presence has been felt ever since was Dr. Fred Murphy. Fred came from a family of lawyers but, like his older brother Pat, decided on a medical career. He was born in Moncton on April 26, 1929, and obtained a BSc from University of New Brunswick in 1950. He went to McGill where he obtained his MD, CM in 1954 and interned at the Montreal General Hospital from 1954 to 1955. He then embarked on a residency program in general surgery at the Montreal General Hospital from 1955 to 1956 and the Lancaster Veterans Hospital from 1956 to 1957. From 1957 to 1958 he did a research year at McGill and was rewarded with an MSc degree. He continued further training in the clinical field at the Royal Victoria Hospital from 1958 to 1959 and Saint Mary's Hospital from 1959-1860. He was certified in general surgery in 1959 and obtained his FRCS(C) and also his FACS in 1964. He soon established a busy general surgical practice but also became active in vascular surgery at its forefront and made this his sub-speciality during his years of practice. In 1983, he became certified in vascular surgery when this became recognized as a separate speciality by the Royal College of Physicians and Surgeons of Canada. In September 1988 he became president of the Canadian Association of General Surgeons, a rare honour for someone practising outside of a university environment. There is an art to being a critic, and Fred was born with a gift for criticism manifested by a tongue that can turn litmus paper red. No performance is ever excellent, of course, but any bad performance around Fred had better be cautioned against, as many a tearful nurse can attest to. Nonetheless, Fred can always cut to the core of any argument or discussion and offer a reasoned opinion or solution to a problem.

Dr. D.I. MacLellan took a leave of absence from the staff to pursue postgraduate studies in orthopaedics and his general practice was taken over by Dr. William Dennis. Bill was born in Brookfield, Nova Scotia, on August 4, 1934, and obtained a BSc from Acadia in 1956 and an MD from Dalhousie in 1961. He served his pediatric internship at The Moncton Hospital and did not require a lot of persuasion to settle in Moncton. In 1964, he was joined in practice by Dr. W.R. Gillis and they established an office on Mountain Road in a drug store owned and operated by David H. MacDonald. They were later joined in practice by Dr. E.A. Macleod, Dr. Gary Chesser, Dr. Donald Geldart and Dr. Hanford Brace. In partnership with Mr. MacDonald, the doctors added a second storey to the drugstore for offices and this became the nucleus of the Moncton Medical Clinic. Dave MacDonald later joined the Shoppers Drug Mart Chain and his business acumen was soon recognized. He became president of the Atlantic Division of Shoppers Drug Mart and then moved to Vancouver to head up the Western Division. Dave's drug store on Mountain Road, by the way, was conveniently located opposite the New Brunswick Liquor Commission Store and Dave had many a frantic call on a Saturday afternoon from a harried physician asking him to make a purchase since the doctor couldn't get away from the office before the store closed at 5 o'clock. Bill Dennis was recognized as an excellent general practitioner and served many years as a teaching preceptor for third and fourth year medical students and postgraduate trainees in family medicine in the Dalhousie Integrated Intern Training Program. He has always been an avid fisherman and has a house on the banks of the Miramichi, where he will, undoubtedly, spend a lot of time after retiring in 1995.

Including patients treated in the Annex, and 1,504 newborns, there were 10,220 patients admitted to The Moncton Hospital in 1961, 4,000 operations were performed and 10,473 visits were made to the outpatient department, of which 3,103 were classified as emergencies; 807 general anaesthetics were given in the outpatient department for minor surgery and fracture reductions. The physiotherapy department carried out 14,833 treatments on 2,171 patients; 2,459 electrocardiograms and 362 basal metabolism tests were performed. The X-ray department carried out 16,766 examinations and 1,335 X-ray treatments on 159 patients. The Cancer Clinic continued to function with 325 new patients registered and 1,115 patients rechecked.

On September 12, 1962, the official opening of the new wing of the hospital took place. Dr. John C. MacKenzie, a former consultant to The Moncton Hospital and recently administrator of the Touro Infirmary, New Orleans, was chief speaker. He unveiled two bronze plaques naming the older wing, the Parlee Wing, and the new wing, the Joyce Wing, in honour of two former mayors of Moncton. Barbara Trenholm, president of the Nurses' Student Council, had the honour of cutting the ribbon to officially open the new wing. Also present at the opening were Hon. Dr. Georges-L. Dumont, the minister of health; Dr. A.J. McInerney, administrative consultant, Hospital Services Division; Dr. A.M. Clarke, the executive director of The Moncton Hospital; Leonard Lockhart, chairman of the board; J.B. Langley, architect; and G.J. Gaudet, associate architect. The capacity of the hospital was now 366 beds and 71 bassinets but by December 31, 1962, only 310 beds and 53 bassinets were in use. The dietary department was undergoing an extension and alterations, and it was impossible to supply food for a greater number of patients. It was also impossible to get additional professional nursing staff that would look after all the new beds. By February 1963, all the new patient areas, with the exception of the nursery, were in use. In addition to the new wing, other renovations were carried out and completed by December 31, 1962. These included: the boiler room, laundry, outpatient and emergency area, X-ray department, operating and delivery room suites,

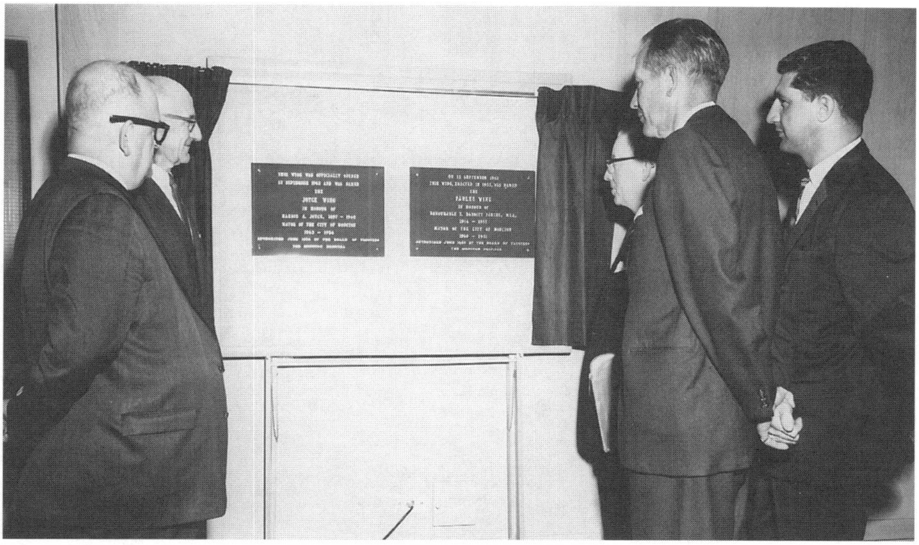

The opening of Joyce Wing in 1962. From left to right: Hon. Dr. Georges-L. Dumont, Minister of Health; Dr. John C. MacKenzie, guest speaker; Mr. Leonard Lockhart, Chairman of the Board; Mr. J.B. Langley, architect; and Mr. G.J. Gaudet, architect.

physiotherapy department, administration wing. The only alterations left to be done in 1963, were to the formula room and nursery, and the kitchen and snack bar. The total cost of the construction and equipment to December 1, 1962, was $2,455,365.36.

With the opening of the new addition, the psychiatric department was moved back to the main hospital in September 1962, after being banished to the Annex in 1960. The new 22 bed psychiatric unit included a kitchenette, dining area, and lounge for the social therapy of these patients. Offices were also provided for psychiatrists and paramedical staff. In this year, a psychologist and a psychiatric social worker brought in and the organization of a teaching program in psychiatric nursing was introduced.

An innovation in the new wing was the provision of a five-bed Intensive Care Unit for the treatment of critically ill patients who needed continual supervision by a nursing staff specially qualified and trained in emergency life-saving procedures. As we will see, the next decade, with its introduction of new technology, would give rise to a marked expansion in the provision of intensive care and the phasing out of private duty nurses.

In July 1962, William A. Kilpatrick became assistant administrator, non-medical, at the hospital, being hand-picked for the job. He graduated from Mount Allison University in 1960 with the degree of Bachelor of Commerce and in the autumn of 1960, at the request of The Moncton Hospital, he entered the Department of Hospital Administration School of Hygiene at the University of Toronto for a two-year course in hospital administration which included a year at the new Mount Sinai Hospital, Toronto. He received his diploma in hospital administration from the University of Toronto in 1962. At that time, John Dingle became personnel director.

An addition to the anaesthetic staff in 1962, was Dr. Kenneth Jennings, but his sojourn on the staff was to be short. He was born in Bathurst on December 2, 1929, received a BA from Mount Allison in 1950 and an MD, CM from McGill in 1954, and interned at the Millard Fillmore Hospital in Buffalo, New York, from 1954 to 1955. He then did residencies in anaesthesia at the Buffalo General Hospital (1956-57), the Los Angeles County Hospital (1957-58) and the Montreal General Hospital (1959-60) and worked at the Brookside Hospital, San Pablo, California, from 1958 to 1959. He lost his driver's license for speeding in July 1963, refused to come to the hospital because of lack of transportation and was not reappointed to the staff in 1963, by which time, however, he had already moved to California.

An addition to the surgical staff in 1962 was Dr. J.H. Rich. Harry was born in Moncton on November 29, 1929, and received a BSc from St. F.X. in 1950 and his MD, CM from Dalhousie in 1956 after interning at the Victoria General Hospital. After two years of general practice in Fredericton, he served as a resident in surgery at the Royal Victoria Hospital in Montreal from 1958 to 1960 and at Southampton General Hospital in England from 1960 to 1961. After another year as a teaching fellow in pathology at the Royal Victoria Hospital, he obtained his certification in general surgery and joined the staff of The Moncton Hospital. He retired in 1991 and was appointed to the honorary staff, and since then, can be seen on the golf links in Moncton and Florida. He was made a senior member of the Canadian Medical Association in 1995.

The Department of Psychiatry again became a two-man department with the appointment of Dr. Philip Michel in December 1962. By the next year, this was again reduced to a one-man department, however, with the departure of Dr. Houston. Philip (Papa Doc) was born on August 13, 1913, in Port-au-Prince, Haiti. He obtained his BA from Saint-Louis-de-Gonggere-College, Port-au-Prince, and his MD from the university of Port-au-Prince, in 1942. He came to Canada and served residencies in psychiatry at St. Michel Archange Hospital, Quebec City, from 1946 to 1949, the Psychosomatic Institute, Quebec City, 1951-52, and the Allan Memorial Institute in Montreal from 1952 to 1954. After working at the Provincial Hospital in Campbellton, he came to The Moncton Hospital and became the first psychiatrist to remain in the community for more than a couple of years attesting to his popularity with his patients and medical colleagues. He retired on May 30, 1986, and moved to Montreal. During his practice, he had the misfortune to undergo shock therapy without the benefit of anaesthesia. On July 2, 1965, an intern brought to the attention of Dr. Michel that one of the electroshock machines was not working. When Philip took the electrodes in his hand, however, the intern pressed the button and the machine came to life, and, as a result, Dr. Michel sustained fractures of both humeri. He had the distinction of being the first patient in Moncton to have a Neer shoulder prosthesis inserted.

Dr. Myer Herman was appointed to the Department of General Practice in his position as Regional Public Health Officer. He was born in London, England, on March 21, 1914, and was educated in Ireland, receiving a BA, from Trinity College, Dublin, and then an MB, BCl, BAO from Dublin University in 1939. He served in the Royal Army Medical Corps from 1939 to 1945 and then had ten years of public health practice before immigrating to Canada in 1960, after which he served two years as assistant director, Maternal and Child Health Division, New Brunswick Department of Health. He was only on the staff for two years, leaving in 1963 to join the public health department of one of the New England states.

Two appointments to the Department of General Practice in 1962 were Dr. T.E. Atkinson and Dr. J.L.G. Melanson. Ted Atkinson has remained a stalwart of the Department of General Practice (later changed to Department of Family Practice) to this day. He was born in Moncton on September 27, 1934, attended University of New Brunswick, where he obtained a BSc in 1957 and then proceeded to Dalhousie. After graduating in 1962 with his MD, he started a general practice in Salisbury but later moved to Moncton. When he is not working one of his regular sixteen-hour days, he can be found attending car shows or travelling to some distant location in the world. He has always shown a keen interest in teaching and has served as Chairman of the Intern Committee and has been very active in the teaching program for interns in the family practice program at Dalhousie University. He was made a Fellow of the College of Family Physicians of Canada in May 1985 and has served as an examiner for the Medical Council of Canada and served on the Examination Committee of the College of Family Practice of Canada.

Dr. John Lewis Guy Melanson was born in St. Anselem, New Brunswick, on October 25, 1933, and received a BA from St. Joseph's in 1956 and an MD from University of Ottawa in 1961. He interned at Grace Hospital and Columbia Medical Hospital in Detroit from 1961 to 1962. He practised mostly at l'Hôtel Dieu and left Moncton in 1965.

Two doctors who stayed in the community only a short period of time were the Blanchard brothers, who were admitted to the active staff in the Department of Orthopaedics but practised mostly at l'Hôtel Dieu. Both were born in Edmonton, Alberta; Bernard on March 10, 1931, and Guy, on May 29, 1932. Both obtained BAs from the University of Montreal. Bernard obtained his MD from the University of Montreal in 1956 and Guy, from the University of Ottawa in 1956. Bernard did a surgical rotation at l'Hôtel Dieu, in Montreal, from 1956 to 1959. Guy did a general surgery residency at Wyanotte General Hospital and Detroit Receiving Hospital from 1957 to 1959. Both then served as residents in orthopaedics at Sacred Heart Hospital, Cartierville, Montreal, from 1959 to 1962, and both obtained their FRCS(C).

There were 10,180 patients, including newborn, admitted to The

Moncton Hospital and Annex during 1962. There were 3,906 operations performed; 18,247 X-ray examinations were carried out and 1,018 X-ray treatments were given to 143 patients; 13,003 physiotherapy treatments were given to 2,036 patients; 3,057 electrocardiograms and 341 basal metabolism tests were carried out; 12,259 visits were made to the outpatient department including 4,693 classified as emergencies; 2,668 minor operations, 1,479 fracture cases and 300 dentistry cases were treated in the outpatient department with 936 general anaesthetics given.

On October 3, 1963, Ralph Belyea succeeded Leonard Lockhart as chairman of the board. Mr. Lockhart had resigned as chairman but agreed to remain as a member of the board. Except for a ten-month period from April 1, 1959, to February 1, 1960, Mr. Lockhart had served as Chairman of the Board since 1947, and had guided the construction of the new hospital and the subsequent addition of the Joyce Wing. Very few men, if any, in our community could boast of spending so many hours of their life without recompense, for the benefit of their fellow citizens.

In 1963 the hospital was inspected by the Canadian Council on Hospital Accreditation and given full accreditation for another three years.

That year also saw the Ladies' Hospital Auxiliary take on two major projects. Firstly, they furnished a lounge and cloakroom to be used by the clergy as headquarters for their hospital visitation work. An up-to-date list of patients identified by church affiliation was kept in this room to help the clergy identify members of their congregations admitted to hospital. Secondly, a coffee shop was opened in the cafeteria so that staff and visitors could obtain light snacks during those periods when the cafeteria was not serving meals. In the main lobby of the hospital, the Nurses' Hospital Auxiliary operated the hospital gift shop and from the proceeds was able to donate $1,000 to the hospital. The operation of the coffee shop was taken over by the School of Nursing Alumnae in February 1964.

This year marked the inauguration of a formalized volunteer service at the hospital. These volunteers were asked to give an afternoon or an evening a week, with hours and activities arranged to suit their schedules. The volunteers worked in the admitting department as escorts for patients being admitted, at the reception desk and in the hospital coffee shop. In addition, teenage girls helped out in the physiotherapy and occupational therapy departments in the summer.

The addition of the Joyce Wing somewhat relieved the demand for beds with the waiting list dropping down to 960 in December 1993, from 1,370 in December 1962.

During the year, Dr. Ian MacLennan resigned as director of laboratories and was succeeded by Dr. Alfred Bastarache. Other departures from the staff included Dr. Fred Houston, Dr. Kenneth Jennings, Dr. Myer Herman and Dr. Colin Ibbotson. New members appointed to the staff included Dr. W.R. Gillis to the Department of General Practice, Dr. R.C. Valdez to the active staff in the Department of Surgery. Dr. Dollard Cormier returned from a leave of absence to join the active staff in the Department of Obstetrics and Gynaecology.

Dr. Romula C. Valdez was born on February 29, 1924, in Barso, Quezon City, Philippine Islands. He took his premed at Philippine Union College, Manila, and obtained his MD from Manila Central University in 1956. From 1955 to 1956 he served an internship at St. John's Hospital, Tulsa, Oklahoma. He then did a general surgery residency at Deaconess Hospital, Buffalo, from 1956 to 1957 and at Colorado State Hospital, Pueblo, California, from 1957 to 1959 and at St. Mary Corwan Hospital, Pueblo, California, from 1959 to 1960. Since his medical degree from the Philippines was not recognized by the Medical Council of Canada, he had to serve two years of an internship in Canada before he became eligible to write the LMCC exams. He was appointed as a resident in pathology at The Moncton Hospital in 1960, a resident in surgery in 1961 and as an OPD resident in 1962. His appointment to the surgical staff was with the provision that he have a member of the surgical department assist him until he passed his certification exams in surgery. He was unsuccessful in passing the exam on two tries and did not apply the third year. Under the by-laws, therefore, he lost his surgical provisions until such time as he obtained his certification. As a result of these events, he subsequently moved to one of the New England states. Because of the difficulties these rules and regulations posed in denying surgical privileges to a surgeon when he had worked in the community for over two years but had failed to pass his exams, the regulations were amended in April 1966 so that surgical privileges would only be granted to those who had already passed the examinations of the Royal College or their equivalent.

An addition to the anaesthetic staff was Dr. Carlos Arranz, who was born on October 7, 1926, in Madrid, Spain. He obtained a BSc at Institito San Isidro, Madrid, in 1946 and a Licentiate in Medicine and Surgery from the Medical School of the University of Madrid in 1952. He interned at the Madrid Provincial Hospital and did a residency at the Madrid Medical School from 1952 to 1955. He took a residency in anaesthesia at Madrid Medical School from 1957 to 1958 and then came to Canada, completing his anaesthesia training at the Ottawa General and the Ottawa Civic Hospitals from 1959 to 1960. He completed his training at the Royal Victoria and the Montreal Children's Hospital from 1961 to 1963. He was well liked and a popular anaesthetist but he resigned from the staff in July 1967 to join the staff of the new Riverside Hospital in Ottawa.

There were 11,448 patients, including 1,622 newborns, admitted to the main hospital in 1963 with 781 admitted to the Annex, for a total of 12,229 admissions. There were 4,548 operations performed in addition to 3,211 minor operations and 2,037 fracture cases seen in the outpatient department where 908 general anaesthetics were given. The outpatient and X-ray departments were experiencing increased usage with 15,429 visits to the outpatient department while the X-ray department performed 20,842 examinations. The X-ray department also performed 1,522 treatments on 190 patients.

Physiotherapy performed 18,803 treatments on 3,510 patients including 86 at the Annex. The new occupational therapy department performed 1,792 treatments on 267 patients. There were 3,813 electrocardiograms performed and 409 basal metabolism tests done. The Cancer Clinic continued to operate with 341 new patients registered.

It was during this time that the government commissioned a study on the future of hospitals in New Brunswick and in 1964, the Byrne Report was released. Unfortunately, it caused some uncertainty for the board of the hospital in trying to formulate future plans for the hospital. As noted in the statistics for 1963, the use of the X-ray and outpatient departments had increased two and a half times in the preceding five years so plans were drawn up for changes to the casualty reception area and the X-ray department.

An important innovation in 1964 was the opening of the Department of Inhalation Therapy. An inhalation therapy technician, Foster Greenlaw, returned from training and it was not long after the department was established that the need for a second technician was obvious. A Bennett respirator and a hypothermia unit were purchased for the Intensive Care Unit as well as a Bird respirator and two Electrodyne monitoring units for the operating theatres. The supervision for the use of this equipment as well as the inhalation service fell to the Department of Anaesthesia.

At this time, it came about that patients would no longer be subjected to being pricked with a used, dull, or barbed needle for injections and no longer would syringes and needles have to be honed and sterilized after each use. The era of disposable needles and syringes arrived in 1964, and their use continues to this day. Some of the paper work done by nurses was also lessened at this time with the introduction of a name plate identification system so that

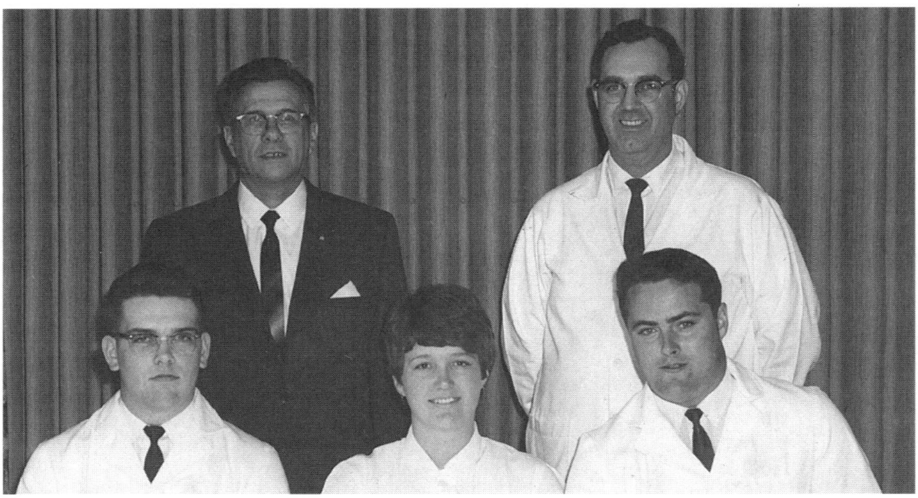

The new department of Inhalation Therapy in 1964. From left to right—top row: Dr. George Parsons, Foster Greenlaw; bottom row: Dennis Shaffer, Connie Colpitts, and Richard Silk.

requisitions for the lab and for X-ray could now be made out with much less writing. Another change ensured that a child could no longer use illness as an excuse for falling behind in his or her schoolwork because the pediatric department gained the full-time services of a school teacher in the person of Martine Nowlan, sponsored by the Department of Education.

There were four additions to the medical staff in 1974: Dr. J.T. Edgett joined the staff in the Department of Internal Medicine, Dr. E.S. Keller, in the Department of Pathology and Dr. W.R. Gillis and Dr. J.S. Noonan to the Department of General Practice. Dr. A.W. Ross retired from the active staff. Dr. F.W. Desmond was killed in an automobile accident.

Dr. Thomas Edgett was born in Moncton on January 15, 1928, the son of Guerney Edgett, a local druggist. He obtained his BSc from Mount Allison in 1949 and his MD, CM from Dalhousie in 1955 after interning at the Victoria General Hospital from 1954 to 1955. He practised as a general practitioner in Digby from 1955 to 1959. He then did a residency in internal medicine at the Victoria General Hospital from 1959 to 1962 with a further year at Sunnybrook Hospital in Toronto from 1962 to 1963, becoming certified in internal medicine by the Royal College in 1963. Tom continued to practise general internal medicine until his retirement in 1996. His kindly disposition and common-sense approach to problems has endeared him to both patients and his fellow colleagues. He has had an interest in arthritis and established the Arthritis Clinic in 1966 and continued as its director until recently. He served as president of the medical staff from 1983 to 1984.

Dr. Edward Sullivan Heller was born on March, 16, 1924, in Pittsburgh, Pennsylvania. He obtained a BA from Johns Hopkins University and an MD, CM from McGill in 1955. He interned at Queen Elizabeth Hospital in Montreal from 1955 to 1956 and then served in the US Army Medical Corps from 1957 to 1960. He had previously served in the US Army Air Force from 1942 to 1947. He did postgraduate training in pathology at Brook Army Hospital from 1958 to 1959 and continued at Medical College of Georgia, 1960-61, Queen's University, 1961-62, Ottawa University, 1962-63 and Norwalk Hospital, Norwalk, Virginia, 1963-64. He was considered a good pathologist, but apparently had difficulty with interpersonal relationships with the nursing staff and his colleagues and left the staff in early 1966.

Dr. W.R. Gillis was appointed to the staff in the Department of General Practice in December 1963, and began practice in Moncton in January 1964 and, with Dr. W.F. Dennis, played a role in starting the Moncton Medical Clinic. He was born in Halifax on April 13, 1936. He obtained a BSc from St. Dunstan's in 1961 and an MD degree from Dalhousie in 1961 after interning at the Victoria General, the Children's Hospital and the Saint John General Hospital. He practised in Summerside, Prince Edward Island, until he moved to Moncton in January 1964. "Bunny" Gillis was always in a rush and on arriving at any meeting he would burst into the room like Kramer on Seinfeld. He took an active part in the Family Practice Program at Dalhousie

University and, subsequently, left Moncton in 1970 to establish a Family Practice Program at the University of Mississippi.

Dr. James Stanislaus Noonan was born in Summerside, Prince Edward Island, on March 10, 1936, and received a BSc from St. Dunstan's University in 1957 and an MD from Dalhousie in 1962 after interning at the Victoria General Hospital from 1961 to 1962. He then established a general practice in Sackville, New Brunswick, in 1962 but moved to Moncton in 1964. While in general practice he served as medical doctor at Dorchester Penitentiary and relates how he would be greeted by duck-like sounds as he walked across the courtyard on his way to the doctor's office. This was at a time when corporal punishment was still meted out in our prisons and he relates how it was the doctor's duty to be present when the strapping was applied. Although an unpleasant task, Jim states that he never saw a prisoner come back a second time. Jim asked me to serve as orthopaedic consultant to Dorchester Penitentiary and this is a task that I have performed ever since, and have found, for the most part, that the men are appreciative of their medical treatment they received while serving their sentences. In 1967 Jim took a leave of absence from the staff and served as a resident in diagnostic radiology at the Royal Victoria Hospital from 1967 to 1971 and received his Fellowship in Radiology in 1971. He then returned to join the radiology staff where he has been a prominent fixture ever since. In the early morning and at noontime, he can be found holding court in the doctor's lounge. Jim sees all, knows all and tells all. One senior physician made the comment at one time that Jim would like to be the bride at every wedding and the corpse at every funeral. He certainly knows how to play to an audience and is often asked to be the master of ceremonies at medical staff functions. His most recent task was master of ceremonies at the ceremony marking the 100th anniversary of the hospital. He served as Chief of Radiology from 1979 to 1989 and as president of the medical staff in 1993 and 1994.

In 1964, 12,024 patients were admitted to hospital including 1,675 newborns; 4,431 operations were performed with 2,297 of them being classified as major operations. The X-ray department carried out 22,780 examinations and rendered 1,047 X-ray treatments on 159 patients. The physiotherapy department carried out 21,596 treatments on 4,099 patients and the occupational therapy department carried out 3,761 treatments on 544 patients; 4,075 electrocardiograms were done as well as 354 basal metabolism tests. There were 17,243 visits to the outpatient department including 3,281 minor operations and 1,777 fracture cases. 7,619 of the visits were classified as emergencies and 1,012 anaesthetics were given in the outpatient department. 313 new patients were registered in the Cancer Clinic.

When we look at the statistics for 1965, we find that The Moncton Hospital, now seventy years old, is not showing its age but rather is growing like a teenager. By this time, it is now the third largest employer in Moncton, employing on average at both the main hospital and the annex, 942 people. The medical staff now numbers 109, including 53 active staff, 2 honorary staff, 20 consulting staff, 15 courtesy staff and 19 members on the dental staff. With this growth, we also see an expansion of the administration staff and auxiliary services. The hospital executive staff numbers 19, including the Radiologist in Chief and the Pathologist in Chief with another five on the executive staff of the Annex. The graduate nurses now outnumber the student nurses, with the average for the year being 209 graduate to 164 student nurses. There were also 32 orderlies, 62 nursing assistants, 61 ward aids, 15 cooks and food supervisors, 73 clerical staff, 32 tradesmen, 132 maids and 42 utility men.

At this time, the Medical Service Departments numbered 16.

1. the Medical Library, rebuilt after the fire, contained over 800 volumes with subscriptions to 40 journals.
2. The Medical Record Department supervised by Janet Mooers with a staff of eight. Since 1964, the staff has participated in the Professional Activities Study initiated by the American College of Surgeons. Every chart on a discharged patient was reviewed and coded and the information then sent to Ann Arbor, Michigan, where the data was computerized with the printed sheets sent back to the hospital providing a summary that compared the level of treatment with accredited hospitals of similar size. Every phone in the hospital was also connected to the records room at this time, so that histories and discharge summaries could easily be dictated by the medical staff for transcription.
3. The Social Service Department had one employee, Margaret MacDonald, who was available to any member of the medical staff to review the home and financial situation of any patient and to arrange for the patient's future care after discharge.
4. The Physiotherapy Department remained a one-woman department in the capable hands of Jean Owens with a treatment load of 3,900 patients. This was, of course, an impossible task for one woman but she had trained a very capable group of nursing assistants and aides to assist her in her work.
5. The Occupational Therapy Department was run by Dorothy Stewart but under the supervision of Mrs. Owens.
6. The Pharmacy Department now had a staff of three pharmacists, Harry Wade, Don Hartley and Gilbert Surette, as well as Tim Murphy, a certified drug clerk. There was also a clerk typist, Myrna Langille. In 1965, the Pharmacy and Therapeutics Committee of the medical staff, with the help of Mr. Wade, produced a Hospital Formulary.
7. The Central Sterile Supply Room, run by Miriam Bulmer and Mildred Caldwell RN, was staffed by 15 people responsible for repackaging and sterilizing the multitude of sterile trays and instruments used on the floors as well as the issue of many of the dispos-

able items and the intravenous fluids. A gas autoclave was added to the bank of steam sterilizers, allowing for the sterilization of delicate instruments which would be damaged by the use of steam.

8. The Radiology Department, with three radiologists, now had four diagnostic rooms of which two were equipped with the latest in image amplifiers, TV viewing screens and cine camera. There was also a cystoscopic unit across from the X-ray department, and adjacent to this was the fracture room also equipped with an X-ray unit. All development of films was now done by mechanized developing units. Two modern radiotherapy units one for superficial and one for deep therapy, were also in use. The department continued to run a School for Radiological Technicians with the chief technician being Ruth Duffy. During the year Miss Duffy was awarded a Fellowship in Radiologic Technology, the only one to have been awarded in Canada. Her talents were well recognized by the hospital administration and she has gone on to be one of the vice-presidents of the corporation.
9. The Emergency and Outpatient departments, in the charge of Leonara Flemington RN, was now servicing 50,000 patients a year with a staff of 20, including nurses, orderlies and office personnel and providing 24-hour coverage. Two members of the medical staff were assigned in rotation to provide 24-hour coverage with the speciality services also providing an on call schedule.
10. The Admitting Office, staffed by Jessie Barnett RN and Hazel Fraser RN and a staff of six, provided a 24-hour admitting service.
11. The Electrocardiographic Service was headed by Frances Cudahy and her three technicians, Gwen Ronalds, Peggy McKinley and Barbara Gay and in 1965 they did 4,818 tracings. During the night the task was performed by an intern or the attending physician.
12. The Cancer Diagnostic Clinic, under the guidance of Mrs. G. Leaman, was responsible for the registration under the Provincial Cancer Program of all persons referred for the investigation of possible cancer and for the follow-up of all persons who had undergone treatment.
13. The new Electroencephalographic Department established in 1965 was under the charge of Camille Richard who continued in this post until his recent retirement. These brain tracings served to aid in the diagnosis of epilepsy and other brain diseases and tumors. At this time there was no neurologist to read the tracings and they were sent elsewhere for the official report.
14. The new Inhalation Therapy Department, established in 1964, was presided over by Foster Greenlaw and was already proving its worth, with over 4,678 treatments within a six-month period in 1965, so that it was necessary to provide two student technicians to assist Mr. Greenlaw.

15. The operating suite was under the supervision of Aline Forsythe RN who ran a tight ship with four operating rooms open and a fifth one available. Surgeons had no assigned time in the operating room and all cases had to be booked through Mrs. Forsythe. At this time the operating rooms ran from 8 am to 1 pm with doctors then proceeding to their offices for afternoon office hours. Emergency surgery could, of course, be done at any hour of the day or night.
16. In the old hospital on King Street, patients had been returned to the wards for recovery from surgery but now in the new hospital there was a recovery room with a staff of nurses under the charge nurse, Irene Leger, so that patients could recover from anaesthesia before returning to the ward.

There were, of course, many other departments that are necessary to support the provision of medical services and to keep the "ship" running in good order. These departments were under the supervision of W.A. Kilpatrick, assistant administrator, non-medical, and were six in number at this time:

1. The Dietary Department, that in 1965 served 335,935 meals to the patients, of which 40 percent were special diets ordered for therapeutic reasons by the doctor. The director of Dietetics, Heather MacLean, had a staff of 80 in addition to the dieticians. In 1963, the department began assembling the trays on a centralized "trayveyor" system. With this system an empty tray was placed in a moving conveyor belt with the menu chosen by the patient or prescribed by the doctor and as the belt passed various stations cutlery, dishes and food were added. With this method all the patients could be served in 30 to 45 minutes.
2. The housekeeping staff with 70 employees under Mrs. C. Bannister, maintained an environment which was not only cosmetically clean but also bacteriologically clean.
3. The Laundry Department under the supervision of Joseph Lombard with 30 employees processed about 7,000 pounds of laundry each day and operated 7 days a week.
4. The Maintenance and Repair Department was headed by Austin C. Geldart and employed 20 persons to look after the maintenance of the building and equipment using a preventative maintenance system. In addition to employing plumbers, electricians, refrigeration specialists, groundskeepers, boiler engineers and carpenters, it was necessary to employ an electronics technician to look after all the additional complex equipment.
5. The Purchasing and Stores Department under M.O. Stiles, kept an inventory of 2,000 different articles and was responsible for keeping these items continuously in stock.

6. The hospital maintained an ambulance service with four ambulance drivers, each of which was required to have completed the St. John Ambulance Brigade First Aid Training Course. On each trip, the ambulance driver was accompanied by a hospital orderly to act as helper. The hospital maintained two ambulances, each of which was equipped with stretchers, oxygen, a resuscitator, a complete first aid kit and a radio telephone.

The Nursing Staff Office now consisted of eight individuals:

1. Katherine Wright, Director of Nursing,
2. Marion Wilbur, Assistant Director of Nursing,
3. Betty Ann Ward, Nursing Office Assistant,
4. Evelyn Atkinson, Intravenous Nurse,
5. Irene MacKenzie, In-Service Program Director,
6. Hilda Stultz, Night Supervisor,
7. Kay MacLeod, Night Supervisor and
8. Hilda Welling, Health Service Nurse.

By this time, the student nurses were no longer the main care providers. The nursing staff was planned so that a ratio of 65 percent professional to 35 percent non-professional staff would give direct patient care and each nursing unit was staffed by registered nurses for each of the three periods of work.

The Faculty of the School of Nursing now totalled 16:

1. Katherine Wright, RN—Director of Nursing, Certificate of Teaching and Supervision, McGill
2. Elsie Steeves, RN—Certificate of Teaching and Supervision, McGill
3. Barbara Taylor, BscN, RN—University of Saskatchewan
4. Elizabeth MacDonald, RN—Certificate of Public Health, McGill Certificate Teaching and Supervision, Dalhousie
5. Edith Warman, RN—Certificate of Public Health, Dalhousie
6. Beryl Balser, BscN, RN—University of Western Ontario
7. Irene MacKenzie, RN—Certificate of Nursing Education, University of Western Ontario
8. Marion Wilbur, RN—Assistant Director of Nursing
9. Hilda Welling, RN—Health Nurse
10. Isabel Wallace—Librarian
11. Harriett Hayes, BN, RN—McGill University
12. Shirley MacLeod, BN,RN—McGill University
13. Judith Spence, RN—Diploma Teaching and Supervision, Dalhousie
14. Florence Akerly, Pdt, BSc—Mount Allison, Victoria General Hospital
15. Paula Hunter, RN—Certificate in Nursing Education, University of Ottawa

16. Patricia Dixon, RN—Diploma in Teaching and Education, University of Ottawa

Although a part of The Moncton Hospital, the Annex maintained its own business office and dietary, physiotherapy and housekeeping departments, with other services being supplied by the main hospital.

Although space was limited, the X-ray department was able to add a second image intensifier and a new X-ray machine in 1965. Fortunately, plans were also proceeding for new additions to the X-ray department and the outpatient department and the opening of a radioactive isotope laboratory. Other equipment purchased during the year were additional cardiac monitoring and pacemaking devices for the anaesthesia department.

Changes to the medical staff saw the retirement of Dr. Paul Melanson, the departure for greener fields of Dr. W.F. Normandeau and the return of Dr. D. I. MacLellan to the staff of the Department of Orthopaedics, which had been reduced to a one-man department under Dr. O.J. White, as a result of the illness of Dr. E.W. Ewart. New additions to the staff included Dr. R.G. Crandall to the Department of Psychiatry, Dr. Roland Maurice to the Department of Otolaryngology and Dr. O. J. Hunter to the Department of Radiology.

Gordon Crandall was born in Moncton on February 14, 1928, and received a BA from Acadia University in 1950 and an MD, CM from Dalhousie in 1956 after interning at the Victoria General Hospital from 1955 to 1956. He took postgraduate work with a psychiatry residency at the Lafayette Clinic in Detroit, Michigan, from 1960 to 1964 and received an MSc with a major in psychiatry from Wayne State University in Detroit in 1965. He was certified in psychiatry by the Royal College of Physicians and Surgeons of Canada in 1964. He developed a busy psychiatric practice in Moncton but resigned after five years to go to Charlotte, North Carolina, in 1970. He has always kept close ties to his home city, returning each year to his cottage at Point du Chene. He is remembered as much for his piano playing as for his psychiatric expertise. During his high school and university days he played in local orchestras and was especially noted for his jazz and boogie renditions.

James Oliver Hunter was born on July 16, 1926, in Londonderry, North Ireland, and was educated in the Republic of Ireland, receiving his BA and then his MB, BCh, BOA from Trinity College, Dublin, in 1950. He interned at Walton Hospital, Liverpool, England, and Redworth Hospital, Redworth, England, from 1950 to 1952. He then worked at Redworth from 1952 to 1953 and subsequently emigrated to Canada and worked at the Yarmouth Hospital from 1956 to 1961. He took a residency in radiology at the Victoria General Hospital from 1961 to 1964, completed his last year of residency at The Moncton Hospital from 1964 to 1965 and became certified in diagnostic radiology in 1965. He joined the radiology staff of The Moncton Hospital but resigned in July 1967, to return to Yarmouth where he practised until he died suddenly of a massive coronary on October 14, 1973, at the age of 47.

Roland Maurice was born in Central Falls, Rhode Island, and received his BA from the University of Montreal in 1949, followed by his BSc in 1950 and an MD in 1955. From 1954 to 1955 he interned at l'Hôtel Dieu, Notre Dame, St. Justine and Misericorde Hospitals in Montreal. He then engaged in a general practice in Shediac from 1955 to 1961. He pursued a residency in ENT at the Hospital of the University of Pennsylvania and the Albert Einstein Medical Centre in Philadelphia from 1961 to 1965, becoming certified in otorhinolaryngology in 1965. He carried on an active practice at both the Moncton and Dr. Georges-L. Dumont hospitals and was responsible for introducing stapedectomy and typanomastoid surgery to the area. He has pursued his hobby of woodcarving since his retirement.

During 1965 there were 10,213 adults and children admitted to hospital in addition to 1,531 newborns; 4,582 operations were performed. The radiology department carried out 29,650 examinations and was still quite active in radiotherapy with 1,147 deep therapy treatments and 251 superficial therapy treatments given. There were 65,908 outpatient visits, of which 20,892 were to the emergency department; 1,262 anaesthetics were given in the emergency department, 1,503 fracture cases were treated and 3,763 minor operations were performed; 4,809 electrocardiograms and 328 basal metabolism tests were done. 1,096 inpatient and 1,170 outpatient electric shock treatments were given. The inhalation therapy department gave 4,858 treatments and the electro-encephalography department saw 166 patients for readings. The relatively new Arthritic Clinic had 119 visits. The Cancer Clinic saw 358 new patients registered.

The last five years had seen many demands on the hospital facilities and there seemed to be no letup, despite the opening of the Joyce Wing in 1963. The X-ray department examined 28,739 inpatients and outpatients in 1966 compared with 26,739 in 1965. The electrocardiographic service did 6,085 tracings in 1966 compared with 4,809 in 1965. The inhalation therapy department had a phenomenal growth, with 10,665 treatments compared to 4,858 in 1965. By this time, there were three student technicians in the department and they were expected to graduate in 1967, providing more personnel for the department. The outpatient department was also outstripping its facilities with 23,193 visits in 1966 compared to 20,594 in 1965.

To help alleviate this problem, tenders were called in December 1965 for additions and alterations to the radiology department with the building of a radioisotope laboratory and a casualty receiving area. In January 1966 the contract was awarded to Century Construction Company with a bid of $479,150. Mechanical work would be done by Moncton Plumbing and Supply and electrical work by Acadia Electric in the amount of $83,620. The total cost of the project would be $681,195. Construction began in February 1966 and by December, the project was 65 percent completed. At the same time, the provincial government undertook to enlarge the facilities of the regional laboratory so that its space would be doubled. In addition to auxiliary services, the need for more beds was apparent and in April 1966, the board met with provincial government authorities to request a 300-bed addition. In July 1966 the government gave approval for 100 beds with provision for another 100 beds in the future. A functional study of the hospital's needs was carried out in July by the hospital staff and the architects, Gaudet and Roy, and in September 1966, the board urged the Government to reconsider its previous response and requested an immediate start on planning for a 200-bed addition. This met with success and in December approval was granted by government authorities to proceed with planning for a 200-bed addition.

In the fall of 1965, a committee was appointed by the board to bring in a completely revised and updated set of by-laws. These by-laws provided for a number of new committees to spread the work more evenly among the board members. The committees now numbered seven:

1. Executive Committee;
2. Building and Grounds Committee;
3. Equipment Committee;
4. Finance Committee;
5. Public Relations and Personnel Committee;
6. School of Nursing Committee; and
7. School of Nursing Advisory Committee.

Members of the Administration distinguished themselves in 1966 with Mrs. Wright being appointed president of the New Brunswick Association of Registered Nurses and W.A. Kilpatrick being appointed vice-president for New Brunswick in the Atlantic Province Hospital Association and president-elect of the New Brunswick Hospital Association.

The citizens of Moncton and vicinity have always been willing to make donations to the hospital to care for their less fortunate fellow citizens but there was no established fund to which they could contribute. Moreover, the need did not now seem as essential since government had taken over the funding of hospitals. Nonetheless, there were, and continue to be many needs which government has been unable or unwilling to fund and only through donations is it possible for the hospital to provide care beyond the lowest common denominator. For several years, the board of trustees of The Moncton Hospital considered the feasibility of having an outside agent to receive and control trust funds. The board believed that the establishment of a foundation for this purpose would encourage people to make donations and leave bequests. In 1964, the board, therefore directed its legal advisors to prepare an application for letters patent. Consequently, Friends of the Moncton Hospital Foundation Incorporated was created by letters patent approved by the Provincial Secretary on February 15, 1965, with G.W. Stewart, S.G. Stratton and Kathleen Wheaton as provisional officers. G.W. Stewart was the brother of Dr. John Stewart, a former member of the medical staff and Stewart Stratton was later to become Chief Justice of New Brunswick. On September 30, 1966, members and officers of the board of trustees of The

Moncton Hospital were named the pro tem officers and board of directors of the foundation. The provisional officers resigned and the by-laws of the foundation were adopted at this meeting. The pro tem board of Directors subsequently appointed a nominating committee and on December 1, 1966, the report of the nominating committee was accepted and the following persons were appointed as the first officers and board of Directors:

H.P Tait, President
Eric Cormier, Vice-President
Dorothy Flemming, Secretary
R.R. Rice, Treasurer
R.W. Belyea
Ray MacLellan
Mrs. Walter Buxton
Mrs. Ranolph Parker
F.P. Driscoll
Frank Lutes
Leonard Lockhart Sr.
Dr. R. B. Eaton
Ralph Lockhart
Fred Forbes
Dr. William Webster
Mildred Hanley
Aurele Arsenault
G.R. Spencer
Reuben Cohen
Mark Yeoman
Mrs. W.V. Creaghan
Mrs. F.J. Godfrey

Under its by-laws the foundation may not have capital stock, but it may acquire real and personal property of a value not exceeding $500,000. The board of directors hold the assets of the foundation in trust and may utilize capital and income either by grant or loan for the following purposes:

1. Construction projects for the erection, extension, or alteration of buildings of The Moncton Hospital
2. Provision of care for patients in the hospital
3. Education and training of professional, non-professional, and teaching personnel
4. Purchase of equipment
5. Research

During its first year of operation the foundation had total receipts of $14,535, a far cry from the $3,600,000 it would raise in the centennial campaign of 1995.

This was again an inspection year for the hospital and it again received full accreditation from the Canadian Council on Hospital Accreditation.

Dr. R.B. Eaton and Dr. S.A. Hopper retired from the active staff to join the consulting staff. New additions to the staff included Dr. G.D. Surette, Dr. A.G. Haché and Dr. Ben Bacongallo to the Department of General Practice; Dr. Y. Lee to the Department of Radiology; Dr. D.A. MacLeod to the Department of Urology and Dr. C.Y. Hong to the Department of Pathology. Dr. D.S. Inglis and Dr. A.M. MacKay were admitted to the courtesy staff. Because of the beginning of cobalt therapy and the imminent centralization of radiotherapy in Saint John, Dr. J.A. Caskey, Dr. G.D. Smith and Dr. H.G.

Whiston of Saint John were appointed to the consulting staff in radiotherapy.

George Surette was born in Moncton on May 11, 1938, and after taking premed at St. Francis Xavier, he received his MD Degree from the University of Ottawa in 1965. He then interned at the Montreal General and Montreal Children's Hospital and began a general practice in Moncton in partnership with Dr. Alban Haché. He returned to Montreal in 1971 to take a residency in radiology at the Royal Victoria, Montreal Neurological Institute, Montreal Children's and Jewish General Hospitals. He obtained his Fellowship in Diagnostic Radiology in 1974 and joined the radiology staff of the Dr. Georges-L. Dumont Hospital and the consulting staff of The Moncton Hospital.

Alban Haché was born in Bathurst on March 31, 1938, obtained a BA from Sacred Heart University, Bathurst, in 1960, went on to obtain his MD from the University of Ottawa in 1965 and interned at the Ottawa General Hospital from 1965 to 1966. After four years of general practice he went to the Royal Victoria Hospital for a one-year residency in general surgery and then three years in orthopaedics, obtaining his FRCS(C) in 1974. He subsequently returned to Moncton and has played a prominent role in the orthopaedic department of the Dr. Georges-L. Dumont Hospital. In 1974 he was appointed to the associate staff of The Moncton Hospital.

Ben Bacongallo was born on January 15, 1931, at Patnongara, Antique, Philippines, and he can tell many stories of growing up in the Philippines under Japanese occupation. He attended Manila Central University and was awarded an Associate in Arts Degree in 1952. He then graduated with his MD from the Far Eastern University in Manila in 1957 and interned at the Far Eastern University Hospital. After two years of general practice in the Philippines, he emigrated to Canada. Following a year of internship at St. Joseph's Hospital in London, Ontario, he did a residency in internal medicine at St. Joseph's Hospital, London, as well as at the Victoria Hospital in London from 1961 to 1964. His postgraduate education was cut short by the death of his wife which left him with the challenge of being a single parent to his two young daughters, a task that he performed admirably. He came to Moncton in 1954, but had to undertake additional training before receiving his LMCC. He interned at The Moncton Hospital from 1964 to 1965 and served as a resident in the OPD of l'Hôtel Dieu from 1965 to 1966. He obtained his LMCC in 1966 and then joined the staff of the Department of General Practice and has continued in this post for the past 29 years. He quickly became recognized as a very competent assistant in the OR where his services have always been in great demand by the surgeons. He has always had the ability to anticipate the surgeons' moves and needs so that any surgery in which he assists usually goes very smoothly. Ben is not only smooth in the OR, that adjective can also be used to describe his attire. He can combine colours of clothing superbly. On some days he looks like a strawberry sundae, on others, like a banana frappé and sometimes like a bowl of licorice all-sorts—but always smart.

Young I. Lee was born in Gilgoo, Korea, on May 4, 1927. He took his premed at Seoul University, South Korea, and obtained his MD from the Medical College of Seoul University in 1953. He came to North America in 1958 doing an internship at the Seattle General hospital from 1958 to 1959. He then embarked on a residency in radiology at several hospitals including the following: Creighton Memorial, St. Joseph's Hospital, Omaha, Nebraska, 1959-60; Shaughnessy Hospital, Vancouver, 1960-61; University of Alberta Hospital, Edmonton, 1961-62; St. Joseph's Hospital, Toronto, 1962-63 and The Moncton Hospital 1963-64. He obtained his LMCC in 1966 and was appointed to the active staff in the Department of Radiology but his stay was short.

Chul Yoo Hong was born on July 11, 1928, in Kyung Gi Do, Korea, and attended Severance Premedical and Severance Medical College in Seoul, Korea, receiving his MD in 1953. After coming to North America, he interned at Mercer Hospital, Trenton, New Jersey, in 1957. He then did a residency in obstetrics and gynaecology at Wychoff Heights Hospital, Brooklyn, NY, from 1958 to 1959 and at Jannish Hospital, New York, from 1959 to 1962. Following this, he changed direction and pursued a pathology residency at the Jewish General Hospital from 1962 to 1963, the Reddy Memorial Hospital, Montreal, 1963-64, Queen Mary Veterans' Hospital, 1964-65 and finally the Pathological Institute of McGill University from 1965 to 1966. He passed the LMCC exams in 1965 and his American Boards in Anatomic Pathology in 1966. He was appointed to the staff in May 1966, but resigned on December 31, 1967.

The appointment of Dr. David A. MacLeod to the Department of Urology raised the number in that department to two. David was born in Rather, Aberdeenshire, Scotland, on October 14, 1932, and retained his Scottish brogue on coming to Canada and Moncton. He took his premed and his medical degree at Aberdeen University, graduating with an MB,ChB in 1956. He then interned at the Royal Northern Infirmary, Inverness, from 1956 to 1957 and after coming to Canada, did a year of internship at University Hospital, Edmonton, from 1958 to 1959. He did a residency in anatomical pathology at Westminster Hospital, London, Ontario, from 1959 to 1961. This was followed by a year of general surgery at the Hamilton General Hospital and from 1962 to 1966 he was a resident in urology at the Royal Victoria Hospital in Montreal. During this time he served a year as a fellow in experimental surgery at McGill University from 1962 to 1963. He received his FRCS(C) in 1965. After marrying a nurse from New Brunswick, he was persuaded to come to Moncton. He liked to relate the story of how on coming to Moncton he surveyed the doctors as to the need for another urologist. He approached Dr. Eaton who told him that he still did the odd prostatectomy. After being in practice for a while he found out that the odd prostatectomy ended up being numbers 1, 3, 5, 7, 9, etc. Dr. MacLeod was instrumental in introducing the Transurethral Resection of the Prostrate (TURP) operation to Moncton. He was well-liked by his colleagues in

Moncton, although to some extent, he was an irascible gentleman and on some days, particularly so. Someone said of him that he was one of those Scots who wore the sporran under his kilt which kept him in a constant state of irritation. He left in 1969 to set up practice in Windsor, Ontario.

Several members of the medical staff spent considerable time and effort during the year on behalf of the Moncton and District Medical Society in its presentation of a brief to the Provincial Medical School Survey Commission, a study committee appointed by the New Brunswick Government to assess the need for a medical school in the Province of New Brunswick. The brief favoured a medical school at the Université de Moncton and offered the facilities of The Moncton Hospital in the event a medical school should be established there. The final report of the Commission, however, concluded that a medical school was not needed in New Brunswick and that Dalhousie University Medical School could continue to supply the manpower needs of New Brunswick.

The Moncton Hospital School of Nursing celebrated its Diamond Jubilee during the year. The number of alumnae now passed the 1,000 mark with the graduation in 1966 of the largest class ever—55 nurses.

There were 11,854 admissions to hospital in 1966 including 1,409 newborn. 4,709 operations were performed in the operating rooms, which were now equipped with electronic monitoring equipment and the use of explosive anaesthetic agents was eliminated. Another 4,230 minor operations were performed and 1,221 anaesthetics given in the outpatient department. Altogether there were 72,980 visits to the outpatient department, with 23,546 classified as emergency visits. There were several Public Health Clinics now operating and 262 patients were seen at the Paediatric Clinic. Ten Orthopaedic Clinics were held with 807 children seen, 47 patients were seen in a Psychiatric Screening Clinic and 186 patients were seen at the Poison Control Centre, 381 new patients were registered in the Cancer Clinic. Including the Annex, 21,080 visits were made to the physiotherapy department and another 6,496 to the occupational therapy department. The radiology department had 31,634 examinations carried out including 1,192 deep and 215 superficial X-ray treatments. There were 6,085 electrocardiograms performed as well as 393 basal metabolism tests. There were also 544 electroencephalograms done and 10,665 inhalation therapy treatments were given and the psychiatric department administered 1,173 electric shock treatments.

The year 1967 was centennial year for Canada, making it only 28 years older than The Moncton Hospital. It was, unfortunately, one of the standstill years for the hospital. Construction of the addition to the X-ray department progressed during the year but was not completed until December and it would be March 1968 before alterations to incorporate the old existing portion of the X-ray department into the new were complete. The standing joke among the medical staff at the time was that we had an X-ray department with a hospital attached to it. We were quite proud of our new facilities, however, which were among the most spacious and modern in Canada. Not only did we have enlarged facilities but also the most modern of X-ray equipment. Diagnostic units had provision for image intensification, cinematography and magnetized tape reproduction. Closed circuit television was also available. A new special procedures room had two new diagnostic units, one for angiography and cardiographic investigative diagnosis and the other for skull and neurological diagnostic procedures. The radioisotope laboratory was completed in December 1967, but alas, there was no trained technician available to staff it. The casualty receiving area and storage and workshop areas were also completed in December 1967. The expansion and renovation to the provincial laboratory concurrently progressed throughout the year and was also nearing completion by year's end.

Although these additional facilities were appreciated, a demand for beds that could not be met continued, and the waiting list climbed to above 1,500. The ultimate capacity of the hospital was approved by government at 850 beds. Although approval had been granted by government authorities in December 1966, to proceed with planning for a 200-bed addition, tenders were not called until November 1967. The contract was awarded to Abbey Landry Limited in the amount of $2,601,316 for completion of 102 beds immediately with 102 beds to be completed in the future. With the awarding of the contract the hospital staff and architects began a functional study on the needs and planning for additions and alterations to the service and paramedical departments to support the additional patient accommodation. To effectively concentrate on the building project, the executive director delegated the supervision of the routine administration to W.A. Kilpatrick, Assistant Administrator. In anticipation of the future staffing needs of the hospital, the School of Nursing, meanwhile, began developing a recruitment program to enrol larger classes. Plans were also being drawn up to erect a joint laundry to service all hospital beds in the Moncton area. In all its previous expansions, the hospital needed to obtain permission from the province to float a bond issue guaranteed by the City of Moncton and the County Councils in order to carry out the construction project. Under the Equal Opportunity legislation of the Louis Robichaud government, however, this was no longer the case, and the new patient tower would be built by the government and would be assets of the Crown in right of the Province.

For their centennial year project, the student nurses raised $200 to buy a mist tent for the treatment of Cystic Fibrosis. It was during Canada's centennial year that nurses from all provinces in Canada staffed the Nurses' Station at the Expo theme Pavilion "Man and His Health." The Moncton Hospital was pleased to be able to supply two of the nurses for this purpose. The School of Nursing Alumnae assisted a senior student nurse, Marie Landry, to attend, and the Nurses' Hospital Auxiliary sponsored a graduate nurse, Judith Spence.

Myrna Sherrard BN, RN, and Helene Dingwell RN, RN, returned to the nursing staff after obtaining their bachelor degrees in Nursing and were employed as Nurse Clinicians, a new designation in the nursing staff hierarchy.

There were a few changes in the administration during the year. R.R. Rice, the comptroller of the hospital since 1954 became seriously ill in January 1967 and died on October 21, 1967. He was replaced by James K. McCafferty, who occupied this post for a good number of years. On January 30, 1967, Pauline Boucher was appointed chief medical record librarian and has continued to hold this post up until the present time. Many members of the administration continued to show leadership in associations related to hospital services. Mr. Kilpatrick, assistant administrator, was elected president of the New Brunswick Hospital Association and New Brunswick vice-president of the Atlantic Provinces Hospital Association. Katherine Wright, assistant administrator-nursing, was re-elected president of the New Brunswick Association of Registered Nurses. Dr. W.B. Stewart was elected president of the Medical Council of New Brunswick. Ruth Duffy, Chief Radiological Technician, delivered the Welsh Memorial Lecture at the annual meeting of the Canadian Society of Radiological Technologists.

The proper utilization of the Intensive Care Unit was the subject of much discussion among the medical staff during the year and in co-operation with the nursing service, progress was made in the planning of a separate Coronary Intensive Care Unit. Dr. C. Arranz, Dr. R.C. Valdez, Dr. J.O. Hunter and Dr. C.Y. Hong all departed for greener pastures during the year. Dr. R.C.E. Bourgeois, a long-time member of the EENT staff, died. Dr. K.W. MacKenzie, having reached his 60th birthday retired from the active staff and joined the consulting staff. There were two new additions to the medical staff during the year: Dr. P. Martenyi and Dr. G. P. Reyes. Each of these men was a graduate of the intern and residency programs carried on at The Moncton Hospital.

Dr. P. Martenyi was born in Budapest. Hungary, on February 25, 1938. He obtained a BSC. at Vovosmarthy Gym., Budapest, and his MD at the University of Louvain, Belgium, in 1964. He interned at St. Pierre Hospital, Louvain, from 1963 to 1964 and at St. Vincent de Paul, Sherbrooke, Quebec, from 1964 to 1965. He then did a residency in pathology at The Moncton Hospital from 1965 to 1966 and a residency in medicine at The Moncton Hospital from 1966 to 1967 and obtained his LMCC in November 1966. He joined the active staff in general practice in January 1967 but transferred to the courtesy staff in 1971. He remained on the active staff at the Dr. Georges-L. Dumont Hospital where he carried out the majority of his practice.

Dr. Gerry Reyes was born on January 8, 1927, in the Philippines and received an Associate in Arts Degree in 1949 at the University of Santo Tomas in Manila and an MD from Manila Central University in 1955. In 1959 he emigrated to North America and did an internship at St. Francis Hospital, Wichita, Kansas, from 1959 to 1960 and a residency in general practice at the same institution from 1960 to 1962. He then did a residency in internal medicine at Sedgewick County Hospital, Wichita, Kansas, from 1962 to 1964. Following this, he came to Canada and after doing further rotating internships at Regina Grey Nuns' Hospital from 1964 to 1965 and

The Moncton Hospital from 1965 to 1966, he was able to obtain his LMCC and remained in Moncton, joining the active staff in general practice, and continued to enjoy a busy practice until his retirement in 1996.

The early part of the year 1968 looked promising for the hospital when on January 23 the sod was turned for the new 200-bed tower by Hon. R. Doucett, minister of public works and the Hon. Norbert Theriault, minister of health and welfare. The project was not without its difficulties, however. There was some delay in getting supplies to the site, and in July there was a strike by tradesmen in the Moncton area which delayed work on the tower and set the project back about five months. A contract was awarded during the year to Abby Landry Ltd. for the replacement of a 10,000 pounds of steam per hour boiler by a 30,000 pounds per hour boiler. At the end of the year this contract was about 55 percent completed. A functional program for the development of all hospital departments and services was completed during the year and presented to the government with no immediate decisions forthcoming. The new X-ray department was officially opened in the spring with Dr. Howard Ripley doing the honours in a ribbon cutting ceremony. Quite appropriately the new wing was named "The Ripley X-ray Wing" in honour of Howard Ripley who had been the Chief of Radiology for the previous 24 years. Dr. Ripley resigned as Chief Radiologist and Director of the Department of Radiology on March 31, 1968, but remained on staff on a part-time basis as therapeutic radiologist. Dr. W.B. Stewart assumed the

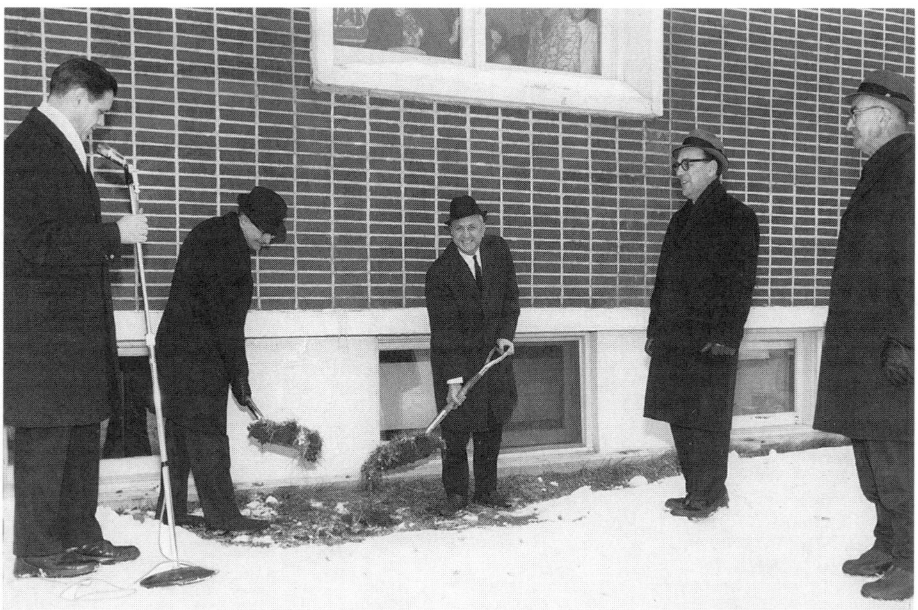

Sod-turning for the new Clarke Wing in 1968. From left to right: Mr. Ralph Belyea, Chairman of the Board; Hon. Georges-L. Dumont; Hon. Norbert Theriault, Minister of Health; Mr. J. Roy Gaudet, architect; and Dr. C.W. Kelly, Deputy Minister of Health.

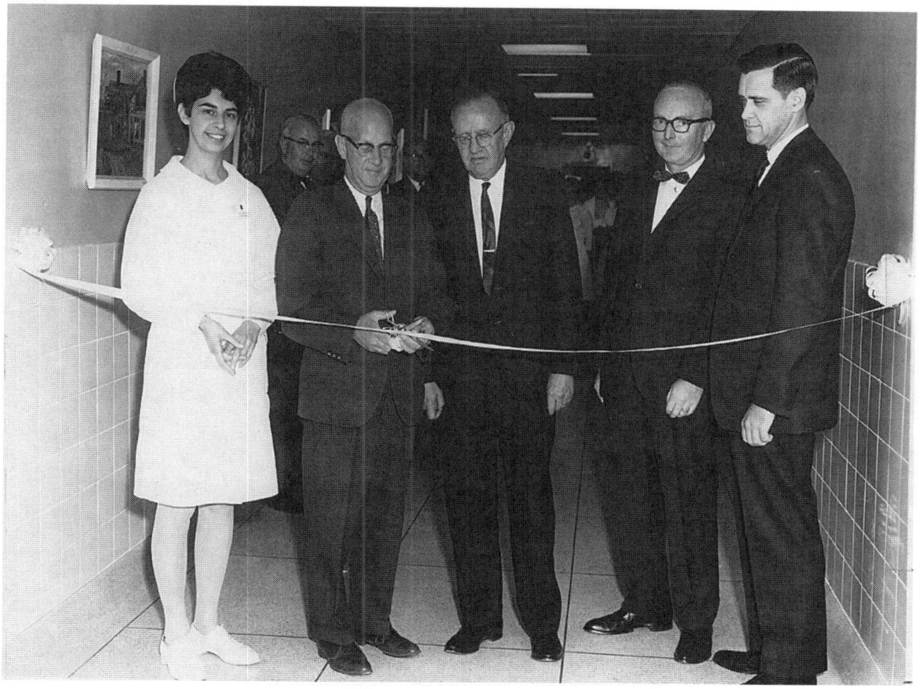

The opening of the new X-ray department in 1968. From left to right: Ruth Duffy, Dr. Howard Ripley, Dr. Austin Clarke, Dr. Brenton Stewart, and Mr. Ralph Belyea.

position of Chief Radiologist and Head of the Department. Another photo opportunity occurred in the fall of 1968 when the hospital was visited by His Excellency Governor General Roland Michener and Mrs. Michener.

The hospital was successful this year in obtaining the services of a radioisotope technician and this new service was inaugurated with Dr. W.A. Turner serving as Clinical Director. The supervision of the organization and operation of the laboratory was performed by Dr. J.A. Caskey, Chief of the Radiotherapy Department of the Saint John General Hospital.

The plans announced in 1967 to create a Cardiac Intensive Care Unit separate from the Surgical Intensive Care Unit bore fruit and they now became two separate units in February 1968. Dr. W.A. Turner, returning from postgraduate work, took an active part in planning for the cardiac unit and assumed the directorship of the unit. With a growing waiting list, the need for more O.R. time was recognized and the operating schedule was changed to allow more afternoon surgery. At the same time, all but emergency surgery was eliminated on Saturday mornings. A Zoning Committee was formed in January to study the feasibility of zoning the hospital to better utilize the beds available. Following the production of recommendations in September, a zoning program was undertaken with a specific allotment of beds to medicine, surgery, EENT, urology and orthopaedic surgery.

For some years the hospital had been approved for a rotating internship

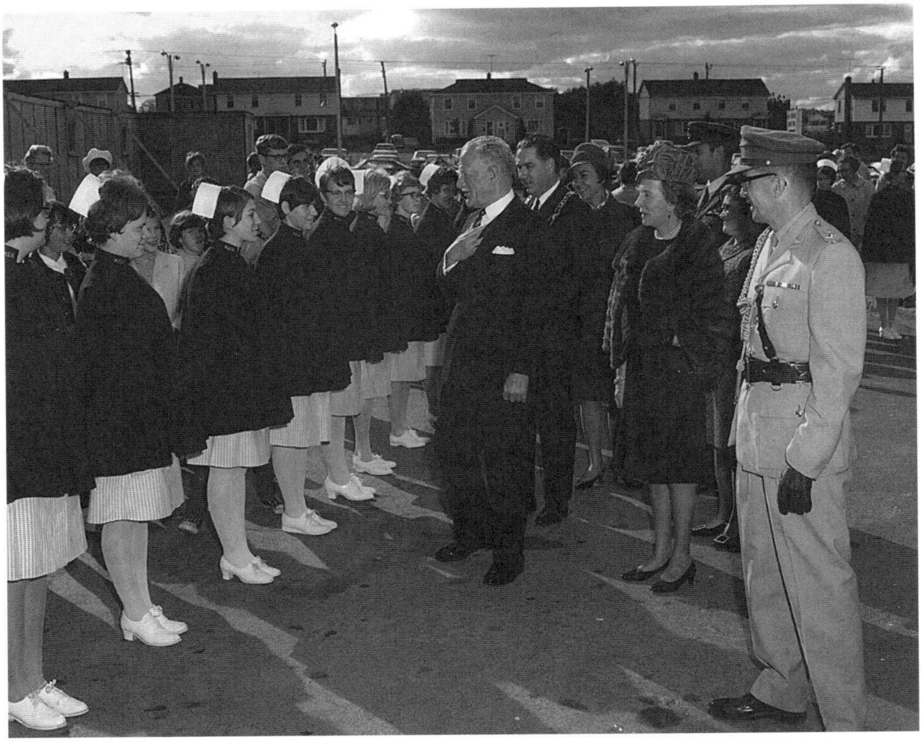

Governer General and Mrs. Roland Michener visited The Moncton General Hospital in the fall of 1968.

by the Canadian Medical Association and for residents in radiology, anaesthesia and pathology by the Royal College of Physicians and Surgeons of Canada. The program was run mostly with foreign medical graduates. In 1967 the hospital was notified that it would be required to develop a university affiliation if it were to continue the residency program and negotiations were carried out with Dalhousie University, but with disappointing results.

On the occasion of the hospital's completion of seventy years of service to the community, the *Moncton Times* and the *Moncton Transcript* issued a special "70th Anniversary Moncton Hospital" edition.

Dr. H.E. Britton, a long-time member of the surgical staff of The Moncton Hospital, died in 1968. Two doctors at the hospital received special recognition during the year. Dr. A.M. Clarke, the Executive Director, was made an honorary member of the New Brunswick Association of Registered Nurses at their annual meeting, and at the annual meeting of the New Brunswick Medical Society, Dr. E.W. Ewart was presented with a life membership in the Canadian Medical Association. The medical staff saw many additions in 1968: Dr. O.J. Messenger, Dr. H.G. Brace, Dr. D.B. Geldart, Dr. E.A. MacLeod, Dr. J.L. Sapp, Dr. R.W. Allanach and Dr. W.G. Chesser to the Department of General Practice; Dr. J.A. Gagnon to the Department of Pathology; Dr. M.T. Stephen to the staff as Public Health Officer; Dr. C.A.G. Armstrong to the Department of Anaesthesia; Dr. C.M. Brown to the

Department of Radiology and Dr. W.A. Turner to the Department of Internal Medicine.

In any organization there are those who go about their tasks and render valuable service but there are also those who are the movers and shakers and seen to be at the forefront. Bill Turner was such an individual. He joined the Department of Internal Medicine at a time when vast changes were taking place in the medical field and especially in the field of cardiology. Bill was at the forefront of making sure that all the latest innovations would be available at The Moncton Hospital. He was born in O'Leary, Prince Edward Island, on August 24, 1926, and received a BSc from Mount Allison University in 1951 and an MD, CM from Dalhousie in 1957. He interned at the Victoria General Hospital and the Halifax Infirmary. He spent his pediatric rotation at The Moncton Hospital and Dr. C.M. Leighton noted in his evaluation that Bill was one of the best interns to have been on the service. In 1957, he began a general practice in Salisbury and joined the courtesy staff but switched to the active staff in 1959. He took a leave of absence in 1963 and undertook training in internal medicine at the Victoria General Hospital in Halifax and the Toronto Western Hospital and received his certification in internal medicine in 1967. He then began his career in internal medicine at The Moncton Hospital in 1968. Tragically, he and his daughter, Sally, were killed in an automobile accident in 1972 but in his four short years on the staff he left a lasting legacy. He was, of course, known to the staff from his general practice days and in his last year of residency his opinion was sought on the setting up of a pulmonary function lab and the required equipment, and he had been asked to become the clinician in the new radioisotope laboratory. He made his mark, however, in the new Coronary Care Unit. Freshly trained in the newly developing coronary units in Halifax and Toronto, he brought with him and effected here a highly developed system of care for the acute coronary patient. He undertook to give courses to the nurses serving in the coronary unit and his enthusiasm soon led to his being given the chairmanship of the Intern Committee. He was appointed Chief of the Department of Medicine in 1969 and held this post until his death on May 13, 1972.

The esteem in which Bill was held was demonstrated on May 5, 1976, when the Coronary Care Unit was named the William A. Turner Coronary Care Unit with a suitable plaque placed in the unit. At that time, his friend and fellow internist, Dr. J.T. Edgett, addressed the gathering and his comments that I quote, best exemplify the man: "Most obvious to us all, Bill Turner was a strong man, strong physically, strong of will and purposiveness, firm of opinion, and a tower of personality strength. His physical energy alone displayed an endless pattern of endurance and stamina, the degree of which would later cause vocal concern among his friends. The force of his motivation was clearly astonishing to those about him and others were often swept along by it, including his patients. Primarily a practical person rather than the academic, I think he got more satisfaction in his practice from his patients, and in getting results rather than in the demonstration of the remote or obscure physical finding. In this regard he had a keen sensibility towards his patients, and never did he evade a responsibility to them. A pleasant, positive personality, but hardly tranquil, the humorous side of otherwise serious work rarely passed him. Usually explicit in course of thought and course of action, sometimes of a one-mindedness in argument, these same characteristics of self-will and tenacity usually led him clearly and rapidly to his objectives. His personality was well suited and well adapted to the life of being a physician. His philosophy I am sure, was that of simple hard work, and he measured his work by his results with his patients. Those who knew him well also recognized an equanimity towards illness and sick people, and his interest in his patient continued long past the point where treatment ceased to be effective. On the other hand his philosophy towards urgent situations was that of a challenge, and to say that the diagnosis of 'sudden cardiac death' became his personal enemy, has a strange ring of truth to us who knew him well."

Dr. Donald Blair Geldart and Dr. Hanford Brace were brothers-in-law and joined the active medical staff in the Department of General Practice in 1968. Donald Geldart was born in Moncton on October 5, 1940, and after taking premed at Atlantic Union College, So. Lancaster, Massachusetts, he went to Dalhousie and obtained his MD in 1968 after interning at the Victoria General and Saint John General Hospitals in 1967-68. Hanford Brace was born in Moncton on May 29, 1939, and also attended premed at Atlantic Union College for two years with a third year at Dalhousie and then obtained his MD from Dalhousie in 1968 after interning at the Victoria General Hospital from 1967 to 1968. Although both were competent and successful general practitioners, they became entrepreneurs, running a sporting store and building a clinic and were known as the "golddust twins". Their entrepreneurial enterprises, however, did not have a happy ending financially for them, and they both left Moncton in October 1976 to establish practices in Florida.

Dr. Brace and Dr. Geldart along with Dr. W.G. Chesser and Dr. E.A. MacLeod joined Dr. W.F. Dennis and Dr. W.R. Gillis in general practice and in their practice together the Moncton Medical Clinic was born. Gary Chesser was born in Moncton on February 13, 1942, and received his BSC. from Mount Allison in 1963 and his MD from Dalhousie in 1968 after interning at the Victoria General and Saint John General Hospitals from 1967 to 1968.

Edgar MacLeod was born on November 15, 1937, in Port Philip, Nova Scotia. After receiving his premedical education at Dalhousie University he obtained his MD from the same institution in 1968 after interning at the Victoria General, Halifax Children's Hospital and the Aberdeen Hospital from 1967 to 1968. He remains on staff at the hospital after being transferred to the senior active staff in 1990, because of ill health.

Dr. John Sapp and Dr. W.R. Allanach both set up a general practice in Shediac and were admitted to the courtesy staff. Dr. Sapp left Shediac a short time after to take post graduate work in rehabilitation medicine. Dr. Bill

Allanach was the son of Dr. Lea Allanach, the first child born by caesarean section at The Moncton Hospital and a prominent member of the dental staff, who for years looked after treatment of mandibular fractures. Bill was born in Montreal on February 9, 1941. He took his premedical education at Mount Allison and received his MD from Dalhousie University in 1968 after interning at the Victoria General and Saint John General hospitals from 1967 to 1968. Bill has remained in general practice in Shediac but transferred to the active staff in April, 1990. He has played a prominent role on the Provincial Committee of Physicians at Risk and has earned the gratitude of many doctors in helping them to return to a productive professional life.

In June 1968, Dr. Orville Messenger was admitted to the staff in the Department of General Practice, taking over the practice of Dr. Joyce Boillat. Orville was born in Windsor, Nova Scotia, on October 17, 1942, and received his BSC. from McGill in 1962 and his MD, CM from McGill in 1966. He then served a two-year internship at the Montreal General Hospital before coming to Moncton. Although he had a distinguished career as a general practitioner, his main love was surgery and he took a leave of absence from the staff in 1972 and from 1972 to 1975 pursued a general and thoracic surgery residency at the University of Toronto and a fellowship in cardiothoracic surgery at Baylor University Medical Centre from January to June, 1972. He received his Fellowship in both General and Thoracic Surgery from the Royal College of Physicians and Surgeons of Canada and rejoined the staff of The Moncton Hospital in these departments. Although thoracic surgery had been a department of The Moncton Hospital for some time under the guidance of Dr. R.B. Eaton, Dr. Messenger was the first to possess a Fellowship in Thoracic Surgery and introduced newer diagnostic equipment to the hospital allowing for such procedures as Flexible Fiberoptic Bronchoscopy and Mediastinoscopy. He was made a Fellow of the American College of Surgeons in 1979. He was a tireless proponent in trying to promote improvement in the facilities of The Moncton Hospital. On October 23, 1978, he addressed the Moncton Rotary Club on the treatment of cancer, stressing the role of smoking in the etiology of cancer of the lung and the need to improve our diagnostic facilities for early cancer detection and the need for a new chest X-ray unit at the hospital. In the course of his address he made the following statement: "Despite these days of financial restraint and the present government policy of splitting health care along language lines there are some things we cannot do without. Please lend your support in any way you can. The regional laboratory here has excellent people whose contribution is stifled by a budget which has been frozen too long. We must elicit the support of this community in assuring that our English community is not neglected. As one who has been involved in health outside New Brunswick, our system is not quite second to none." He also asked for support to encourage government to permit a Comprehensive Cancer Centre, including radiotherapy, to be established at the hospital. I am afraid that his speech was not helpful, however, as at a Christmas cocktail party which I attended that year, the Minister of Health, at the time, the Hon. Brenda Robertson, gave me an earful of what she thought of The Moncton Hospital and she had no kind words for Orville Messenger. After only nine years, his surgical career was cut short when he had a massive coronary and underwent bypass surgery in Halifax. He resigned from the medical staff in November 1985 to take a position with the Canadian Medical Protective Association where he established an Educational Department to make doctors more aware of malpractice suits and their prevention. At the time of his leaving Moncton, the medical staff was unaware of the tragedy that would haunt him for the remainder of his life. During his coronary by-pass surgery he had received HIV positive blood and was informed of this fact in December, 1985. This has all been revealed and described in his book "Borrowed Time, a Surgeon's Struggle with Transfusion Induced AIDS", which was published in 1995, the year of his death due to AIDS complications.

Dr. Carl Brown was born on July 8, 1931, in Charlottetown, Prince Edward Island. After taking the premed course at Prince of Wales College, he entered Dalhousie University and obtained his MD, CM in 1958 after interning at the Victoria General Hospital from 1957 to 1958. After a general practice in Moose Jaw and Charlottetown, he undertook a residency in radiology at the Ottawa Civic Hospital from 1962 to 1966 and obtained his certification in radiology from the Royal College of Physicians and Surgeons of Canada. Although he enjoyed an excellent reputation as a radiologist, his heart was not in the medical field, and he resigned from the staff in May, 1980, to take up farming in Prince Edward Island.

Dr. Joseph A. Gagnon was born in Dupuis Corner on August 19, 1928. He obtained a BSc from Saint F.X. in 1953 and an MD, CM from Dalhousie in 1958. He interned at the Victoria General, the Halifax Infirmary and The Moncton Hospital from 1957 to 1958. While in general practice in St. Antoine, he was appointed as a member of the courtesy staff in general practice in 1959. He left general practice in 1965 and took postgraduate work in pathology at the Pathology Institute, McGill University, from 1965 to 1966, the Montreal General Hospital from 1966 to 1967, the Montreal Children's Hospital and St. Mary's Hospital from 1967 to 1968. He was awarded a diploma in anatomic pathology from the American Board of Pathology in 1969. His career on the pathology staff spanned 26 years, with some of those years spent as Chief of Pathology. He was appointed to the senior active staff in 1989 and retired on July 1, 1994, and thereby became a member of the honorary staff.

In would seem that one of the prerequisites for joining the anaesthetic staff in 1968 was to have the Christian name of "Arthur." Dr. C.A.G. Armstrong joined the staff that year making three "Arthurs" on the anaesthetic staff. Arthur Armstrong was born in Ballymena, Ireland, on January 24, 1924. He took his premedical education at Royal School, Dungannon, and received his MB, BCh, BAO in 1947 from the Queen's University of Belfast. He interned at the Royal Belfast Hospital for Sick Children and the Waverly

Hospital, Ballymena, from 1947 to 1948. He then did residencies in anaesthesia at the Royal Halifax Infirmary (1948-49), Bradford Royal Infirmary (1949-50) and the City General Hospital, Sheffield (1950-52). He was awarded a diploma in anaesthesia by the Royal College of Physicians and Surgeons in 1950 and also the Faculty of Anaesthesia of the Royal College of Surgeons in Ireland. He worked at South Tyrone Hospital, Dungannon, from 1952 to 1967 and then emigrated to Canada, receiving his LMCC in 1967. He was appointed to the staff of The Moncton Hospital in March, 1968. He received his FRCP(C) in 1980. Arthur is a very intelligent man and suffers fools poorly. Any surgeon who might try to book a case as an emergency which obviously did not fit into this category would certainly hear Arthur's opinion on the matter. On the other hand, if a situation, although not exactly an emergency, was explained to him without embellishment, he could be quite cooperative in meeting the surgeon's needs. In 1982, he took umbrage with statements made by the executive director, William Kilpatrick, that the waiting list could be solved by the hiring of two anaesthetists. Dr. Armstrong, along with the other anaesthetists, responded by sending a letter to the editor of the *Moncton Transcript* which was published on December 8, 1982. This resulted in a feature article in the paper by Charles Perry which stated "Armstrong pointed to deficient operating room space, a frequency of double shifts by operating room nurses and increased tension due to inadequate rest areas for certain staff as examples of the predicament." The article stated also that Dr. Armstrong pointed out that the anaesthetists were not hired by the hospital but were free spirits who chose to come to the hospital and would only be induced to come with increased facilities. Arthur obviously did not endear himself with the administration or the board of Trustees with his public statements but the matter was soon forgotten. In 1988, a day surgery unit was set up at the Sackville Hospital and Dr. Armstrong moved to Sackville. He continued to work at The Moncton Hospital a couple of days a week until February, 1989, when the day surgery unit at the Sackville Hospital was expanded to five days a week. He was appointed to the senior active staff in 1985 and retired from practice on December 31, 1993, when he was made a member of the honorary staff. To stimulate his intellectual curiosity, Arthur took advantage of the presence in the city of the Université de Moncton where he enrolled in courses and continued this practice at Mount Allison after moving to Sackville, receiving a degree from Mount Allison, and graduating at the top of the class.

During 1968 there were 9,926 adults and children admitted to the main hospital and another 362 adults to the Annex. There were 1,369 newborns admitted to the nursery, and 5,032 operations were performed in the main operating rooms. In addition, 1,458 anaesthetics were given in the emergency department for minor operations and fracture cases. There was a total of 95,732 visits to the outpatient department, of which 30,345 were classified as emergencies. In the Public Health Clinics, 249 patients were seen in the Paediatric Clinic and 835 children in the Orthopaedic Clinic. One hundred seventy patients made visits to the Poison Control Centre and 438 new patients were registered in the Cancer Clinic. In the radiology department 33,876 visits took place, including 1,105 visits for deep therapy and 411 for superficial therapy. The physiotherapy department had 26,194 visits recorded with another 6,076 to occupational therapy. There were 8,591 electrocardiograms read and 278 basal metabolism tests performed, 742 electroencephalography tracings were done and 7,304 inhalation treatments were given. Electric shock treatments were given to 348 inpatients and 471 outpatients. The ambulance service travelled 22,970 miles while making 2,062 calls.

On March 5, 1969, the Minister of Health and Welfare met with members of the boards of Trustees of various hospitals. The purpose of the meeting was to announce to hospital boards, in advance, that there would be no new hospital construction approved in New Brunswick for the next year, but that present contracts would be honoured. The new patient tower for The Moncton Hospital was already under construction and hence was approved, but authority had been received to finish only three of the six patient floors—the third, fourth and sixth were those selected. By December 31, 1969, the work was approximately 85 percent completed and the new boiler room was finished. However, no authority had been received to have the service tunnel built which would convey steam from the boiler room to the new patient tower and would carry lines to provide electrical, oxygen and air conditioning services to it.

As a follow up to the meeting of March 5, 1969, representatives of provincial hospitals were called to a meeting in Fredericton on May 12, 1969, at which the Minister of Health and Welfare announced that the firm of Llewellyn-Davies, Weeks, Forestier-Walker and Bor had been retained by the province to do a study of Health Services Facilities for the Province of New Brunswick. During the year the medical staff prepared an excellent brief which was presented to the hospital consultants.

After administering the Annex for nine years, Jean Lyons resigned on September 1, 1969, on account of ill health. She was replaced as administrator by Roberta Perry. Other resignations during the year were: Miss E.R. Johnson, Chief Physiotherapist; Mrs. R.M. MacDonald, Occupational Therapist; and R.E. Theriault, Psychologist; and George Geldart, Plant Superintendent at the Annex. The physiotherapy department was enhanced during the year with the hiring of four physiotherapists from Australia and one from Wales.

Among the medical staff, Dr. David MacLeod left for Ontario and Dr. Joyce Boillat, on leave of absence at the time, decided to remain in Montreal. Dr. A.W. Ross died during the year. The medical staff, however, continued its growth with several new additions to the staff: Dr. Alan Covert and Dr. John Curtis to the Department of General Practice; Dr. Loyola LeBlanc to the Department of Paediatrics; Dr. Kenneth Tulle and Dr. Louis Gaudet to the Department of Radiology; Dr. M. Britton and Dr. E. Steven and Dr. R.

Sunaric to the Department of Ophthalmology and Otolaryngology; Dr. C. Dyack to the Department of Obstetrics and Gynaecology; and Dr. G. Dumo to the Department of Anaesthesia.

Alan Covert was born in Halifax on June 8, 1944, and received his premedical and medical education at Dalhousie obtaining his MD in 1969. After a short time in general practice, he left to specialize in radiology.

Dr. John Curtis served in the Department of General Practice for an even shorter period of time. He was born on November 6, 1942, in Toronto, but received his post secondary education in Nova Scotia, obtaining a BSc from Dalhousie in 1964 and an MD in 1969. He interned at the Victoria General Hospital from 1968 to 1969. After practising in Bath, New Brunswick, for five months he moved to Moncton and was appointed to the active staff in general practice in November. In 1970, he took a leave of absence to take postgraduate work in psychiatry at McMaster University but did not return to The Moncton Hospital.

Dr. Loyola LeBlanc was a New Brunswick native born on September 11, 1922, and received a BA from St. Joseph's in 1943 and an MD from the University of Montreal in 1949. He interned at l'Hôtel Dieu, Ste. Justine and Misericorde hospitals in Montreal from 1949 to 1950 and then pursued postgraduate work in pediatrics at Pasteur Hospital 1950-51 and the Montreal Children's Hospital from 1951 to 1953. He then did private practice in pediatrics in Edmundston, New Brunswick from 1953 to 1957. He obtained certification in pediatrics from the Royal College of Physicians and Surgeons of Canada in 1956. From February 1967 to March 1969, he was Director of the Mental Retardation Department, Providence Hospital, Montreal, but then returned to the private practice of pediatrics in Moncton in 1969. He remained on the active staff of both hospitals but was taken off the call schedule of The Moncton Hospital in September 1982, for health reasons. He was subsequently killed in a motor vehicle accident.

Kenneth Tulle was born on January 4, 1934, in Charlottetown, Prince Edward Island. He took his premedical course at Prince of Wales College and then went to Dalhousie where he received his MD, CM in 1958 after interning at the Victoria General and Halifax Infirmary Hospitals. He did a year of internal medicine at the Victoria General Hospital (1962-63), followed by a stint of general practice in Dalhousie, New Brunswick, from 1963 to 1966. This was followed by two years of residency in radiology at the Ottawa Civic Hospital, after which he spent his final year of residency at The Moncton Hospital and became certified in radiology in 1969. He replaced Dr. W.B. Stewart as Chief of Radiology in 1974 and held this post until 1980. He found this a frustrating job and had difficulty in accepting the limitations placed on the Department of Radiology by budget considerations regarding the acquisition of new or replacement radiographic equipment as well providing adequate technical staff for his department. He could be quite vocal at times in defending his department, sometimes leading to shouting matches with the Executive Director, Mr. Kilpatrick, at Medical Advisory Committee meetings. He resigned in 1981, hoping to find a more serene atmosphere at Saint Martha's Hospital in Antigonish.

Dr. Louis Camille Gaudet also joined the radiology department the same year, 1969, and, in marked contrast to Kenneth Tulle has always gone about his work in a quiet unassuming manner. If anything gets him angry, the world would never know. Louis was born on December 10, 1939, in Yarmouth, Nova Scotia. He received a BA from St. Anne's College in 1960 and an MD from Laval in 1965. He interned at St. Sacrement Hospital, Quebec City, in 1964-65, with a year of internal medicine residency at the same hospital from 1965 to 1966. This was followed by a residency in radiology for one year at St. Sacrement and two years at Charity Hospital in New Orleans. He received his Fellowship in Radiology in 1969 and was qualified for nuclear medicine procedures and hence was able to take over supervision of the radioisotope laboratory. He received his diploma from the American Board of Nuclear Medicine in 1972. He remains a mainstay of the Department of Medical Imaging and his opinion in any phase of the department's work is highly valued.

Michael Britton was born in Moncton on October 17, 1938, the son of Dr. H.E. Britton. He obtained his BSc at University of New Brunswick in 1960 and his MD, CM degree from McGill in 1965. He interned at the Royal Victoria Hospital from 1965 to 1966 and then did a residency in ophthalmology at the same hospital from 1966 to 1969, becoming certified in ophthalmology in 1969. After practising his specialty for eighteen years he elected to confine his practice to his office and stopped doing surgery and taking calls. As a result, he was not reappointed to the staff in 1988.

Dr. Eric Steven, the other addition to the ophthalmology staff in 1969, has continued to practice at the hospital ever since. Eric was born on October 6, 1934, in Hamilton, Scotland, and has kept the Scottish brogue throughout his life. He took his premedical training at Hamilton Academy and received his MB,ChB from the University of Glasgow in 1959. He interned at the Glasgow Royal Infirmary and the Easter District Hospital, Glasgow, from 1959 to 1960. He then pursued postgraduate studies in ophthalmology at Bangour General Hospital (1961-62), Aberdeen Royal Infirmary (1962-63), Bangour General Hospital (1963-65), Royal Infirmary of Edinburgh (1965-68). He received his FRCS(E) and DO(England) and after coming to Canada, he became certified by the Royal College of Physicians and Surgeons of Canada in 1968. In 1974, he began doing laser surgery at the Dr. Georges-L. Dumont Hospital but this particular surgery was not performed at The Moncton Hospital until 1990, after the purchase of a Yag Laser.

The Department of Ophthalmology and Otolaryngology was still one department in 1969, although the newer members of the staff confined themselves to practising in only one branch. Dr. Radomir Sunaric was born on November 1, 1922, in Vrasenica, Yugoslavia. He received a diploma from the

Gymnasium in Sarajevo in 1941 and an MD and ScD from the University of Zagreb in 1952. He interned at Sarra Jero Hospital in 1953 and then did one year of general surgery and three years of EENT postgraduate work at the University Hospital, Zagreb, from 1955 to 1960 and became certified with a Fellowship in EENT in Yugoslavia. On immigrating to Canada in 1968, he served a residency at the Victoria General in Halifax from 1968 to 1969. He received a provisional 21-month appointment to the EENT staff in October, 1969, but by June, 1971, he had failed to become certified by the Royal College and his appointment had to be terminated because of the prevailing by-laws for appointment to the surgical staff. By all reports he was a technically capable surgeon and it was felt that it was his difficulty with the English language that posed the problem for him during the course of examinations.

Colin Dyack was born in Kakamega, Kenya Colony, on December 25, 1937, but was educated in Scotland, where he received his premedical and medical education culminating in the awarding of his MB,ChB in 1961. He interned at East Suffolk Hospital (1961-62) and then did residencies in obstetrics and gynaecology at Royal Berkshire Hospital, Reading (1962-63), Central Middlesex Hospital, London, in 1966 and then came across the ocean to finish up at the Victoria General and Grace Maternity Hospitals in Halifax from 1966 to 1969. He was appointed to the staff in the Department of Obstetrics and Gynaecology in 1969, but only remained on staff for three years before returning to England in 1972, where he began working at Central Middlesex Hospital.

Dr. Gonopoti Dumo was born on October 4, 1929, in Margis, Portugal. He received his BSc in 1950 from Coimbra University and his MD from the Faculty of Medicine at the same university in 1956. Dumo, as he is called, even by his wife, came to Canada in 1961 and took postgraduate training in anaesthesia at Grace Hospital, Winnipeg, in 1961, St. Boniface Hospital, Winnipeg, (1961-61) and Winnipeg General Hospital and Winnipeg Childrens' Hospital (1962-63). He was awarded a specialist certificate in anaesthesia in Portugal in 1964 but then returned to Canada to spend the rest of his life in this country. From 1964 to 1966 he served as an intern at the Regina Grey Nuns Hospital and then did a fellowship in anaesthesia at l'Hôtel Dieu de Sherbrooke from 1966 to 1967. He then became a resident in anaesthesia at The Moncton Hospital from July 1967 to January 1969, with the exception of the period from January to July 1968, when he did a fellowship at Boston University Hospital. He joined the active staff of the Department of Anaesthesia at The Moncton Hospital in 1969 where he has remained a fixture ever since, with his no nonsense approach to getting the work done.

The year 1969 saw continued growth in the use of hospital facilities with 10,689 patients admitted to the main hospital and annex, an increase of 401 over 1968. In addition, 1,428 newborns were admitted to the nursery; 5,245 operations were performed; 40,909 visits were made to the X-ray department for diagnostic purposes and radiotherapy was still an available service with 1,179 deep and 437 superficial treatments given. The radioisotope laboratory had 368 visits. The outpatient department showed over 10,000 more visits than the previous year with 107,602 visits recorded. Of these, 33,377 were classified as emergencies with 1,434 general anaesthetics given. 4,455 minor operations were done in the outpatient department, and 2,274 fracture cases attended to and 633 dental cases were cared for. Outpatient clinics continued to operate with 225 patients seen in the Arthritic Clinic and 390 new patients were registered at the Cancer Clinic. Clinics operated by the Public Health Service saw 262 patients at 46 Paediatric Clinics, 744 children at 11 Orthopaedic Clinics and 179 patients at the Poison Control Clinic. There was a reduction in the number of electroshock treatments given with 619 performed; 9,878 electrocardiograms, 42 basal metabolism tests and 564 electroencephalography tracings were done. The reduction in number of basal metabolism tests signified the beginning of the end for this test with the opening of the radioisotope laboratory. The physiotherapy and occupational therapy departments showed a reduction in their workload with 25,048 and 2,497 visits respectively. Inhalation therapy treatments continued to rise, with 7,719 given.

Chapter Nine

The Seventies— Technology and Specialization Take Over

The onset of the 1970s heralded greater departmentalization and the introduction of new services such as plastic surgery and neurosurgery. The introduction of newer diagnostic tools and new methods of treatment arose partly because of new technology associated with the space age. The decade saw the departure of the general practitioner as an entity only to re-emerge as the family physician. It also saw the hospital-trained nurse replaced by university-trained nurses with bachelor degrees and by nurses trained in two-year community college-type programs.

Construction on the new wing of The Moncton Hospital was continuing, and was still not ready for occupancy. As yet, no word had been received from the government concerning the additions and renovations required to service the increased patient load once the new wing was opened. On May 31, 1970, Dr. Austin M. Clarke retired as Executive Director. On May 22, 1970, about 400 friends and associates attended a reception and dinner in his honour at which the Honourable Norbert Theriault, minister of health and welfare, announced that the new patient tower would be named the Clarke Wing and unveiled a bronze plaque to be placed in the new wing. Mr. Theriault paid tribute to Dr. Clarke for his outstanding work with the Department of Health and his capable leadership as Executive Director of The Moncton Hospital. The Llewellyn-Davis Weeks Report had not been released as yet but Mr. Theriault stated that the consulting firm had reported that The Moncton Hospital was the most efficiently operated hospital in the Province of New Brunswick.

The report from the consulting firm of Llewellyn-Davis, Weeks, Forestier-Walker and Bor of London, England, entitled "Study of Health Facilities in New Brunswick," was published during the year. The report proposed a system of delivery of health care services which tended to shift the emphasis from very expensive hospital-based acute curative care to a program which increased the emphasis on a number of less-expensive and perhaps more effective alternative techniques. Some alternatives that were proposed were home-care programs, chronic-convalescent hospitals and nursing homes, and specialized geriatric and rehabilitation programs. As mentioned above, the report was very flattering to The Moncton Hospital, and stated in Section 14.11: "The executive direction of The Moncton Hospital was found to be above average. This is due in large measure to the personal qualities and abilities of the executive director and his senior staff, who, together with the medical director and the director of nursing, constitute a strong and effective top management team."

With the retirement of Dr. Clarke and the appointment of Mr. Kilpatrick to the position of executive director, the position of assistant executive director was filled with the appointment of Lloyd D. Secord to the post on June 1, 1970. Mr. Secord, a native of New Brunswick, graduated in science from the University of New Brunswick in 1968 and received his diploma in hospital administration from the University of Toronto in 1970. Albert J. Levesque was appointed as psychologist to the hospital and has continued in this post for the past 25 years, giving valuable service to the Department of Psychiatry not to mention fishing advice to those members of the medical staff engaged in this sporting activity.

Developments with the nursing staff included the resignation of Betty Ann Ward RN, as Nursing Supervisor after seventeen years of service. Myrna Sherrard, BN, RN, began her climb up the nursing hierarchy ladder resigning her position as nurse clinician to become associate director of Nursing Service. Miss Harriett Hayes, BN, RN, associate director of Nursing Education for some years was elected president of the New Brunswick Association of Registered Nurses. Several changes were made to the pediatric nursing program during the year. Andrew Williams, an orderly with artistic talent, created a number of nursery rhyme wall murals on the sixth floor Parlee pediatric ward and the nurses' station was converted to a Little Red School House. In an effort to ease the difficulties some young children experience in the hospital, visiting restrictions for parents were completely removed and an organized afternoon play program was initiated by Charlotte Duncan.

On May 31, 1970, Dr. Howard Ripley passed away suddenly after a few weeks of failing health. Since he was the only radiologist on staff qualified in therapeutic radiotherapy and given the government's intention, with the introduction of cobalt therapy, to concentrate all radiotherapy at the Saint John General Hospital, his death also spelt the death knoll for radiotherapy services at The Moncton Hospital.

A pulmonary function laboratory was set up during the year in conjunction with the Department of Respiratory Technology. It was planned under the direction of Dr. J.T. Edgett of the Department of Internal Medicine. The opening of the laboratory would not have been possible without the Friends of the Moncton Hospital Foundation, as it was responsible for purchasing the equipment needed for the laboratory. The Isotope Service took a large step forward with the acquisition of a Gamma Camera and another technician. During the year, Dr. Louis Gaudet obtained his license from the Atomic Energy Commission and took over the supervision of the department. The Department of General Practice took over responsibility for providing 24-hour coverage in the outpatient department. It was also at this time that the hospital joined the rest of Canada in adopting the metric system. This did not present too much of a problem because over the previous few years the metric system had been gradually creeping unofficially into general use in medical parlance. Changes were made in the organization of the various services in the hospital with the zoning of beds to the various services. For the surgical services, this was combined with a program of prebooking and pre-admission work-up of elective surgical cases.

Dr. Gordon Crandall resigned at this time from the Department of Psychiatry to accept a position in North Carolina. There were, however, several additions to the staff, including Dr. Denys R. Wilcox and Dr. M. Majka to the Department of Pathology, and Drs. Michael T. Johnson, Isak Kohener, and Robert L. Frizzell to the Department of General Practice. A Medical Manpower Committee consisting of members of the medical staff and the board of trustees was formed to review manpower needs and to actively seek out trained personnel to fill these needs.

Dr. Denys R.C. Wilcox was born in London, England, on April 28, 1916, and received his MRCS, LRCP degrees from Guys Hospital Medical School, University of London, in 1939. After interning at Guys Hospital from 1939 to 1940, where he served as house physician and house surgeon, he did a residency in pathology at Guys Hospital in 1948. His Fellowship from the Royal College of Pathology (UK) was received in 1969. He was appointed to the Department of Pathology in November 1970, but resigned on June 1, 1971. The other member to join the pathology staff in 1970, would leave a much more lasting impression. Dr. Mieczslaw Majka, referred to usually as "Mike", was born on December 20, 1921, in Poland. He graduated from the Lyceum in Tarmow, Poland, in 1939 and received his MD in 1951 from Leopold Frazeus University in Innsbruck, Austria. He immigrated to Canada and interned at St. Joseph's Hospital, Hamilton, from 1951 to 1953. He did a residency in pathology at St. Joseph's Hospital from 1953 to 1958, followed by assistantships at Westmorland Hospital, Hamilton, from 1958 to 1959 and 1960 to 1961 and also at the University of Western Ontario from 1959 to 1960. He then moved to New Brunswick where he was employed at the regional laboratory on a ministerial letter in 1961, remained on the staff of the laboratory following this and then joined the active staff of The Moncton Hospital in the Department of Pathology in 1970. He remained on staff until his retirement in December 1993, when he was appointed to the honorary staff. Outside his well respected professional career, Mike and his wife, Mary, established reputations as naturalists and have been prominent residents of Albert County, first on Caledonia Mountain and then at Mary's Point.

Michael T. Johnston was born in Toronto on March 9, 1945, and after premed at St. Francis Xavier, obtained his MD degree from Dalhousie in 1970. He established a good reputation as a family physician in Moncton and became certified in family medicine by the College of Family Physicians of Canada in 1975. In 1980, he developed a wanderlust and moved to Dawson, Yukon, but he has since moved back to New Brunswick, where he has a busy family practice in Dalhousie, New Brunswick.

The other two members to join the Department of General Practice in 1970 had shorter stays in the community. Isak Kohener was born in Istanbul, Turkey, on January, 28, 1941, and graduated with his MD degree from the University of Istanbul in 1966. He then immigrated to Canada and interned at the Saint John General Hospital from 1967 to 1968, followed by a residency in anaesthesia at the Saint John General Hospital from 1968 to 1969 and another year in psychiatry at the Provincial Hospital from 1969 to 1970. He obtained his LMCC in 1970, established a general practice in Shediac and was appointed to the courtesy staff but became a member of the active staff in 1971 when he moved to Moncton. In 1977, he made a further move, this time to Houston, Texas.

Dr. Robert L. Frizzell was born in Summerside, Prince Edward Island, on May 23, 1929, and, after taking premed at Prince of Wales College, he attended Dalhousie, graduating with his MD, CM in 1958. He interned at the Victoria General Hospital from 1957 to 1958. Bob was another doctor affected by the wanderlust and served the staffs of the Greater Niagara General Hospital in Niagara Falls from 1959 to 1963, the Scarborough General Hospital in 1964 and the Los Angeles County General Hospital from 1965 to 1970. He joined the staff of the Moncton Medical Clinic in October, 1970, and proved to be an able general practitioner. He departed the following year, however, to pursue postgraduate training in anaesthesia.

For the previous six years, Dr. White and Dr. MacLellan had the unenviable task of being on call every day for a month each during the summer. Since these months are busy ones for the orthopaedic service, some help was sought. They were fortunate to obtain the services of Dr. Alan Gross to serve as a locums for the months of July and August while each went on vacation. Although it is not intended to include in this history every doctor who did a locums, Dr. Gross deserves special mention. Alan was born in Toronto on January 12, 1938, and received his MD from the University of Toronto in 1962. He did a residency in general surgery at the Toronto General Hospital from 1964 to 1966 followed by residencies in orthopaedics at the Toronto General Hospital (1966-67), Hospital for Sick Children, Toronto (1967-68), and Toronto Wellesley Hospital (1968-69). He obtained his Fellowship in Orthopaedics from the Royal College in 1969. He was appointed to the staff of the Toronto General Hospital from 1969 to 1970. In the fall of 1970 he had planned to do a year of research at Oxford University before returning to an assured position on the staff of the new Mount Sinai Hospital in Toronto. To fill in his summer, he accepted our call for a locums and had an enjoyable summer where he states he saw and treated more trauma than during his years as a resident in Toronto. The use of total hips had just come into use in Canada and the United Kingdom, but was still only approved for use on an experimental basis at certain centres in the United States by the Food and Drug Administration. Dr. Gross had been trained in this surgery in Toronto and he brought some instruments with him from Toronto. With his teaching, Dr. White and Dr. MacLellan were able to introduce this revolutionary new surgery for arthritic hips to the Moncton community. Since his short stay here, Dr. Gross has gone on to become the Chief of Orthopaedics at Mount Sinai Hospital in Toronto and Head of the Department of Orthopaedics at the University of Toronto.

In 1970, 11,044 patients were admitted to the main hospital along with 366 to the Annex and 1,523 newborn; 3,223 major and 2,395 minor operations were performed. Visits to the X-ray department totalled 46,126, including 603 deep therapy treatments and 212 superficial therapy treatments. There were also 691 patients seen at the radioisotope laboratory. There were 33,269 visits to physiotherapy and another 2,719 to occupational therapy; 11,966 electrocardiograms were done and 773 electroencephalograms. The inhalation therapy department saw 9,013 patients. There were 113,408 visits recorded in the outpatient department and of these, 38,289 were classified as emergencies. Among the clinics, 283 were seen at the Arthritis Clinic, 355 at the Paediatric Clinic, 664 at the Orthopaedic Clinic and 401 new patients at the Cancer Clinic. 194 patients were seen in poison control and 477 patients received electroshock treatments.

On January 18, 1971, the 34-bed unit on the third floor of the Clarke Wing was opened. The other two floors, the fourth and fifth, were not to be opened until September 20, 1971. The staffing of the wing was aided by the fact that 65 percent of the 1971 graduating class of the School of Nursing chose to join the nursing staff of the hospital. The ribbon cutting ceremony for the opening of the wing was performed by Dr. Austin Clarke for whom the new wing had been named. Participating in the ceremony was the Hon. Paul S. Creaghan, minister of health in the Hatfield Conservative government which had defeated the Liberal government of Louis Robichaud in the 1970 provincial election. No word had yet been received from the new government on the enlarging of the support services or on the opening of the other three floors of the Clarke Wing. Instead, it took the usual course of government by studying a problem to death and appointing a Toronto firm of hospital architects to act as co-ordinators of hospital construction in the province. Since the beginning of government-paid hospitalization, there had been increased usage of facilities. By 1971, with the introduction of Medicare in New Brunswick, increased patient loads for physicians were increasing along with the attendant increased demand for diagnostic facilities. Medicare also brought about another change. Doctors began to get paid for all their work, so the profile of the community doctor changed from that of being a humanitarian. Dr. A.W. Ross once remarked that one of the worst aspects of

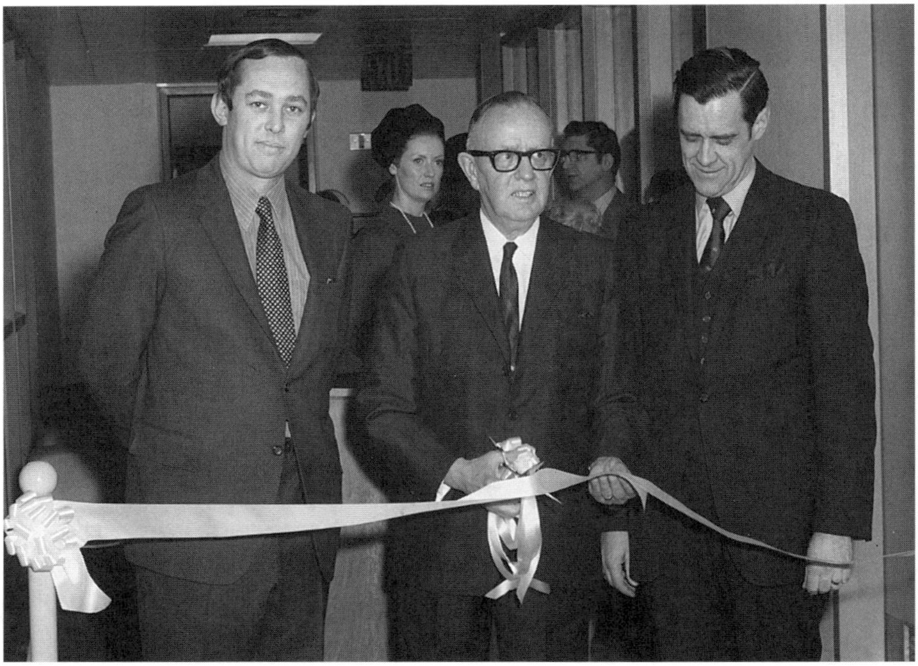

The opening of the Clarke Wing in 1971. From left to right: Hon. Paul Creaghan, Minister of Health; Dr. Austin Clarke, and Mr. Ralph Belyea, Chairman of the Board.

Medicare was that it took away the privilege of the doctor of doing something for nothing. Health costs had been rising on average of ten percent a year, with one-half of the cost being borne by the federal government. In November 1971, the Honourable John Munro, minister of national health and welfare, proposed a change in financing with a new policy in which the increase in federal payments for health care would be allowed to increase only in proportion to the increase in the gross national product, which at that time was four to five percent a year. To assist in the development of new approaches for the provision of health care a special $640 million. "Trust Fund" would be made available to the provinces by the federal government to help them reorganize their health care systems. By 1971, the expense of operating The Moncton Hospital, including the Annex, had risen to $8,503,345.

With government funds becoming increasingly limited, the Friends of the Moncton Hospital and other volunteer organizations came to the rescue. During the year, the Friends purchased a diffusion module for the inhalation therapy department of the hospital at a cost of $5,800. The Ladies' Hospital Auxiliary purchased paintings worth $1,000 from the Moncton Art Society for the patient rooms in the new Clarke Wing.

There were several changes in the hospital's administrative field in 1971. Given the extended operating room hours at the time, Dr. W.A. Oatway resigned from his position as medical director to devote his full time to the practice of anaesthesia. John Dingle resigned from his position as director of the hospital's Personnel and Public Relations Department to become director of personnel and training with the provincial Department of Welfare. His position was filled by Geoffrey W. Lodge. An important promotion within the hospital family was that of Ruth Duffy from being the chief radiological technician to the position of administrative assistant for the hospital. She has continued to play an important role in the administration of the hospital ever since, and the manner in which she has conducted herself is attested to by the fact that she has never been the object of criticism by Dr. Fred Murphy.

Among the nursing administration, Miss Harriett Hayes, BN, RN, associate director of nursing education, took a leave of absence to study for a Master's Degree in nursing at Boston University. Meanwhile, the School of Nursing could no longer provide accommodation for all students and the Anne Street residence was closed, leaving only the main West Lane residence. This was able to accommodate only 120 first and second year students, and the remaining second and third-year students were required to obtain their own accommodations in the community. A Provincial Study Committee on Nursing Education was formed during the year, and the School of Nursing Advisory Committee, under the chairmanship of Barbara Steeves, prepared and presented at a public meeting a brief outlining the hospital's beliefs regarding nursing education. A six-week reorientation program at the hospital continued, with the result that the hospital was provided with a source of experienced and reliable nurses for the Moncton area. Many of

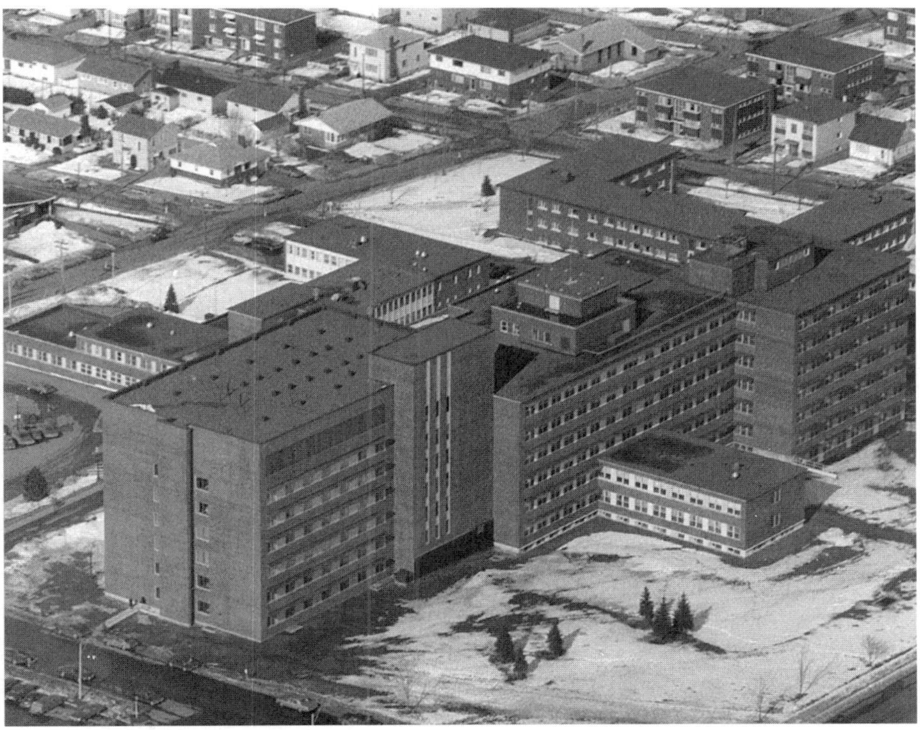

The Moncton Hospital—after the addition of the Clarke Wing.

these nurses had been out of the nursing field for several years while raising their families and they welcomed the opportunity to become "retreads" to regain their nurse's registration and start working again in their chosen field. It was difficult to keep up a supply of trained nurses in the operating room but it was also recognized that not all tasks in the operating room theatres needed to be carried out by registered nurses. The hospital established New Brunswick's first formal training course for operating room technicians and five registered nursing assistants were enrolled in this six-month course which was under the direction of Joan Donald. She did a good job of teaching and obviously had good students as many on graduation became employed in our operating rooms and have supplied exemplary service since.

With the increased emphasis on continuity of care, members of the Public Health Nursing Services, the Victorian Order of Nurses and the Hospital Nursing and Social Service staffs collectively developed a home care planning guide for patients of the orthopaedic service. With the implementation of this program, it was possible to begin active discharge planning on or before the admission of the patient, with the result that the discharge and subsequent care of the patient would take place with greater patient and family co-operation and understanding and an ensured program of home supervision. The program represented the first few hesitant steps in what the hospital hoped would become a full-scale home care program. Such a program would be available to all members of the community and might provide nursing, physiotherapy, homemaking and other services in the home, and thereby decrease the number of patients who must be cared for in the hospital.

The hospital's intern program continued under approval granted by the Canadian Medical Association. Medical students from Mexico supplied the services in the program and they were hand picked by the Chairman of the Intern Committee after visiting Mexico and conducting interviews with the candidates to obtain good quality interns. Dalhousie University continued to use our hospital but only sent one intern on a bi-monthly rotation to the Department of Obstetrics and Gynaecology. Agreement for affiliation for the training of residents was reached during the year with Dalhousie University. With this agreement, the Royal College of Physicians and Surgeons would continue to approve our programs but before any programs were implemented, agreement had to be reached between the medical staff of the department concerned and the appropriate department at Dalhousie University. No agreements were ever signed, however, and training of residents at The Moncton Hospital ceased.

The death of Dr. E.W. Ewart occurred on April 1, 1971. On June 23, 1972 a play therapy unit was opened on the pediatric floor and was named The Ewart Play-Therapy Unit in recognition of Dr. Ewart's contribution to the care of crippled children.

During the year, three doctors, Dr. R.L. Frizzell, Dr. D.R. Wilcox and Dr. R. Sunaric departed from Moncton but their departures were outnumbered by eleven new additions to the staff. Also Dr. James S. Noonan

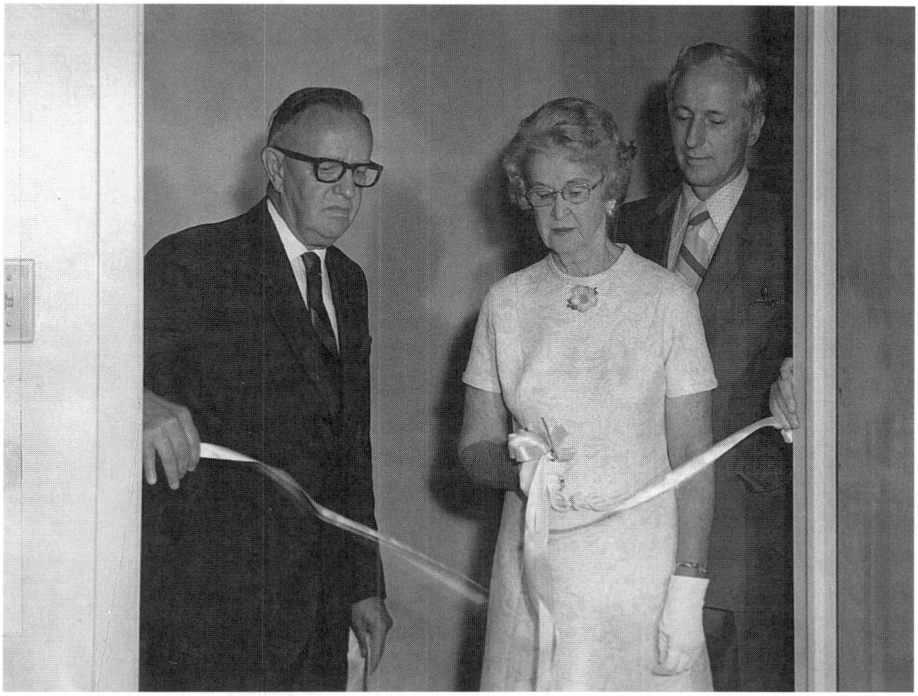

The opening of the Dr. E.W. Ewart Playroom. From left to right: Dr. A.M. Clarke, Mrs. E.W. Ewart, and Dr. O.J. White.

returned from postgraduate work to join the staff in the Department of Radiology.

Dr. Cuthbert J. Pinto, was born in Basra, Iraq, on March 20, 1933. He obtained a BA degree from the University of Madras in 1952 and his MB, BS degree in 1960 from Kasturba Medical College, Kanatah University, India. He interned at Kasturba Medical College from 1959 to 1960 and then interned another year in surgery at the Christian Medical College, Velure, India, from 1960 to 1961. He immigrated to Canada in 1966 and took the McGill diploma course in anaesthesia, receiving his diploma in 1970 and was certified in anaesthesia by the Royal College of Physicians and Surgeons. He then joined the staff of The Moncton Hospital where he has been a valuable and conscientious member of the anaesthetic staff ever since, becoming a member of the senior active staff in 1994.

There were two additions to the Department of Surgery: Dr. S. Guergawi and Dr. R. Orvoine. Sam Guergawi was born in Egypt on April 28, 1925, and went to medical school at Kasr-el Aini School of Medicine at Cairo University, graduating with an MB, BCh. degree in 1949. He did postgraduate work in surgery in the United Kingdom and obtained his FRCS (Edinburgh) in 1957. After being in private practice in general surgery in Cairo from 1957 to 1967, he immigrated to Canada. To obtain his Canadian qualifications, he served as an intern at The Moncton Hospital from 1967 to 1968 as well as a resident in surgery from 1968 to 1969. He then served as a resident at the Ottawa General Hospital from 1969 to 1971 and received his Fellowship in General Surgery from the Royal College in November 1971 and joined the active staff in general surgery. He was a well-thought of surgeon with excellent judgement and the staff was sad when he departed for the warmer climate of Florida in June 1979.

Dr. R. Orvoine, the "whistling doctor", did not gain the confidence of his confrères as Sam Guergawi did. Dr. Orvoine was born on May 14, 1926, in Lanester, Morbihan, France, and received a SPCN degree from the Faculté des Sciences de Paris, and then his MD from the Faculty of Medicine, Paris, in 1956. He interned at Novel Hospital, Amiens, France, from 1956 to 1957 and did postgraduate training in surgery in England and Ireland serving at the Royal Victoria Hospital, Folkstone (1959-60); Royal Surrey County Hospital, Guildford (1960-61); Share Green Hospital, Preston (1961-63), and Westmeath County Hospital, Millingar, Eire, from 1963 to 1965. He received his FRCS from Edinburgh and Ireland. In 1966, he came to Canada on a fellowship at the Institute of Experimental Medicine and Surgery and received an MSc in Experimental Medicine and Surgery from the University of Montreal. He received his LMCC in 1969 and was certified in surgery by the Royal College of Physicians and Surgeons of Canada in 1970. He had set up practice in the Magdalen Islands, Quebec, but moved to Moncton in 1971 and was appointed to the active staff in the Department of Surgery. Despite his excellent credentials, he proved to be a very inept surgeon. In July 1972, the surgical department began restricting his surgical privileges and he resigned from the staff in December 1972.

There were two additions to the Department of General Practice. Dr. Elizabeth Eaton (née Elizabeth Morris) was born on May 29, 1910, at Nantymoel, Glaumorgan, South Wales. She took her premedical and medical education at the London (Royal Free Hospital) School of Medicine for Women receiving her LRCP (London), MRCS (England) in 1934 and her MB, BS in 1935. She did a residency in anaesthesia at Royal Free Hospital, London, in 1935 and served as house surgeon at South Hospital for Women from August to December 1935. Further anaesthetic training was carried out at Hospital for Sick Children, Great Ormond Street, in 1936 and Bristol Postgraduate Medical School, Hammersmith, in 1937. She then served as house physician at Nottingham Children's Hospital from 1937 to 1938. She met Bernie Eaton who was doing postgraduate work in England and following her marriage to him, moved to Canada. After raising their five children, she undertook to become qualified in Canada and obtained her LMCC in 1971 and joined the active staff in general practice.

The other addition to the Department of General Practice this year was Dr. P.C. Stoddard. Peter was born in Halifax on February 11, 1945. After taking his premed at Dalhousie, he entered Medical School and graduated with his MD in 1971. He interned at the Victoria General Hospital from 1970 to 1971, joined the Moncton Medical Clinic on graduation from medical school and has run a busy practice ever since, taking an interest in all aspects of his patients' lives.

There were two additions to the Department of Psychiatry: Dr. C. MacGregor and Dr. M. Wright. Colin MacGregor was born in England on April 29, 1932, and graduated with an MB, BS in 1955 from the University of Durham. He interned at the Preston Hospital, North Shields (1955-56) and at Royal Victoria Infirmary, Newcastle-upon-Tyne, from 1956 to 1957. From 1958 to 1959, he did a residency in medicine at Preston Hospital, North Shields, and psychiatric residencies at the Royal Edinburgh Hospital and the Stabhill General Hospital, Glasgow, from 1959 to 1963. He received a diploma in psychological medicine from the Royal College of Physicians (Edinburgh) and then served as a consultant in psychiatry at Hartwood Hospital, Shotts, Lanarkshire, from 1965 to 1967. For years he enjoyed the confidence of his colleagues and gave good psychiatric advice. He was a delight at parties and could always liven up a discussion by being the devil's advocate. He resigned from the staff in September 1982, and has continued in private practice in Moncton but never rejoined the hospital staff.

Dr. Wright came to Moncton as an employee of the Mental Health Clinic under the Department of Health and Social Welfare. Born in Blandford Forum, Dorset, England, on December 21, 1926, he was educated at the University of Cambridge, receiving a MA, BCh, MB in 1955 and also MRCS (England) and LRCP (London). He interned at Salford Royal in 1955 and pursued training in psychiatry at the same institution from 1956 to 1960. He received a diploma in psychological medicine from the Royal College of Physicians (London) in 1960, worked at St. Andrew's Hospital, Northampton, from 1960 to 1961, and then was senior registrar at the University of Leeds from 1961 to 1965. He was appointed to the medical staff of The Moncton Hospital after he became registered under section 16B of the Medical Act. His privileges were suspended by the MAC in August 1972 because of a mental breakdown. After resigning his positions at the Mental Health Clinic and at Dorchester Penitentiary, a member of the medical staff escorted him back to England to undergo treatment.

Dr. Gabriel Leger was born on February 24, 1938, in Memramcook. He obtained a BSc from St. Joseph's University and then travelled to France where he obtained his MD degree from the Faculté Libre de Médecine de Lille in 1966. He returned to Moncton and served his internship at The Moncton Hospital from 1966 to 1967. From 1967 to 1970, he did postgraduate work in pediatrics at the children's hospital in Halifax, serving as a clinical fellow in haematology in his last year. After another year at Hôpital l'Enfant Jésus at Laval from 1970 to 1971, he obtained his certification in pediatrics from the Royal College of Physicians and Surgeons of Canada in 1971 and returned to practise pediatrics in Moncton. Although principally based at the Dr. Georges-L. Dumont Hospital, he has been on the active staff of both hospitals.

Dr. Robert Caddick was born on April 2, 1943, in Cosley, Wolverhampton, England. He attended Kings College, Durham University, graduating with his MB, BS degree in 1966. He interned at Newcastle General Hospital from 1966 to 1967 and then served as a resident in obstetrics and gynaecology at the same hospital from 1967 to 1969. He immigrated to Canada and finished his postgraduate training at the Ottawa Civic Hospital. After receiving his English qualifications, a diploma in obstetrics from the Royal College of Obstetricians and Gynaecologists, he became certified in obstetrics and gynaecology by the Royal College of Physicians and Surgeons of Canada in November 1971. He then established practice in Moncton where he has remained since. Bob is very musical and can be heard humming or singing a good deal of the time. He plays the piano for many medical functions and serves as organist at St. James Anglican Church. He has taken an active part in the training of interns from Dalhousie and was appointed Clinical Instructor in the Department of Obstetrics and Gynaecology at Dalhousie in 1987. He has been active in the organization of the staff and was elected president of the medical staff in 1995.

Owen Audain was born in St. Kitts, West Indies, on April 13, 1930, and received his premedical education at Grammar School, St. Kitts, Nevis, and then went overseas for his medical education at Edinburgh University, receiving his MB, ChB in 1956. He interned at Rothdole Infirmary, Laner, UK, from 1956 to 1957 and Ryhope General Hospital, England, from 1957 to 1958. He did postgraduate work in general surgery at Bangour General Hospital, West Lathem, from 1965 to 1966 and received his FRCS (Edin.) in 1965. He did a surgical practice at Surgem Basseterre Hospital from 1966 to 1968. He deserted general surgery practice to undergo training in urology at Dalhousie University, serving at the Children's Hospital, the Halifax Infirmary, Camp Hill Hospital and the Victoria General Hospital. He received his FRCS(C) in urology in 1971 and came to Moncton where he has remained ever since with his ever-present smile and easy going manner, as one of the mainstays of the Department of Urology. He became a Fellow of the International College of Surgeons in 1973. In the summer, when he is not working, he can usually be found on the golf course.

Last but not least, Dr. Edwin Douglas Crawshaw made his appearance on the medical scene in Moncton in 1971. "Little Dougie" was born on February 19, 1938, in Calverly, England. He took his premedical and medical education at the University of Edinburgh graduating in 1962 with his MB, ChB degrees. After crossing the ocean he interned at the Saint John's General Hospital from 1963 to 1964 and he served in the Grand Bank Cottage Hospital, Newfoundland, from 1964 to 1965. He returned to England where he served as Registrar at Hexham General Hospital, Northumberland, England, from 1965 to 1966. He subsequently came back to Canada to return to his native England only for visits. His general surgery residency was undertaken at the Royal Victoria Hospital in Montreal from 1966 to 1967, followed by an orthopaedic residency at the Royal Vic from

1967 to 1969, the Shriners' Hospital from 1969 to 1970 and then another year as a research fellow at the Royal Victoria from 1970 to 1971. He obtained his Fellowship in Orthopaedic Surgery in 1970. Since coming to Moncton he can be easily recognized as the small fellow with hair on end and plaster on his shoes and clothing. Everyone driving into the parking lot at the hospital is careful not to park his car next to Douglas's car since it can usually be identified by a dent or two. The story is told that one night as Douglas was leaving the hospital, he discovered that his keys would not open his car door. Somehow he managed to get into the car, hot-wired it and drove merrily home. His serenity was unfortunately short-lived when a nurse who owned a car similar to Douglas's reported hers stolen. Then there is the tale of Douglas and the Saint Bernard. It's been said that one should be aware of Greeks bearing gifts and this should also apply to neurosurgeons. Dr. Harold Tucker had an unruly St. Bernard dog, and very generously gave it to Doug. A neighbour complained of the barking and Doug was charged, and went to court where he put up a spirited defence of his maligned dog. His legal skills failed to impress the judge, however, and he was found guilty. Douglas has established a reputation as a gardener, but his skills in this area do not include weeding or putting away his tools.

There were 11,830 admissions in 1971 as well as 1,654 newborns with an additional 190 admissions to the Annex. There were 3,803 major and 2,758 minor operations performed; 28,005 visits were made to the physiotherapy department and 12,349 inhalation therapy treatments were given; 1,118 shock treatments were carried out. The diagnostic services were kept busy with the following patient visits recorded: radiological examinations (51,935), radioisotope studies (1,760), electrocardiograms (11,862), and electroencephalograms (1,000). The outpatient department saw 49,951 emergency visits. Clinics continued with 372 patient visits to the Paediatric Clinic, 522 to the Orthopaedic Clinic, 458 to the Arthritis Clinic, 396 to the Cancer Diagnostic Clinic and 135 to the Well Woman Clinic which opened on September 28, 1971.

Throughout 1972 there was still no report by the hospital consultants appointed by the provincial government on overall planning for The Moncton Hospital, either on a short-term or long-term basis. Because of the lack of planning, several service departments, such as inhalation therapy, electrocardiology, admitting, booking office, diagnostic clinic, volunteer office and medical records, had to be located either in whole or in part, in temporary offices.

Changes in the administration in 1972 saw the resignation of Geoffrey Lodge as Director of Personnel and Public Relations to be replaced by J. Frederick Rayworth, a Moncton native and graduate of the Université de Moncton. Mr. Rayworth served with distinction in this capacity for several years. Mrs. Pauline Boucher, Chief Medical Record Librarian, was elected to the presidency of the Canadian Association of Medical Record Librarians.

The big event of the year was the opening of the Department of

Neurosurgery under the direction of Dr. H.H. Tucker. This department would soon serve the eastern half of New Brunswick as well as the northern part of Nova Scotia and Prince Edward Island. Although the hospital already had a good reputation for the treatment of multiple trauma, the addition of the neurosurgery service allowed for the additional handling of those cases with severe head injury which otherwise would have to be transferred to Saint John or Halifax. To help equip the new department, the Nurses' Hospital Auxiliary donated $24,000 towards the purchase of operating room instruments. The department has continued to flourish ever since, and with the money raised by the Friends of the Moncton Hospital during the Centennial Campaign, will continue to flourish in the years to come, offering first-rate diagnostic and treatment facilities second to none in Canada. Of course this is also only possible with the well-trained and dedicated neurosurgical staff that have followed in Dr. Tucker's footsteps. With the opening of twenty additional beds for the Department of Neurosurgery, the rated capacity of the hospital grew to 489 beds plus 85 extended care beds giving a total of 574 beds, a figure which would never be reached again.

Dr. Herbert Harold Tucker was born in West Newbury, Massachusetts, in 1924. During the Second World War he showed his leadership capabilities, serving as Company Commander of the First Special Service Force, a combined Canadian and American Force nicknamed "The Devil's Brigade." After the war he received his premedical education at Mount Allison and graduated in medicine from Dalhousie University with an MD,CM degree in 1951. He interned at the Victoria General Hospital from 1950 to 1951, and pursued postgraduate work in neurosurgery, serving a year of general surgery at the Victoria General Hospital from 1951 to 1952 and a year of neurosurgery from 1952 to 1953. This was followed by a year at the University of Toronto in neuropathology from 1953 to 1954 and further clinical training in neurosurgery in Boston at the Children's Medical Centre and the Peter Bent Brigham Hospital from 1954 to 1955. He received his FRCS(C) in Neurosurgery in 1956 and then joined the neurosurgery staff at the Victoria General Hospital, where he remained until coming to Moncton in 1972. He became a Fellow of the American College of Neurosurgeons in 1960. Despite suffering a massive coronary while in practice in Halifax, he took on the task of developing the Department of Neurosurgery in Moncton.

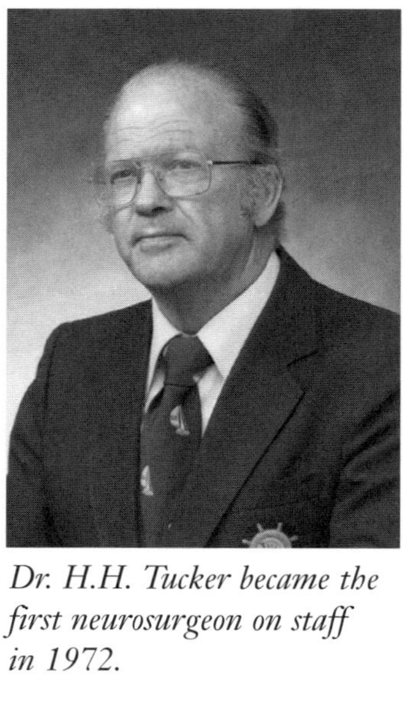

Dr. H.H. Tucker became the first neurosurgeon on staff in 1972.

Possessed of boundless energy and good surgical skills, with confidence to match, he soon made his mark on the Moncton medical scene. He was a man who got things done and was not above stretching the truth or arguing fervently for anything that was going to benefit his department. He was possessed with a gift of the gab. In any argument, he always remained calm and would press his point without ever once showing signs of losing his temper. Hal was an enthusiastic sailor and was a member of the Shediac Bay Yacht Club, serving as Commodore of the Shediac Club in 1978. He also was a member of the Royal Nova Scotia Yacht Squadron and used to participate in the Halifax to Marblehead races. Even in his leisure pursuits, he was an extremely competitive person and members of the medical staff, who served as crew on these races, fondly referred to him as "Captain Bligh."

The New Brunswick Telephone Company has long been recognised as being on the leading edge of technology in the communication field and an early glimpse of this could be seen in 1972. It installed special equipment to permit the direct transmission of electrocardiographs from the Miramichi Hospital to The Moncton Hospital, along with a direct telephone line to allow doctors and technicians at the two hospitals to communicate quickly and easily.

During the year, the Friends of the Moncton Hospital Foundation Inc. began construction of a six-story Professional Arts Building adjacent to the hospital and connected to it by a short passageway. The ground floor was designed to contain a branch of the Royal Bank of Canada and other public services and the other five floors were designed to be leased, with priority given to members of the health care professions and health care agencies.

During the previous year, a major undertaking by the medical staff was a revision of the by-laws under a committee chaired by Dr. V. McLaughlin. These were passed and accepted by the medical staff and the board of trustees in 1972. One of the major changes was the provision for a chief of staff in addition to a president of the medical staff. The chief of staff is nominated by the medical staff but is appointed by the board of trustees and is chairman of the Medical Advisory Committee and through the executive director, is delegated responsibility for the quality of medical care. The president is elected by the medical staff and is their representative in matters affecting each individual's hospital practice. The president would no longer chair the Medical Advisory Committee but remained a member of it and would chair the quarterly staff meetings. He also served as director and co-ordinator for social functions of the medical staff. Dr. McLaughlin was appointed the first chief of staff at the hospital.

The deaths occurred during the year of three prominent members of the medical staff: Dr. George A. Lyons, Dr. H.M. MacLean and Dr. William A. Turner. Dr. Turner was killed, along with his daughter, in an automobile accident. Again there was an influx of new doctors with the addition of Dr. G.W. George to the Department of Internal Medicine; Drs. W.R. Dykeman, G.M. Antle, Mary Klein, Carolyn Rideout and W.H. Scholz to the Department of General Practice; Dr. M. Zahir to the Department of Pathology; Dr. Mary

Mitton to the Department of Psychiatry; Dr. G. Nanjundan to the Department of Ophthalmology and Otorhinolaryngology; and Dr. H.H. Tucker to the Department of Neurosurgery.

William George was born in Windsor, Ontario, on December 6, 1940. He obtained a BA at the University of Western Ontario in 1963 and an MD from the University of Ottawa in 1967. He interned at Harper Hospital in Detroit from 1967 to 1968 and then spent a year in internal medicine at the Ottawa Civic Hospital from 1968 to 1969. Following this, he embarked on a residency in dermatology at the Royal Victoria and the Montreal Children's Hospital from 1969 to 1972. He subsequently came to Moncton as the first specialist in dermatology in Moncton. He built up a large dermatology practice but left Moncton in 1969. There has not been another dermatologist on the active staff since but the hospital has been fortunate to receive excellent dermatology coverage from the dermatologists on staff at the Dr. Georges-L. Dumont Hospital.

Mary Cameron Mitton was born in New Glasgow, Nova Scotia, in December 1940. After premed and medicine at Dalhousie, she received her MD degree in 1966 after serving a rotating internship at Victoria General Hospital. Following a year of general practice in Saint John from 1965 to 1966, she pursued a career in psychiatry, taking one year of postgraduate work at the Royal Ottawa Hospital and three years in the Dalhousie program at the Victoria General, the Halifax Infirmary and Camp Hill Hospital from 1968 to 1971. She was a teaching fellow at Dalhousie and the Victoria General from 1971 to 1972 and obtained her Fellowship in psychiatry in 1972. After joining the associate staff in 1972, she resigned in 1974, and from 1974 to 1983, she was on the staff of the Halifax Infirmary but returned to Moncton in 1983, rejoining the staff of The Moncton Hospital. She has remained on staff ever since, except for a short period from December 1984 to September 1985 when she confined her practice to the Mental Health Clinic.

Gopal Nanjundan was born on July 19, 1936, in Coimbatore, India. He attended premed at Madras University, India, and then Madras Medical College, receiving his MB, BS in 1962. He interned at the Government General Hospital, Madras, from 1962 to 1963. He immigrated to Canada and took a year of residency at the Ottawa General Hospital from 1965 to 1966 and completed his training in otorhinolaryngology at University Hospital, Edmonton, from 1966 to 1970 and served as a teaching fellow at the University of Alberta from 1970 to 1971. He received his fellowship from the Royal College and also passed the American Board of Otolaryngology examinations and practised in Sault Ste. Marie for one year before coming to Moncton. He was a quiet, very soft spoken man who did excellent work in his specialty. He had a large waiting list for surgery and found the workload in Moncton quite oppressive, however, and in August 1989 he resigned and moved to St. Catherines, Ontario.

Mohammad Zahir was born on November 27, 1936, in Ludhiana, India. He received an FSc degree at the University of Punjab in 1953 and a MB, BS at the King Edward Medical School, University of Punjab in 1958. He interned at Mayo Hospital, Lahore, Pakistan, from 1958 to 1959. As a Rhodes Scholar, he studied pathology at Radcliff Infirmary, Oxford, from 1962 to 1965, and received a DPhil from Oxford. He then travelled to the United States where he served as assistant professor of pathology at University of Maryland Medical school in Baltimore from 1968 to 1972. He became a Diplomate of the American Board of Pathology in 1972 and also received his Fellowship from The Royal College of Physicians and Surgeons of Canada in the same year. Why such a brilliant scholar would come to Moncton is anybody's guess. His appointment to the associate staff in 1972 and the active staff in 1973 was apparently only a stepping stone in his odyssey, as he resigned in 1974 to go to British Columbia.

Of the four admissions to the Department of General Practice in 1972, only Mike Antle continues to serve at the hospital to this day. George Michael Antle was born in Halifax on August 26, 1946. After receiving a BA at St. Mary's in 1967, he entered Dalhousie Medical School and graduated with his MD in 1972 after interning at the Victoria General from 1971 to 1972. On graduation he joined the Moncton Medical Clinic where he has remained ever since. With others at the clinic, he has taken a prominent role in teaching residents in the Family Practice Program at Dalhousie and has served as an examiner for the College of Family Practice. While at Dalhousie, he played goalie for various hockey teams and has continued to play hockey since coming to Moncton. He has also served as team doctor for American Hockey League teams in Moncton.

Winston Dykeman has played a prominent role in the medical scene since coming to Moncton in 1972. He was born in Campbellton, New Brunswick, on September 27, 1941, and received a BSc from Mount Allison in 1963 and his MD, from Dalhousie in 1971. He interned at the Victoria General and served from 1971 to 1972 as a resident in the emerging family practice program at Dalhousie from 1970 to 1971. Upon moving to Moncton, he took over the general practice vacated by Orville Messenger. In September 1976, he wished to confine his practice to the care of geriatric patients at his office and home and gave up his hospital responsibilities. In June 1978, he moved to Elsa, Yukon, where he served as company physician for United Keno Hill Mines. He returned, however, to New Brunswick in June 1979 and opened up an office in Hillsborough and joined the active staff of the Albert County Hospital with courtesy privileges at The Moncton Hospital. In March 1983 he terminated work at the Albert County Hospital and changed to active staff privileges at The Moncton Hospital but continued to practice in Hillsborough. He has been on the leading edge of the applications of clinical computer technology in patient care and has devised a prototype computer program called CUPID to follow patients with their risk factors for coronary artery disease. In 1994, he was awarded the "Literary Award" by the College of Family Physicians of Canada.

Carolyn Rideout was born in Grand Falls, New Brunswick, on December

21, 1945. She obtained a BSc at St. Francis Xavier in 1967 and an MD at Dalhousie in 1972 after serving an internship at the Victoria General Hospital from 1971 to 1972. She joined the Moncton Medical Clinic and was appointed to the associate staff in 1972, but departed for Ontario in May 1973.

Dr. Wolfgang Heinz Scholtz was born on July 13, 1943, in Germany, and was educated in Canada receiving his BSc from McGill and his MSc from the University of Montreal before entering medical school at Dalhousie and obtaining his MD in 1972. He set up private practice in Moncton joining the associate staff in general practice, but moved to British Columbia in 1979.

Nine hundred and fifty-seven more patients were admitted in 1972 than in 1971, with an occupancy rate of 82.5 percent and an average stay of 11.5 days. In addition, there were 1,664 newborns admitted to the nursery. The admissions to the Annex were down with 160 admitted versus 190 in 1971. There were 7,471 operations performed, 910 more than in 1971. There were 55,507 visits to the emergency unit, 58,053 radiological examinations, 2,098 radioisotope studies, 13,239 inhalation therapy treatments and 27,428 physiotherapy visits; 12,835 electrocardiograms and 1,318 electroencephalograms were done; 1,405 shock treatments were given, 345 more than the previous year. The outpatient clinics continued to flourish with 322 visits to the Paediatric Clinic, 503 to the Orthopaedic Clinic, 416 to the Arthritis Clinic and 731 to the Well Women Clinic, which had only just started on September 28, 1971. Since all radiotherapy treatments were now given in Saint John, regular follow up Radiotherapy Clinics were now held at the hospital, staffed by the radiotherapists from Saint John, and 1,460 visits were made to this clinic. Including calls to the Dr.Georges-L. Dumont, the ambulance service made 2,983 calls. Including students, the hospital and annex now boasted having 1,158 employees with a budget of $9,806,689. The cost per patient day was now $56.91, more than twice the cost of $23.07 in 1960.

Ever since construction had begun on the Clarke Wing, it was recognized that new space would be required for support services to service the new beds. The government had already done a study of bed requirements in the province, including The Moncton Hospital. As governments are prone to do, it was determined that another study of The Moncton Hospital was to be carried out to determine the requirements for the support services. In June 1973 the Minister of Health authorized a study of the hospital's facilities to develop an updated program including immediate, short-term, and long-term space requirements. The firm of Agnew Peckham and Associates Limited, Health Care Planners and Consultants, was engaged and the final report for Phase One was received in October 1973. Lo and behold, the report found the existing number of beds adequate but recommended additional space for many of the supporting services. At least now the hospital was able to get down to the nitty gritty, and the second phase of the consultants report was planned. This would consist of preparing a Master Plan showing how the various hospital services could be accommodated given the limitations imposed by the existing structures and the availability of space for additions. This Master Plan was to be completed by the end of April 1974 and then, if accepted by both the hospital and government, a process called "Functional Program Planning" was to be proceeded with to determine in detail the functions to be carried out in the areas identified in the Master Plan. Subject to further agreement by the hospital and the provincial government, detailed architectural plans and specifications would then be prepared for the actual renovations and construction.

The Master Program Report, as presented by Agnew Peckham and Associates Ltd., consisted of 73 pages and had 15 main recommendations. The study team included Ruth M. Duffy (Moncton Hospital representative), M.J. Poirier (provincial government representative) and Peter F. Hart, MD, CM, DHA, vice-president of Agnew Peckham. Although the recommendations in the report numbered fifteen, they are best summarized as eleven recommendations in the annual report of 1974:

1. Moncton Hospital should continue in its present role as a regional hospital with a provincial referral role in selected fields. It will need to consolidate existing thinly covered areas of service and to add additional services where appropriate.
2. While the number of acute beds available or planned is likely sufficient, these will not be adequate if the capacity of the longer stay bed services is not increased.
3. We believe it is vitally necessary that effective administration arrangements be made between The Moncton Hospital and hopefully a single large nursing home organization so that there be no impedance in the transfer of patients from the more expensive and less appropriate acute general hospital setting to the less expensive, more appropriate nursing home setting.
4. There is an urgent and priority need to develop and renew the facilities of The Moncton Hospital.
5. The number of anaesthetizing locations should be reduced through provision of a single larger operating and recovery service.
6. A dental clinic is required to serve the dental needs of longer stay patients.
7. Nursing units for rehabilitation and extended care should be provided with larger patient rooms and washrooms and additional support areas for patient dining activity and physiotherapy.
8. Coronary Care Unit—The present unit of five beds is very undersized in terms of support areas.
9. Intensive Care Unit—The present unit of six beds has totally inadequate support services.
10. Psychiatric Unit—Because of the shortage of psychiatric beds and related facilities in the community, we believe this service at The Moncton Hospital should receive a high priority. The psychiatry service should be expanded and include the day care and outpatient

services as well as the inpatient service. Administration co-operation between these modalities of care is essential.

11. Rehabilitation Unit—A general rehabilitation service has recently been established at the hospital. A chief of service is being appointed. Ideally, a unit of forty beds should be provided. Because of the dearth of rehabilitation beds and services in the Moncton area, we strongly recommend establishment of a unit in Moncton.

The opening of the remaining 50 beds in the Clarke Wing was authorized, but with the provision that the Annex be closed and 50 beds be made available in the main hospital for extended care patients. The Annex patients were transferred to The Moncton Hospital and local nursing homes, including the newly opened Villa de Repos Nursing Home, with the last patient transferred on September 1, 1973. The Annex staff were re-located to The Moncton Hospital. Including active treatment and extended care beds, The Moncton Hospital now had a rated bed capacity of 539 beds.

During 1973, the board chairman, Ralph Belyea, retired after serving 11 years on the board and 10 years as chairman. His position as chairman was taken by Howard C. Grayston. Arrangements were completed in early 1973 for a one-year exchange of administrative personnel between The Moncton Hospital and the Royal Free Hospital in London, England. Ruth Duffy, administrative assistant at The Moncton Hospital, went to London at the beginning of October. Miss Juliet LeFanu, a graduate of Trinity College, Dublin, with studies in Hospital Services Administration and a senior administrative assistant at the Royal Free London Hospital, arrived in Moncton to take Miss Duffy's place.

With the opening of the new beds in the Clarke Wing, 18 the extended care beds were located on 1-Parlee to serve as a special Extended Care/Rehabilitation Unit. A multidisciplinary committee with representation from medicine, nursing, physiotherapy, occupational therapy and social services was established to decide on all admissions to the unit and to assess progress at regular intervals. To be admitted, patients had to have the potential to be rehabilitated to home care or at least to nursing home level. A further innovation was the opening on 3-Joyce of a six-bed Day Surgery Unit. On April 4, 1973, an $80,000 project was completed and put into operation to provide facilities for a neurosurgical operating room, induction area and adjacent neuro-radiographic room. In addition, the four-bed Neurosurgical Intensive Care Unit on 3-Clarke was renovated and expanded to six beds in March, 1973.

The influx of new physicians continued during the year with fifteen additions to the medical staff and three new specialities established: neurology, gastroenterology and plastic surgery.

With the opening of the Department of Neurosurgery, it made sense to have a neurologist on staff and the hospital was fortunate to have Dr. Michael A. H. Robertson answer the advertisement in *The Canadian Doctor*. Robertson was born on July 30, 1938, in Inverkeithing, Fife, Scotland. He received his medical degree, an MB, ChB from Edinburgh University in 1960. From 1960 to 1963 he studied internal medicine at Eastern General Hospital, Edinburgh; Deaconess Hospital, Edinburgh; Victoria Hospital, Fife, Scotland; and St. Bartholomew's Hospital, Rochester, England. He then undertook subspecialty training in neurology at Northern General Hospital, Edinburgh, from 1963 to 1964, and Midland Centre for Neurology and Neurosurgery, Birmingham, England, from 1964 to 1965. He received his MRCP in Neurology (Edinburgh) in 1965. He then practised neurology on the staff of the Institute of Neurological Sciences, Glasgow, Scotland, from 1965 to 1967, and at the Royal Infirmary, Dundee, Scotland, from 1967 to 1971. He immigrated to Canada and started practice at the Manitoba Clinic, Winnipeg, in January, 1972, but his love of the sea made him an eager respondent to the ad in *The Canadian Doctor*. Mike was an able neurologist but he liked to tell it "like it is" and kept a Kleenex box on his desk for all the patients that he told, in no uncertain terms that there was no organic cause for their symptoms. He always seemed to need a challenge, and after only five years on the staff, returned to Scotland, but in a most unusual manner. He resigned from the staff and took his 25-foot yacht, *Fuinary*, and sailed across the Atlantic Ocean with his wife and children. He set sail from Norfolk, Virginia on May 14, 1977, arriving in the Azores 28 days later.

Dr. Peter Bright-Asare was born in Ghana on March 26, 1938. After pre-university education in Ghana, he came to Canada in 1960 on a Commonwealth Scholarship and attended Dalhousie for his premed and medical education, obtaining his MD in 1967, after serving a rotating internship at the Victoria General from 1966 to 1967. Postgraduate studies in internal medicine at the Halifax Infirmary and the Victoria General from 1968 to 1969 were followed by two years as a fellow in gastroenterology at the Victoria General from 1969 to 1971, resulting in his obtaining an MSc in biochemistry. He served as a research associate in medicine at Yale University from 1971 to 1972, and as a post doctorate clinical fellow in gastroenterology at Yale New Haven Hospital from 1971 to 1972. He obtained his FRCP(C) in 1972 and then another FRCP(C) in the newly evolved speciality of gastroenterology. After starting practice in Glace Bay in July, 1972, he moved to Moncton and was appointed to the associate staff in May, 1973. On arriving in Moncton, he set up the first Endoscopic Room and GI Functional Laboratory at the hospital. Although there was some initial concern among the staff that maybe the results of endoscopic exams did not correlate well with radiological findings and the pathological findings at surgery, the new method of diagnosing gastrointestinal disorders soon became a routine procedure in the investigation of GI disorders. He was appointed to the Medical Advisory Board of the Canadian Foundation for Ileitis and Colitis in March 1977. Peter was very interested in research and as a result of his research he was able to get valuable equipment donated by drug companies. Equipment for a GI Motility Lab was donated in March 1979, and a paediatric panendoscope was donated to the

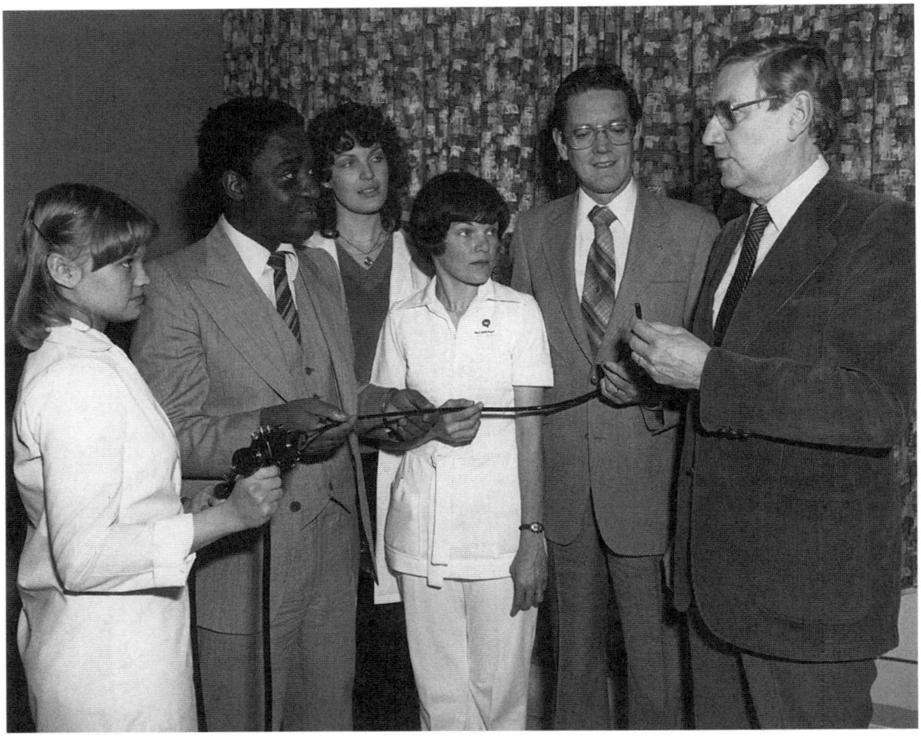

Dr. W.A. Oatway makes a presentation of a gastroduodenoscope to Dr. Peter Bright-Asare on behalf of the Friends of the Moncton Hospital. From left to right: unidentified, Dr. Peter Bright-Asare, Jean Ann MacDonald, Carolyn Lewis, Robert MacQuade—Chairman of the Board, and Dr. W.A. Oatway.

hospital in 1980 by Smith, Kline and French Company. This equipment was used in a study of Peter's entitled "Placebo versus Meloclopramide versus Cimetidine in Gastrointestinal Reflux Disease," the results of which were published in the *Journal of Clinical Gastroenterology*. The *Moncton Transcript* of September 9, 1978, reported on a research paper of his on "Biomechanics of Low Back Pain due to Manual Handling of Materials," co-authored with M. El Bassoussi, Associate Professor of Engineering at the Université de Moncton, and R. Cadela, PhD, another professor at the Université de Moncton. This work would seem a little far removed from the world of gastroenterology. Peter's forte, however, seemed to be the world of research and academia and in March 1980 he left Moncton to assume the post of chairman of the Division of Gastroenterology at Cook County Hospital, University of Chicago. After a five-year stint at this institution, he moved to Los Angeles.

Douglas Stewart Inglis was born in Saint Thomas, Ontario, on January 29, 1941. He obtained a BA from Mount Allison in 1961 and an MD from Dalhousie in 1966. He was appointed to the courtesy staff in general practice in 1966 while he practised in Shediac, but he deserted general practice to take up plastic surgery in 1968. After training at the Victoria General Hospital in Halifax, the Peter Bent Brigham in Boston and the Victoria Hospital in

London, Ontario, he obtained his Fellowship in Plastic Surgery and was appointed to the staff in November 1973. He was the first plastic surgeon on the staff but was assigned to the general surgical staff as it was not felt practical from an administrative standpoint to have a one-man department.

Although started as a one-man department, the Department of Neurosurgery was expanded to two people in 1973. Kail Habib Kazi was born on October 18, 1937, in Satara, Bombay, India. In 1955 he received a BSc from D.J. Sind Government Science College, Karachi, and then in 1960, an MB, BS degree from Don Medical College, Karachi, Pakistan. He moved to North America in 1960, interning at Our Lady of Lourdes Hospital, Camden, New Jersey, from 1962 to 1963. He then served a residency in neurology at the Philadelphia General Hospital from 1963 to 1964 and a year of general surgery at Presbyterian Hospital, Philadelphia, from 1954 to 1965. This was followed by a three-year residency in neurosurgery at the Hospital of the University of Pennsylvania from 1966 to 1969 and two years at University Hospital, Saskatoon, from 1970 to 1972. He became certified by the American Board of Neurosurgery in 1970 and obtained his Canadian Fellowship in 1971. After all the specialist training, he obtained his LMCC in 1972. He first started working at The Moncton Hospital as a resident in neurosurgery in October 1972, until he was appointed to the active staff in March 1973. He proved to be a proficient neurosurgeon and got along well with his colleagues on staff. Although a good operator, he was somewhat slow at first, and seemed to lack confidence and while able to give a good consultation, would often have to consult with Dr. Tucker before committing himself to a course of action. During his stay, he went to the University of Western Ontario in London to learn the technique and became quite expert in the temporal-cerebral artery by-pass surgery which enjoyed a place in the neurosurgeons armamentarium until later studies showed the surgery had no benefit in preventing strokes. As he grew in stature as a neurosurgeon in his own right, I think he found his association with Dr. Tucker too suffocating and moved to the Regional Hospital in Saint John where he was able to work in a less confining environment. There he established a reputation as an excellent neurosurgeon, but, unfortunately, his surgical career has been cut short because of visual problems.

With the addition of new surgeons, one of the most pressing needs was in anaesthesia and the department was fortunate to obtain the services of Dr. Juliet Gill (née Matthews). Juliet was born in Llandeila, Wales, on February 16, 1941. She graduated from St. Bartholomew's Hospital Medical College, London, with an MB, BS in 1964 and interned at Bethnal Green Hospital, London, from 1964 to 1965. After serving as an obstetric house surgeon from July to December, 1965, at Edgware General Hospital, London, she took anaesthesia training at University College Hospital, London, and Westminster Hospital, London, from January 1966 to December 1968 and was awarded a Fellowship of the Faculty of Anaesthetists Royal College of Surgeons, England, in 1968. She served as a registrar in anaesthesia at the

Hospital for Sick Children, Great Ormond Street, London, from June 1967 until March 1971. She then immigrated to Canada and served on the anaesthetic staff of the Isaak Walton Killam Hospital from 1971 to 1972. She received her FRCP(C) in anaesthesia in 1972. After moving to Newfoundland for a very short period, she came to Moncton along with her husband, Darshan Gill. She was a very personable woman but only stayed on staff until June 1975 when she left on a leave of absence with her husband who wished to take postgraduate work in urology in Toronto. After their stint in Toronto, the pair departed for south of the border to the good old USA.

Juliet's husband, Darshan Gill, was born in Nasrala, India, on June 21, 1936, and was educated in the United Kingdom, taking his premedical work at Aberdeen University from 1956 to 1957 and his medical education at London Hospital Medical College receiving his MB, BS in 1962. He interned at London Hospital and Whippe Cross Hospital from 1962 to 1963 and served as a surgical resident at several London hospitals from 1963 to 1971, receiving his FRCS (England) in 1970. In 1971 he was a research fellow in surgery in the liver unit of Royal Free Hospital, University of London. On coming to Canada, he served another year as a resident in surgery in the Dalhousie program from 1971 to 1972 and obtained his FRCS(C) in 1972 along with his LMCC. He initially went to Newfoundland to start a surgical practice, but when his wife answered the call for an opening in the anaesthetic department in Moncton, he was accepted on the general surgical staff. After serving on the staff for a two-year period, he took a leave of absence to study urology in Toronto but after this additional training, he headed for the United States.

In September, 1971, Dr. MacLellan had a coronary thrombosis which put the Orthopaedic Department back to a two-man call schedule for a six-month period of time. Consequently, the department felt it was a good time for another orthopaedic surgeon on staff. Attempts to obtain a recent Canadian graduate were unsuccessful but Dr. W.S.B. Loosmore responded in May, 1972, to an ad placed in the *British Medical Journal*. Brian Loosmore was born on September 18, 1932, in Neath, Glamorgan, Wales. After premedical education at the University of Wales, he received his medical degree MB, BCh from Welsh National School of Medicine in 1956, and his MRCS, LRCP (London). He interned at the United Cardiff Hospital and the Merthyr General Hospital from 1956 to 1957. He did national service with the Royal Army Medical Corps from 1957 to 1959 in Malaya. Between 1959-1962, his surgical training consisted of a stint as senior house officer in general surgery, Swansea Hospital, senior house officer in orthopaedic surgery at Cardiff Royal Infirmary and senior house officer in thoracic surgery at Sully Hospital, Cardiff. From 1962 to 1967 he served a short service commission in the Royal Army Medical Corps as specialist and senior specialist in surgery and received his FRCS (Edinburgh) in 1967. From then until he came to Canada, he served as a locums at various hospitals in England both as an orthopaedic surgeon and as a general surgeon. At the time of his appointment

the new by-laws stated that qualifications for surgical appointments required certification by the Royal College of Physicians and Surgeons of Canada or its equivalent. The Credentials Committee questioned whether or not his training was equivalent but the Medical Council of New Brunswick accepted him for registration as a specialist and licensed him to practise under Section 16B of the Medical Act. Brian was a very religious and caring person. Although he responded to the ad in May 1972, he did not appear on the scene until the spring of 1973, because he had to fulfil a missionary obligation in Bangladesh. During this trip to Bangladesh he brought a little girl back to England for adoption and this resulted in further delay as he had to wait for the adoption to come through before coming to Canada. I suspect his wife was a little more of a religious persuasion than Brian as no television or newspapers were allowed in their home. Brian, nevertheless, always managed to buy and read a paper at the hospital. Unfortunately, later events were to prove that the misgivings of the Credentials Committee should have been heeded. Although he seemed to be well versed in the treatment of trauma, it subsequently became apparent that his knowledge of treatment of adult and children's orthopaedic problems was not up to the standards of orthopaedic practice in North America. The Worker's Compensation Board criticized the clinical work of Dr. Loosmore and the Medical Advisory Committee, thereafter, requested a review of his privileges by the Department of Orthopaedics and the Credentials Committee. This review resulted in a recommendation that an orthopaedic consultation should be required on all cases of spine surgery and he would require an assistant on all WCB cases. In February, 1976, the Royal College of Physicians and Surgeons of Canada ruled that he would require an extra year of approved residency to be eligible to write the fellowship examinations in orthopaedics. With these restrictions on his practice, Dr. Loosmore chose to leave Moncton and go to Alberta.

There were 13 additions to the Department of General Practice in 1971.

Michael Burslem was born on February 7, 1933, in Fyzabad, Trinidad, West Indies. He received his university education in Canada, graduating from McGill with a BSc in 1955. In 1957, he started working with the Canadian Meteorological Service, but resigned in August 1961, and entered King's College to train for the ministry with the intention of serving in the north. After finishing at King's, however, he had a change of heart and entered medical school at Dalhousie and graduated with his MD degree in 1970. He interned at the Victoria General from 1969 to 1970 and did a residency in psychiatry at Dalhousie from 1970 to 1973, but again did not pursue this career and entered into general practice in Moncton, joining the associate staff in April 1973. He continued in general practice until August, 1990, when he moved to Guelph to work in the Homewood Health Centre.

Dr. Kim DeWare was born in Halifax on July 7, 1947, while his father, a Moncton native, was attending Dalhousie. His father, Dr. Ralph DeWare, returned to Moncton on graduation to establish his dental practice and served on the dental staff of the hospital. Kim took his premedical education at Mount Allison and received his MD from Dalhousie after interning in Halifax, which included a stint at The Moncton Hospital. He joined the Moncton Medical Clinic and has been a stalwart of the Department of General Practice ever since. Besides serving on numerous committees and as chief of the department, he has served as the medical staff's representative on the Board of Trustees.

William J. Taylor, another addition to the Moncton Medical Clinic, has continued to practise there until the present. Bill was born in Sydney Mines, Nova Scotia, on August 23, 1946, and received a BSc from St Francis Xavier in 1967 and an MD from Dalhousie in 1972. He interned at the Victoria General and the Halifax Infirmary from 1971 to 1972 and then entered practice briefly in Summerside before coming to Moncton in January, 1973.

Norman Shore was another addition to the expanding Moncton Medical Clinic. He was born in Glace Bay, Nova Scotia, on May 3, 1944, and received his BSc from McGill and his MD from Dalhousie in 1972. He interned at the Victoria General Hospital from 1971 to 1972 and pursued a further year of training in the family medicine program at Dalhousie from 1973 to 1973. He obtained a leave of absence from the staff in July 1975 to take postgraduate studies in radiology but never returned to Moncton.

Dr. J.M. Daley also joined the Moncton Medical Clinic. Michael is a Moncton native, born on December 9, 1946. He went to St. F.X. obtaining a BSc in 1967 and then an MD from Dalhousie in 1972. He interned in the Dalhousie program from 1971 to 1972. After starting practice in Kensington, Prince Edward Island, he returned to his native Moncton, but left in 1974, after only a year on staff, to take postgraduate work in radiology. On his return to Moncton, he joined the radiology staff of the Dr. Georges-L. Dumont Hospital.

In 1973, Drs. Brace and Geldart left the Moncton Medical Clinic and started the Lakeside (Riverview) Medical Centre in a new building and mall complex. Dr. David W. Hiltz was among the first to join them in this new clinic. He was born in Kentville, Nova Scotia, on February 9, 1945, and attended Mount Allison, from which he received a BSc in 1967, and then moved on to Dalhousie, obtaining his MD in 1972. From 1971 to 1972, he interned at various Halifax hospitals in the Dalhousie intern program and then set up practice in Dartmouth, Nova Scotia, but moved to Moncton in April 1973, to join the new Riverview Medical Clinic. He was certified in family practice by the College of Family Practice in 1980. He has continued as a senior partner in the Riverview Medical Clinic and has served a term as president of the medical staff.

Another charter member of the Lakeside Medical Clinic was Eric Pasquet. Eric was born in Montreal on April 10, 1947, and raised in Halifax. He attended Dalhousie where he obtained a BSc in 1968 and an MD in 1973. He interned at the Victoria General Hospital and the Halifax Infirmary from 1972 to 1973. He enjoyed a busy general practice, but even in those days it was apparent that he had lots of patience and enjoyed working with children.

He was certified by the College of Family Practice in 1980, the same year that he was awarded a black belt in karate. In 1981 he embarked on a residency program in paediatrics, serving at the Foothills Hospital, Calgary (1981-1982), the Alberta Children's Hospital (1982-1983 and 1984-1985), with a year at the Isaak Walton Killam Hospital from 1983 to 1984. He then served as a clinical fellow in pediatric emergency medicine at the Children's Hospital of Western Ontario. He received his Fellowship in pediatrics from the Royal College in 1985. We were, indeed, fortunate that he was a Maritimer and married one, as, otherwise, he may have succumbed to the offers to remain in London, Ontario.

A.K. (Khi Kiam) Jong was born in Malaysia on April 24, 1944. His education in Canada was sponsored by the Canadian International Development Association (CIDA) and he settled on Dalhousie University where he obtained his BSc in 1969 and his MD in 1973. He interned at various Halifax hospitals as well as the Saint John General and St. Joseph's Hospital in the Dalhousie rotating internship program from 1972 to 1973. Tony joined Dr. Gerry Reyes in general practice in Moncton. He enjoyed his stay in Moncton, but not the weather, so in 1981, he moved to British Columbia.

Another addition to the staff in 1973 was Roger Leger who was born on March 10, 1942, in Saint John, New Brunswick. He received a BA from the Université de Moncton in 1964 and then spent a year at Saint Mary's University from 1964 to 1965 before entering Ottawa University, from which he received an MD in 1969. After interning at the Saint John General Hospital from 1969 to 1970, he served in the Canadian Armed Forces from 1970 to 1973 including a year from 1972 to 1973, in internal medicine at the National Defence Medical Centre. He continued in general practice and became the penitentiary physician to Dorchester Penitentiary but then stopped general practice to serve as Regional Medical Officer for Correction Services Canada, although still continuing to work assigned shifts in the outpatient department. He found that pushing paper was not his niche, however, and he eventually resigned from the penitentiary service. In 1987, he was again engaged in family practice and part-time in the emergency department, but in 1988 he abandoned family practice and joined the group of emergency room physicians performing full time duties in this newly emerging department. Later he would resume general practice but continue as an emergency room physician on a part-time basis.

Lakhlir Ranjit Nayak (Lucky) was born in Delhi, India, on April 27, 1949. He received a PPC undergraduate degree at the Bangalore University and then an MB, BS degree in 1971 from the Bangalore Medical College. On coming to Canada he interned at The Moncton Hospital from 1971 to 1973, obtaining his LMCC in 1973. He then set up a general practice in Petitcodiac, New Brunswick, and was admitted to the courtesy staff. He has remained in Petitcodiac ever since, but was admitted to the active staff in 1990.

A delightful addition to the medical staff in 1973 was Luella Smith. She was born on November 15, 1948, in Maonils, in the Philippines, where she received her early education and a BSc from the University of the Philippines, Quezon City, in 1968. She came to Canada and received her MD from Dalhousie in 1973 after interning at the Victoria General from 1972 to 1973. Along with her husband, Ed, she was appointed to the active staff of the Albert County Hospital and the courtesy staff of The Moncton Hospital in 1973, and kept this status until 1980. From 1980 to 1982, she served as an emergency room physician at the Victoria General Hospital. She then returned to family practice in Alma from 1982 to 1984, and also served as a part-time emergency room physician at The Moncton Hospital. In 1984, she became a full-time emergency physician at The Moncton Hospital, a role she continues to perform in an admirable manner. Always smiling, she seems unflappable and conscientiously goes about her tasks. Since 1980 she has been an instructor throughout the Maritimes in ACLS courses. She has boundless energy and, besides her busy professional life, has the responsibility of raising six children. Yet, she still finds time for community affairs. Since 1982, she has been a member of the Alma Consolidated Home and School association and since 1986, a member of the District 4 School Board. She has been active in the Scout Movement, serving since 1988 as secretary of the Alma Group Committee, Scouts Canada. She has served as Leader of the Duke of Edinburgh's Award in New Brunswick and since 1992 has been chairman of the Albert, West, Kent, Duke of Edinburgh Awards in New Brunswick. When she finds the time, her hobbies include photography, sailing, and cross country skiing. She also enjoys a reputation as a gourmet cook.

Luella's husband, Willard Edwin Smith, was born on January 15, 1946, in Wolfville, Nova Scotia. He attended Acadia University and CSC Royal Roads, receiving a BSc in 1967. He then entered Dalhousie University, receiving his MD in 1973 after interning at the Victoria General from 1972 to 1973. He was appointed to the associate staff in the Department of General Practice in July 1973 and practised at the Albert County Hospital. In 1980 he returned to Halifax to take up a residency in psychiatry, but never completed it and returned in 1982 to the Department of General Practice at the hospital. During his stay in Albert he gained recognition for his boatbuilding skills when he made a concrete hull sailing boat.

Ernest Douglas Swersky was born in Saint John's, Newfoundland, on February 9, 1944, and received his BSc from Dalhousie in 1968 and his MD in 1973. He interned in various Halifax hospitals as well as The Moncton Hospital from 1972 to 1973 and then set up a general practice in Shediac and was appointed to the associate staff. He resigned in 1978, and moved to Texas.

Admissions to the Annex were down to 137 for the year and would now cease, as a result of its closure. A total of 13,547 adults and children were admitted to the main hospital, as well as 1,771 newborns; 8,198 operations were performed. Emergency unit visits increased by 9,479 over the previous year, but radiological examinations showed a decrease of 5,646 to 52,407 and inhalation therapy had a decrease of 2,612 to 10,627 treatments. These decreases occurred as a result of a six-week strike of technical staff in February and March 1973. Other departments showed small increases in visits, with 28,893 physiotherapy visits, 2,270 radioisotope studies, 1,557 electroencephalograms and 13,976 electrocardiograms; 1,428 shock treatments were given and a new Audiogram Service was started with 10 audiograms performed; 296 children were seen at the Paediatric Clinic, 450 at the Orthopaedic Clinic, 521 at the Arthritis Clinic, 906 at the Well Women Clinic and 1,488 at the Radiotherapy Clinic; 3,383 ambulance calls were made.

The Master Program for the hospital was received from the consultants, Agnew Peckham and Associates Ltd., in October 1973, and by October 1974, they had developed a Master Plan based on the Master Program. The main purpose of the Master Plan was to graphically illustrate the expansion of the Hospital. In general, the plan called for a hospital of about 600 beds with space of about 800 square feet per bed. The existing space was 570 square feet per bed. The plans called for new construction of 160,000 square feet with renovations to 80,000 square feet of the existing space (281,476 square feet). Most of the new construction would be to the south and to the west. This plan had to be approved by the hospital board and the government. Relief was still a long way off as the next step would be to develop a Functional Program. This would involve a detailed determination of the manner in which the services would be enclosed in the space provided for in the Master Plan. Then, there would be the hiring of architects to prepare the necessary plans.

In March 1974 a three-day work stoppage was staged by the non-professional employees of the hospital, marking the first time in the history of the hospital that services had to be curtailed. Similar work stoppages would occur over the next year requiring cancellation of admissions and pressing the medical staff into providing non-medical services.

In November the School of Radiological Technicians was surveyed by representatives of the Canadian Association of Radiologists, Canadian Association of X-ray Technicians, Canadian Medical Association and the Canadian Hospital Association, and received renewed accreditation with high praise for the staff, instructors and facilities of the school. During the year, the Canadian Medical Association carried out an inspection of the hospital's intern program and not only approved the program, but gave approval for the program to be increased from twelve to fifteen interns a year.

Lloyd Secord, who had been an assistant administrator of the hospital since 1970, resigned, to become administrator of the Kings County Memorial Hospital in Sussex.

An innovation in the psychiatric department was the opening of a Psychiatric Day Hospital in the Professional Arts Building adjacent to premises occupied by the Mental Health clinic. Neal Stevens, Administrator of the Mental Health Clinic in Region 1, was also appointed as an assistant administrator for the hospital.

Historically, the function of the Inservice Education Department had been primarily oriented to the Department of Nursing. During the year its responsibilities were enlarged, under the direction of Karen Croll, to include the inservice educational needs of all departments of the hospital.

The hospital had followed the government policy and established a Therapeutic Abortion Clinic at The Moncton Hospital. While complying with the law, the hospital had no desire to serve as an abortion centre for the province, and the board of trustees passed the following policy on abortions at a meeting in October, 1974:

> That applications for therapeutic abortions will not be accepted for patients residing outside of Hospital Region 1 as defined in the 1972 Annual Report of the Deputy Minister to the Minister of Health (defined as the counties of Kent, Westmorland and Albert) and the Sussex area of Kings County, except in unusual circumstances, a procedure may be approved at the discretion of the Therapeutic Abortion Committee.

No new departments were formed, but the influx of new physicians continued in 1974, with additions to the Departments of Internal Medicine, Obstetrics and Gynaecology, Psychiatry and General Practice. Dr. Donald Pelky was the first fully qualified oral surgeon appointed to the dental staff. Dr. Alban Haché and Dr. D. deYturralde joined the orthopaedic staff of the Dr. Georges-L. Dumont Hospital and the courtesy staff of The Moncton Hospital.

1974 saw the recruitment of two new members to the Department of Internal Medicine: Dr. C.D. Douglas and Dr. Peter Lightfoot who have continued to have distinguished careers at The Moncton Hospital since then.

Dr. George David Douglas was born in Halifax on December 29, 1939, and after taking premed and medicine at Dalhousie, graduated with the MD, CM degree in 1965. He interned at the Victoria General and Halifax Infirmary Hospitals (1964-65). He then undertook training in internal medicine with a subspecialty in cardiology. He served as a resident in internal medicine at the Victoria General from 1965 to 1966 and 1967 to 1968 with a year at the Montreal General from 1968 to 1969. He served as a cardiac resident at the Victoria General from 1966 to 1967 and then as a fellow in cardiology from 1969 to 1970. He had further cardiology training as honorary assistant registrar at the National Heart Institute, London, England, from 1970 to 1971. He obtained his FRCP(C) and was made a Fellow of the American College of Cardiology. He served as an assistant professor of medicine and cardiology at Dalhousie University and served on the staffs of the Victoria General, Camp Hill and Victoria General Hospitals from 1971 to 1974 when he was induced to leave the academic life and come to Moncton. When not available for cardiology consults, David can usually be found casting his rod on some salmon stream.

Peter Lightfoot was born in Halifax, June 16, 1943, receiving a BA from Dalhousie in 1965 and an MD (cum laude) in 1970. He interned at the Victoria General and the Isaak Walton Killam Hospital from 1989 to 1970. He did a residency in internal medicine from 1970 to 1974 at the Victoria

General, Halifax Infirmary and Camp Hill Hospitals receiving his FRCP(C) in 1974. He was appointed to the medical staff in 1974 although he did not begin to admit patients until January 1975. Although a general internist, he has had a special interest in gastroenterology. An accomplished musician on both the organ and piano, he is often requested to play at hospital functions.

Dr. Aristotelis Criticos was born on November 30, 1924, in Iasi, Rumania, and received a bachelor's degree at the National Lyceum, Iasi, Rumania, in 1943 and an MD from University of Iasi in 1952. He came to Canada in 1962 and served an internship at Hôtel Dieu of Saint Joseph, Tracadie, from 1962 to 1963. He did a residency in psychiatry at Maisonneuve Hospital, Montreal, from 1960 to 1962, Campbellton Provincial Hospital from 1963 to 1964, Notre Dame Hospital, Montreal, from 1964 to 1965 and at Ste. Justine Hospital, Montreal, from 1965 to 1966. He became certified in psychiatry by the Royal College in 1968 and practised psychiatry on the staff of the Provincial Hospital in Campbellton from 1967 to 1970. After serving on the psychiatric staff of The Moncton Hospital he took a leave of absence in 1978. In 1984, he was serving as a psychiatrist at the Moncton Mental Health Clinic, but he was denied courtesy privileges at The Moncton Hospital.

The two new additions to the Department of Obstetrics and Gynaecology were Dr. Arman Topakian and Dr. Carol Bergquist. Dr Topakian was born in Istanbul, Turkey, on May 6, 1939, and attended the University of Istanbul where he received a BSc and then an MD in 1967. He interned at St. Mary's Hospital, Montreal, in 1967 and did a residency in obstetrics and gynaecology at the Royal Victoria, St. Mary's, Lakeshore, and Queen Elizabeth Hospitals in Montreal from 1970 to 1973 becoming certified in 1973 by the Quebec College of Physicians and Surgeons in obstetrics and gynaecology. He remained on the staff only until October 1975.

Dr. Carol Bergquist was born in Camrose, Alberta, on November 29, 1941, and after premed at Camrose Lutheran College and the University of Alberta, she attended medical school at the University of Alberta, receiving her MD in 1967. She interned at the Royal Alexander Hospital from 1967 to 1968 and then embarked on a residency program in obstetrics and gynaecology. She spent her first year at Morrisania Montifiore Hospital, Bronx, New York, from 1968 to 1969 and then completed her training in Canada at the Royal Victoria Hospital in Montreal from 1970 to 1973, followed by a year as an infertility fellow at the Royal Victoria from 1973 to 1974. Like Dr Topakian, her stay in Moncton was short, departing from the city in the summer of 1975.

It had been nearly twenty years since a husband and wife team joined The Moncton Hospital medical staff and Dr. George Allison Prescott and Dr. Shirley Prescott were only the second husband and wife team to join the staff. Al Prescott was born in Bournemouth, England, on January 5, 1948, but grew up in Canada and received a BSc at University of New Brunswick in 1969 and his MD from Dalhousie in 1974. He interned in the Dalhousie program at the Victoria General, the Izaak Walton Killam, Grace Maternity and St.John's General hospitals from 1973 to 1974. He has continued to enjoy a busy general practice in Moncton ever since.

Dr. Shirley Prescott was born on April 1, 1949, in North Sydney, Nova Scotia, and after taking premed and medical education at Dalhousie, received her MD in 1974. From 1973 to 1974 she served her internship at various hospitals in the Dalhousie rotating internship program. She remained on the active staff of The Moncton Hospital until November 1983, when she relocated to London, Ontario, following her divorce from Al.

Another addition to the Department of General Practice was Douglas Arthur Keith. Doug was born in Campbellton on March 30, 1946. He graduated in pharmacy from Dalhousie in 1968 but then chose to enter the medical profession instead, and continued on at Dalhousie, receiving his MD in 1974 after interning in the Dalhousie rotating intern program from 1973 to 1974. He joined the new Lakeside Medical Clinic. In 1975 he took over as Health Services Physician for The Moncton Hospital and continued with this job until 1983, when, with Dr. David Hiltz, he began working part-time as penitentiary physician for Correctional Services Canada at Dorchester Penitentiary and Westmorland Institutions. He has since given up the penitentiary physician post, but continues with a family practice at the Riverview Medical Clinic.

Dr. Donald Pelky was born on January 31, 1944, in Woodstock, New Brunswick. He received a BSc from University of New Brunswick in 1965 and a DDS from Dalhousie in 1969. He served an internship in oral surgery at the Victoria General Hospital from 1971 to 1972 and a residency in oral surgery from 1972 to 1974 receiving his MSc degree from Dalhousie at the end of his training. He remains the sole oral surgeon on the hospital staff.

The burden to the orthopaedic department of trying to serve both hospitals was helped with the appointments of Dr. Alban Haché and Dr. Daniel deYturrralde to the active staff of the Dr. Georges-L. Dumont Hospital and the consulting staff of The Moncton Hospital. Alban Haché had previously served on the staff in general practice before pursing his orthopaedic training at McGill and the Royal Victoria Hospital. Daniel deYturrralde was born in Montreal on May 14, 1942, and received a BA from St. Francis Xavier in 1962 and an MD, CM from McGill in 1968. He served a rotating internship at the Montreal General Hospital from 1968-69, and then a year of general surgery, followed by three years of orthopaedics at the same hospital. He became certified and received his FRCS in 1973.

Admissions of adults and children in 1974 totalled 13,320 with 1701 newborns also admitted. The cost of running the hospital was $12,900,067 at an average of $76.80 per patient per day. Every service in the hospital showed an increase except for the outpatient department which showed a decrease in number of visits, for the first time. This perhaps, was a reflection on the large number of general practitioners who had joined the staff in the previous three years making it easier to be seen in the doctor's office. Examinations carried out by the various services included electrocardiograms—16,026; electroencephalograms—1,978; physiotherapy—22,660; occupational therapy—3,601; radioisotope studies—2.923; radiological exams—63,872 and gastrointestinal exams—583. There were now nine Outpatient Clinics with the number of patients seen at each as follows: Arthritis—568; Cardiology—55; Diabetes—142; Diet Counselling—260; Hyerlipoproteinemia—53; Obesity—163 with 500 additional obesity weight checks; Orthopaedic—275; Paediatric—253 and Radiotherapy—1,456. The Orthopaedic Clinic was showing a gradual decline. This decline started with the introduction of medicare so that now more patients were seen in the doctor's office and also the decline in the number of post polio patients.

Inflation was roaring in 1974, and with escalating costs, governments were unsure how to cope with its money pit, Medicare, which was demanding ever increasing amounts of money in order to supply the demands of both the users and the providers. Twenty years later, governments continue to struggle with this and have not found a solution to the problem or the political will to tackle it. In the federal election of 1974, many a nurse vowed that she would not vote for Stanfield and have him freeze her wages, so voted for Trudeau, only to have him impose wage and price controls.

The studies for expansion of the hospital were done, but no response was forthcoming from the government during 1975 and no permission was received to proceed with any of the recommendations of the Agnew Peckham and Associates Master plan. In fact, government was cutting the hospital's budget and the hospital was informed by the Department of Health that the plan to provide a new laundry at The Moncton Hospital must be deferred. There was to be no present for the laundry manager, Joe Lombard, who was celebrating his 25 years of service to the hospital. The government approved a capital equipment budget in 1975 which was less than one-third the amount requested. Meanwhile, the cost of running the hospital was escalating with total operating expenses of $15,663,308 ($90.90 per patient day) in 1975, compared to $12,377,846 ($73.70 per patient day) in 1974. One item obtained from the government was a grant of $11,500 towards the purchase of a new ambulance. In addition, the government announced in September a plan to implement a training program for ambulance personnel. Among new equipment obtained was a new centralized medical record transcription service with special telephones hooked up to a bank of recorders in the medical records department. The age of computers also made its appearance in the hospital at this time with the installation of a computerized scheduling system by Teldata, a division of the New Brunswick Telephone Company. Juliet LeFanu from the Royal Free Hospital in London, who had exchanged places with Ruth Duffy in Administration for a year, remained in Canada and went to work with Teldata in developing the computer program. In addition, the hospital's finance department was in the process of becoming computerized.

The hospital was surveyed again this year by the Canadian Hospital Council on Hospital Accreditation and received full accreditation.

Stuart Stratton, long time legal advisor to the hospital was appointed Judge of the Court of Queen's Bench of New Brunswick and was replaced by George Rideout.

The hospital had to contend with a three-day work stoppage in February, when all the nurses in New Brunswick resigned as a result of a labour dispute. August witnessed another change in nursing practice when The Moncton Hospital School of Nursing graduated its last class of hospital based trained nurses. Over the span of 69 years, 1,436 nurses had graduated from this school. The A.J. MacMaster School of Nursing had started in 1974 with its first class, but student nurses were no longer expected to give primary nursing service, although they would use the hospital for clinical training. Mrs. Wright, an assistant administrator of the hospital and director of the School of Nursing from 1953 to 1975, stated that she was a little sad to be graduating the last class, but not completely so, as "nursing education has been due a change for some time. And I've worked quite hard with the New Brunswick Association of Registered Nurses to bring about the change, feeling it would be better." In conjunction with the closing of the school, a four-day alumnae reunion was held with over 450 alumnae members in attendance. Credit for the organization and planning of the event goes to the Alumnae Executive that included the following: Miss A.J. MacMaster, honorary president; Audrey Oke, president; Joan Allain, first vice-president; Karen Johnson, second vice-president; Nancy Bishop, secretary; and Edith Fairweather, treasurer.

With the closing of the School of Nursing, Mrs. Wright gave up her dual role as director of nursing and assistant administrator to serve full time as an assistant administrator. The post of director of nursing was filled by Myrna Sherrard. She graduated from The Moncton Hospital School of Nursing in 1958. Following graduation, she took a three month course in psychiatric nursing at the McLean Hospital School of Nursing in Belmont, Massachusetts. For several years, she served on the faculty of The Moncton Hospital School of Nursing, and in 1965 she took a leave of absence to take her Bachelor of Nursing Degree from the McGill School for Graduate Nurses. Upon her return to Moncton in 1967, she became this Hospital's first nurse clinician and in June 1970 was appointed associate director of nursing.

Despite financial restraints, the medical staff felt the hospital could not stand still but must seek new equipment and services to remain in the forefront of modern medical practice. Strong representation was made to the provincial government for the purchase of a CAT (Computerized Axial Tomography) Scanner. Following a survey of the obstetrical and nursery facilities of the hospital by a team from Dalhousie University, a multidisciplinary Perinatal Intensive Care Committee was formed to study the needs of the hospital for improved facilities in these areas. This committee subsequently recommended a Neonatal Service in the Hospital and the job was on to recruit a neonatologist and convince the government of the need for such a service.

With government supplying less money, the hospital was fortunate to have the assistance of many private organizations. The Friends of the Moncton Hospital Foundation was investigating the feasibility of helping to purchase a CAT Scanner. The Fort Moncton Chapter of the IODE provided $1,500 for the purchase of a fetal monitor and the Sir Charles G.D. Roberts Chapter, IODE, donated $500 for the purchase of a Jobst pressure pump. The Moncton Lions' Club donated a TV set and the West Riverview Rotary Club a ping-pong table for the rehabilitation wing. The Ladies' Hospital Auxiliary provided a television set for the psychiatric ward and the Lions' Club provided five sets for the pediatric ward.

Several changes occurred in the organization of the medical staff. Dr. Victor McLaughlin resigned as chief of staff and was replaced by Dr. C.E. Doyle. Dr. W. Brenton Stewart resigned as chief of radiology and was replaced by Dr. Kenneth Tulle. Dr. Louis Gaudet took over as head of the School of Radiological Technology. Dr. Alfred Bastarache resigned as chief of the laboratory and was replaced by Dr. Aubrey Hudson. There were only six new additions to the medical staff in 1975: Dr. Sheldon Rubin, Dr. Aubrey Hudson, Dr. K. Patel, Dr. George Boyd, Dr. A.C. Bond and Dr. Terry Jones. Of the six, only Dr. Rubin and Dr. Bond have continued to provide for the health needs of the community served by this hospital. Dr. Cynthia Watson was appointed to the courtesy staff after joining her husband, Dr. Trevor Watson, at the Albert County Hospital.

Dr. Sheldon Rubin was born in Moncton on February 10, 1943, the son of Mike Rubin, a prominent merchant. He received his premedical and medical training at Dalhousie University, graduating in 1969 with his MD degree after a rotating internship at Dalhousie (1968-69). He embarked on a residency program at Dalhousie taking internal medicine (1969-71) and then going to Princess Margaret Hospital in Toronto as a research fellow in haematology (1971-73) and returning to Dalhousie for two more years of residency in haematology (1973-75). He received his FRCP(C) in both internal medicine and haematology in 1974. On returning to his native Moncton, he has proved to be one of the hardest working and most dedicated physicians on the staff.

Dr. Aubrey Densmore Hudson was a Moncton native, born on November 28, 1917. After serving in the RCAF during the Second World War, he entered Dalhousie University taking his premedical and medical training, graduating in the class of 1954 with a MD, CM. He interned at the Victoria General Hospital from 1953 to 1954. From 1954 to 1955, he served a fellowship in pathology at Queen Elizabeth Hospital, Birmingham, England. He did a two-year residency in pathology at the Saint John General Hospital from 1955 to 1957 and then another year in England at St. Mary's Hospital, London, from 1957 to 1958, followed by a year at the Montreal Children's Hospital, from 1958 to 1959. He received his FRCP(C) in Pathology in 1959, as well as his Fellowship in Pathology from the Royal

College of Pathologists in Great Britain. He served as pathologist at Soldiers Memorial Hospital in Campbellton from 1959 to 1965. He then moved west, serving as pathologist at the Calgary General and Grace Hospitals from 1965 to 1975. From 1970 to 1975, he was an associate professor of pathology at the University of Calgary. After being appointed to the head of the Regional Laboratory in October 1975, and joining the staff of The Moncton Hospital, he only remained until June, 1976, when he resigned citing personal and family reasons for his departure.

Kanaiyalal Patel also joined the pathology staff in 1975. He was born in Kampala on March 17, 1940, and received premedical and medical training at University of Baroda, receiving an MB, BS degree in 1966. In 1969, he interned at C.S. Wilson Hospital, Fort Wayne, Indiana, and then undertook pathology studies at McGill and the Royal Victoria, Montreal General and Jewish General Hospitals from 1970 to 1974, resulting in his receiving his FRCP(C) in Pathology and his American Boards in Pathology in 1974. He remained on the pathology staff for only two years, leaving in the fall of 1977.

George Boyd was born in River Bourgeois, Cape Breton, Nova Scotia, on May 29, 1939. He received a BSc from St. F.X. in 1959 and an MD from Dalhousie in 1964. He interned at the Victoria General Hospital from 1963 to 1964. He did a general practice at Neils Harbour, Cape Breton, in 1965 and returned to the Victoria General in 1966 where he did a residency in general surgery from 1966 to 1968 and then a residency in anaesthesia from 1968 to 1969, only to decide that the life of an anaesthetist was not for him. He returned to general practice serving on the staffs of St. Elizabeth Hospital, North Sydney and Harbour View Hospital, Sydney Mines, from 1969 to 1972. The bug for further training, however, hit him again and he pursued a residency in otolaryngology at the Royal Victoria, Montreal General, and Montreal Children's Hospital from 1972 to 1975, receiving his Fellowship in the Royal College. His decision to come to Moncton was no doubt influenced by the fact that his brother-in-law, Dr. William Taylor, had established a general practice here, but he again showed his restless streak, and left Moncton in April 1976, after serving on the staff for just a few months.

Anthony Charles Bond was born in England on December 7, 1944, and after pre-medical education at London University he attended Charing Cross Medical School at London University, graduating in 1968 with the degrees MB, BS, LRCP, MRCS. He interned at Kettering General Hospital from 1968 to 1969. He then entered the service of the Royal Army Medical Corps, serving at Cambridge Military Hospital, Aldershot, 1970 to 1973, British Military Hospital, Hammer (1973-74) and British Military Hospital, Rinteln, from 1974 to 1975. While in the service he pursued anaesthetic training and became a Fellow of the Faculty of Anaesthetists Royal College of Surgeons of England in 1973. Coming from Britain, he was registered to practice medicine in Canada under section 16B of the Medical Act and obtained his LMCC in 1977. He has since provided exemplary service to the Department of Anaesthesia earning the utmost respect from his anaesthetic and surgical colleagues. Besides serving as chief of anaesthesia at The Moncton Hospital, he has served as president of the New Brunswick Division of the Canadian Anaesthetist Society in 1992-93.

On November 14, 1974, the psychiatric day hospital was established, and in 1975, Dr. Thomas Terry Jones was appointed as staff psychiatrist at the Moncton Mental Health Clinic and director of the Psychiatric Day Care Hospital and was granted staff privileges at The Moncton Hospital. Terry Jones was born in South Wales on July 2, 1934. He graduated from the Welsh National School of Medicine in 1960 with the degree MB, ChB and then interned at St. David's Hospital, Cardiff, Wales, from 1960 to 1961. He did a residency in psychiatry at the Peter Bent Brigham Hospital, Boston, from 1962 to 1963, and then the Princess Margaret Hospital, Perth, West Australia, from 1965 to 1967. He was on the staff of Lions Gate Hospital, Vancouver, from 1969 to 1973, and Vernon Jubilee Hospital, Vernon, British Columbia, from 1973 to 1974. His stay in Moncton was short, as he left in June, 1976, to become regional director of mental health in Fredericton.

There were 13,254 admissions in 1975 with 1,589 live births. The average length of stay was 12.4 days. Outpatient visits numbered 173,394 with the outpatient special clinics showing the following number of visits: Arthritis—514; Cardiology—164; Diabetic—176; Diet Counselling—287; Hyperlipoproteinemia—118; Obesity—193; Orthopaedic—153; Paediatric—148; and Radiotherapy—1590. All services showed increased use with statistics recorded for the various services as follows: electrocardiography—17,657; electroencephalography—1,745; gastrointestinal unit—995; occupational therapy—7,399; physiotherapy—26,785; radioisotope—3,452 and radiology—66,522.

On May 28, 1976, Howard Grayston stepped down as chairman of the board, although he remained as a member of the board. He was succeeded by Robert A. MacQuade, a member of the board since 1972 and vice-chairman since 1973. Financial problems continued to plague the hospital with the provincial government giving it significantly less money per patient day than it was giving to other hospitals in the province with more than 200 beds. Mr. MacQuade had just settled into his new office, when on June 4 he had to travel to Fredericton to present a brief to the Minister of Health outlining the difficulties faced by the hospital. The main recommendations in the brief were as follows:

Section 1—PHYSICAL FACILITIES

1. That approval in principal be given to the renovation and reconstruction of The Moncton Hospital as proposed by Agnew Peckham and Associates.
2. That approval be given to the timetable for this work with completion of the project in mid-1982.

3. That subject to the approval of the above recommendations approval be given for the hiring of Agnew Peckham and Associates for Functional Programming.
4. That urgently required interim renovations and relocations be started immediately.

Section 2—BED ACCOMMODATIONS IN REGION 1

1. That additional hospital beds be opened in the Region and that these beds be designated for extended or Level IV care. With the opening of these, the patients presently being cared for in nursing homes should be reassessed and those who are, in fact, Level IV patients, should be transferred to the hospitals providing Level IV care.
2. That persons requiring Level III nursing home care be given priority for admission to nursing homes so as to ensure that the greatest possible benefit is derived from the money being spent on the operations of hospitals.
3. That there be close and frequent communication between the Department of Health and the Department of Social Services so as to ensure the co-ordination of government policy toward the objective of better health care for the citizens of New Brunswick.

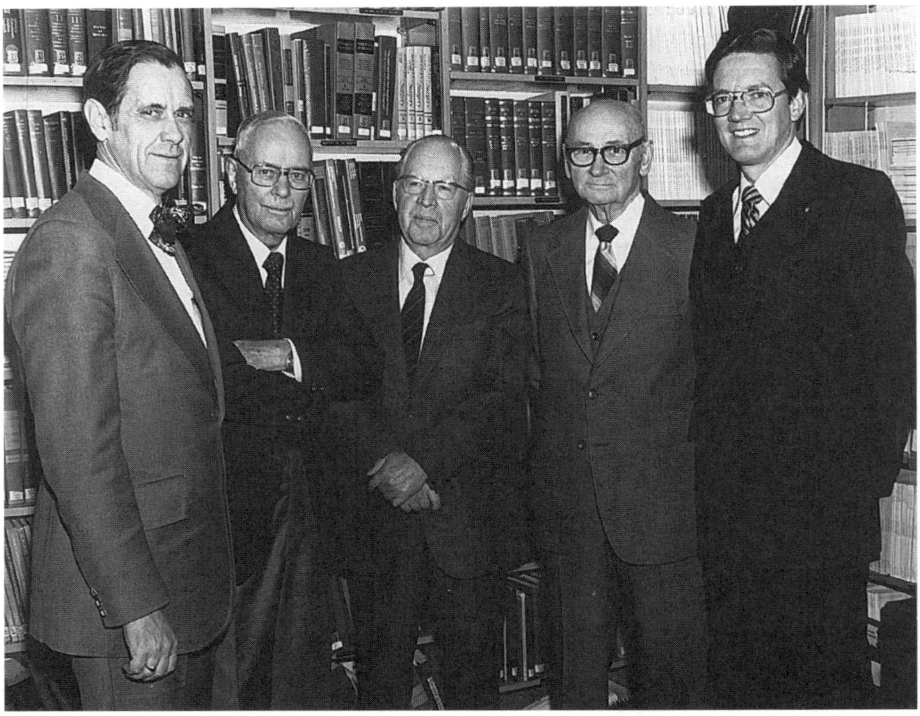

Chairmen of the Board, 1947-1983. From left to right: Mr. Ralph Belyea, Mr. Howard Grayston, Mr. Leonard Lockhart, Mr. Harris Tait, and Mr. Robert MacQuade.

Section 3—FINANCE

1. That The Moncton Hospital be provided with an operating budget which is appropriate to its provision of a broad variety and sophistication of health services. In particular that the per diem rate for The Moncton Hospital be allowed to rise until it is second only to that of the Saint John General Hospital.
2. That more money be allocated for capital equipment purchases and the policies by which the money is to be spent be clarified and adhered to throughout any given fiscal year.
3. That the government's involvement in physical plants be protected through the availability of additional monies either through the Department of Supply and Services or through increased hospital operating budgets to ensure an adequate level of plant maintenance.
4. That the Department of Health move quickly to a conclusion on the installation of a CAT scanner in a hospital in New Brunswick.

A separate brief was also presented to the Department of Health regarding the hospital laundry. In this brief, it was outlined that the laundry was built in 1953 to fulfil the needs of a 210 bed hospital and, although the laundry was somewhat expanded in 1960, the number of hospital beds had in the meantime increased to 539. Moreover, The Moncton Hospital was now providing a laundry service to the Spencer Memorial Home and the Kings County Memorial Hospital. The brief recommended the purchase of new laundry equipment to replace most of the existing equipment, certain changes to the physical layout with minor building renovations, and much improved ventilation.

The Hospital Brief met with partial success in that the government agreed with the proposal to have Agnew, Peckham and Associates proceed with Functional Programming and to the purchase of a CAT scanner.

In 1973, a 19-bed rehabilitation unit had been established on 1 Parlee to serve as an extended care/rehabilitation unit with supervision by a multidisciplinary committee. On January 1, 1976, the physiotherapy, occupational therapy and speech therapy departments were joined to form a Department of Rehabilitation Services. To supervise and run the enlarged department, the hospital was able to recruit the services of a physiatrist or physical medicine specialist in the person of Dr. Renald Simard. Dr. Simard was born on March 29, 1937, in Chicoutimi, Quebec, and after premedical education he entered the Medical School of the University of Ottawa, obtaining his MD in 1962. He served a rotating internship at the Chicoutimi Hospital from 1962 to 1963, began a residency in physical medicine and rehabilitation in 1968 at the Nova Scotian Rehabilitation Centre and then did six months in neurology and neurosurgery at the Victoria General Hospital. He served a year in internal medicine at Hôtel Dieu de Quebec from 1969 to 1970 followed by a year in physical medicine and rehabilitation at the same hospital from 1970 to 1971. He was on the active staffs of the Royal Ottawa, the Ottawa General and Ottawa Civic

Hospitals from 1972 to 1974 and was appointed an Assistant Professor of Medicine in Rehabilitation at the University of Ottawa. He soon became recognized as a competent physical medicine specialist and served a great need in the hospital but he left in December 1977, returning to the position of Assistant Professor at the University of Ottawa. Like many of his counterparts from Quebec, he had found his family could not adapt to life in Moncton and found it difficult to fit in with the social life of the Acadian French.

With the admission to the staff in late 1975 of Dr. Sheldon Rubin, a Chemotherapy Clinic was started in 1976, which, until recently, Dr. Rubin continued to operate single-handedly, providing this valuable service to the entire eastern half of the province. Although sometimes jokingly criticized by the staff for causing a lot of budget problems for the hospital, there has not been a more hard-working, sympathetic man and advocate for his patients than Sheldon Rubin.

Plans were made to expand the Coronary Care Unit to eight beds and install new monitoring equipment. On May 5, 1976, the Coronary Care Unit was dedicated to the memory of the late Dr. William Turner. The Medical and Surgical Intensive Care Units were also physically inadequate and plans were proceeding for revision of this space.

In the orthopaedic department, all members took courses in arthroscopy of the knee and authorization was received to buy the equipment to implement this new diagnostic service although the equipment was not received until 1977.

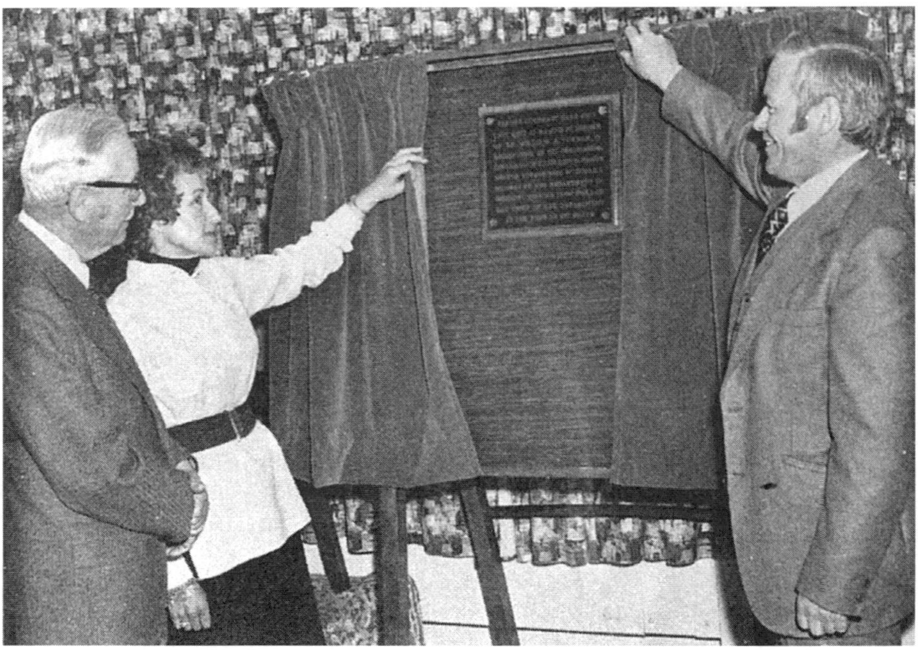

The dedication of the W.A. Turner Coronary Care Unit. From left to right: Mr. Howard Grayston, Mrs. Avis Turner, and Dr. J.T. Edgett.

On July 29, 1976, Miss A.J. MacMaster died at The Moncton Hospital, the institution where she served as Superintendent and Director of Nursing from 1919 to 1947. Less than three weeks before, on July tenth, The A.J. MacMaster School of Nursing had graduated its first class.

In October, The Moncton Hospital's Recreation Centre, a cottage in Shediac Cape, was destroyed by fire. This property had been donated to the hospital by Mr. and Mrs. Leonard Lockhart for use mainly by the student nurses, but had become the main venue for the annual intern's lobster party hosted by the medical staff, as well as other functions connected to the hospital.

Under the guidance of its president, Reuben Cohen, QC, the Friends of the Moncton Hospital inaugurated a Christmas Appeal for funds in 1976, and this has continued to be a yearly event since then. This first campaign was only directed at 450 names, was undertaken late in the year and raised $3,665. The Friends contributed $4,935 for the purchase of equipment during the year, with the larger part of this money used to purchase an Aqua K Thermia Unit for the Neurosurgery Department. Service clubs and other organizations also raised funds for the benefit of The Moncton Hospital. The Elks Club donated $4,000 to the hospital for the purchase of an impedance audiometer and for the training of the staff to operate such equipment. The Nurses' Hospital Auxiliary donated 1) a Doppler stethoscope, 2) a radio for the day-surgery unit and 3) a microphone for the nurses' residence auditorium. The Moncton Aquarium Society donated an aquarium for use in the outpatient waiting room. The Co-Op Book Exchange Centre donated a colour TV for the use of patients in the hospital's psychiatric wing. The Gyrettes donated a master electronic control card for use with one of the hospital's respirators. The IODE continued to help, with the Dr. John Clarence Webster Chapter donating $1,000 towards the purchase of a Jobst Pump, and the Hon. C.H. Blakeny Chapter donating equipment for thoracic surgery. In 1967, the Municipal Chapter of the IODE had developed a patient library as their centennial project, and on February 10, 1976, the library found a permanent home on 3 Clarke. The administration of the library was transferred to the hospital's Volunteer Service Department.

For several years the Dr. Georges-L. Dumont Hospital had been holding an annual dinner at the hospital honouring and roasting those who had given 25 years of service to the hospital. The medical staff felt that The Moncton Hospital should do something in a like manner for members of our staff and chose to have an annual Medical Staff Dinner held at the Beausejour Hotel with members of the staff and their spouses and guests attending. The format chosen for the evening consisted of a dinner and dance. During the evening, those members of the staff who had reached the age of 60 years were honoured with a roasting by the staff and presentation of a silver tray from the Board of Trustees. The first such dinner was held on November 12, 1976, and all those members of the staff over sixty years of age who were both active and retired were honoured this first year. Those so honoured at this inaugural

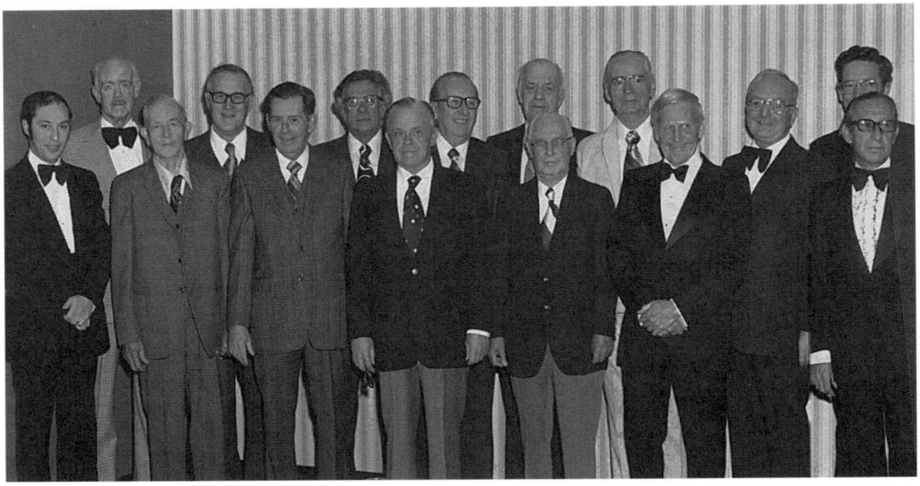

The first Annual Medical Staff dinner was held in 1976. Front row: Dr. E.A. MacLeod—President of Medical Staff, Dr. W.A. Pullin, Dr. R.P. Myers, Dr. R. Murphy, Dr. H.L. McKeen, Dr. R.B. Eaton, Dr. W.B. Stewart and Dr. C.E. Doyle—chief of staff. Back row: Dr. R. Fitch, Dr. C.M. Leighton, Dr. G. Parsons, Dr. L. Ramsay, Dr. S.A. Hopper, Dr. R.I. McKenna and Robert MacQuade—Chairman of the Board.

dinner were: Dr. J.A. Delaney, Dr. C.E. Doyle, Dr. R.B. Eaton, Dr. R. Fitch, Dr. J.A. Fownes, Dr. L.A. Goodridge, Dr. S.A. Hopper, Dr. R.D. Landry, Dr. C.M. Leighton, Dr. E.D. Levittan, Dr. R. M. Murphy, Dr. R. Myers, Dr. H.L. McKeen, Dr. R.I. McKenna, Dr. G.V. Parsons, Dr. W. Pullin, Dr. L.R. Ramsay, Dr. W.B. Stewart and Dr. R.S. Wadup. This dinner has continued to be a social event for the medical staff each November.

In addition to Dr. Orville Messenger returning from postgraduate work in general and thoracic surgery, there were six new additions to the medical staff in 1976: Dr. G. Llewellyn to the Department of Radiology, Dr. R.K. Jones to the Department of Neurosurgery, Dr. George Cobb to the Department of Ophthalmology and Dr. John Leger and Dr. Rita Kahn to the Department of General Practice. Dr. W.J. Walton, who established a general practice in Shediac, was also admitted to the associate courtesy staff and Dr. Julien D'Astous and Dr. William LaPlante were admitted to the active staff of the Dr. Georges-L. Dumont Hospital and the courtesy staff of The Moncton Hospital.

Grant Llewellyn was born on April 12, 1942, in Summerside, Prince Edward Island, and after taking premed at University New Brunswick he obtained his MD from Dalhousie in 1968. He served a rotating internship at the Victoria General, Halifax Infirmary, and Grace Maternity Hospitals from 1967 to 1968. He served a residency in radiology at the Health Sciences Centre in Winnipeg from 1971 to 1975 with a further year of fellowship at University Hospital, London, Ontario, from 1975 to 1976, obtaining his FRCP(C) in Radiology in 1976. With his special interest in neuroradiology, he was a welcome addition to the staff and gave exemplary service to the hospital. Alas, he was enticed to join the radiology staff of the Victoria General Hospital in Halifax in 1983.

Robert Kenneth Jones was born in Chicago on March 11, 1924. He received a BSc from Purdue University in 1943 and an MD from Northwestern University in 1949. He interned at St. Luke's Hospital in Chicago from 1948 to 1949. After taking a year of general surgery at the Illinois Research Hospital from 1949 to 1950, he spent four years from 1950 to 1954 at the Illinois Neuropsychiatric Hospital studying both neurology and neurosurgery. He spent a further year of fellowship at the Peter Bent Brigham and the Children's Hospital in Boston and obtained his American Boards in both Neurology and Neurosurgery. He practised in Philadelphia and served as Clinical Instructor of Neurosurgery at the University of Pennsylvania from 1955 to 1957 and then as Associate Professor from 1957 to 1966. He then served as an associate professor of neurosurgery at Thomas Jefferson Medical School from 1967 to 1975. He moved to Canada in 1975, citing the high cost of malpractice insurance in the United States, and spent a year at the Montreal Neurological Institute, obtaining his LMCC in 1976. Prior to Dr. Jones joining the department, the other two neurosurgeons were paid by a salary, arrangement with the Department of Health but the government would not support paying another salary, so he came under regular medicare reimbursement. Dr. Jones was a marathon runner, often running ten miles a day, and was featured in an article in the *Moncton Transcript* on January 4, 1977. Despite his pleasant personality, his professional work was found wanting and Dr. Tucker, as chief of neurosurgery, invoked a rarely used section of the by-laws to temporarily suspend his privileges. This was upheld at subsequent emergency meetings of the Medical Advisory Committee and Dr. Jones did not contest the matter further, and left Moncton to return to Philadelphia in 1979.

George Mark Cobb was born in St. John's, Newfoundland, on December 3, 1931. He took premedical at Memorial University and then attended Dalhousie, obtaining the MD, CM degree in 1958 after spending a year of rotating internship in the Dalhousie program. From 1960 to 1961 he did a residency in general surgery at the General Hospital in St. John's and then a residency in ophthalmology at the University of Toronto from 1961 to 1964. He set up practice in Guelph, Ontario, from 1965 to 1968 and then moved to Toronto where he was on the staff of the Humber Memorial Hospital, Weston, from 1968 to 1976 and Sunnybrook Hospital from 1972 to 1974. George has a gift at carpentry work and he combined this with his love of sailing to build his own sailboat. On December 31, 1986, he stopped doing surgery and subsequently resigned from the staff on August 31, 1987.

John Leger was a brother to Roger Leger and was born on December 27, 1945, in Woodstock, Ontario. He received a BSc from St. Francis Xavier University in 1967 and an MD from Dalhousie in 1973. After serving a rotating internship at the Victoria General Hospital from 1972 to 1973, he did a three-year stint as a medical officer in the Canadian Armed Forces and was on the staff of the Chilliwack General Hospital from 1974 to 1976. He was appointed to the staff in the Department of General Practice on December 16, 1976, but left in February 1978.

Rita Kahn was born in India on August 9, 1947, and received her pre-medical and medical education at the University of Delhi receiving the MB, BS degree in 1969. She interned at the Irwin Hospital, India, from 1969 to 1970 and worked as a general practitioner in India from 1970 to 1972. After immigrating to Canada, she served as a resident in pathology at the Moncton Regional Laboratory from 1972 to 1974 and an internship at The Moncton Hospital from 1974 to 1975. After obtaining her LMCC in August 1975, she was appointed to the staff in the Department of General Practice. She continued to run a busy general practice until 1987, when she left Moncton.

Dr. William LaPlant joined the active staff of the Dr. Georges-L. Dumont Hospital and the courtesy staff of The Moncton Hospital. Because of a common emergency call schedule with the Dr. Georges-L. Dumont Hospital he played a larger role in the functioning of the staff than is usual in courtesy staff appointments. Bill was born in Bathurst on April 25, 1943, and received a BA from the University of Bathurst in 1964 and an MD from Ottawa University in 1970. He interned at the Ottawa General Hospital from 1970 to 1971 and then did a residency in urology at the Ottawa General, Ottawa Civic Hospitals and the Children's Hospital of Eastern Ontario from 1974 to 1975, receiving his FRCS(C) in urology in 1975.

Although a member of the active staff of the Dr. Georges-L. Dumont Hospital and the courtesy staff of The Moncton Hospital, Dr. Julien D'Astous is a common visitor to The Moncton Hospital in his role as the sole nephrologist in the area. He was born in Dalhousie, New Brunswick, on May 19, 1944. He received a BA from the Université de Moncton in 1965 and an MD from the University of Ottawa in 1970. He interned at the Ottawa General from 1970 to 1971 and pursued postgraduate work at the Ottawa Civic Hospital in internal medicine from 1971 to 1973, followed by six months of gastroenterology and eighteen months of nephrology finishing in 1975. He received his FRCP(C) in 1976. As the sole nephrologist in Moncton he has run a very busy Kidney Dialysis Unit at the Dr. Georges-L. Dumont Hospital, and is very obliging with any request for consultation and arranging for dialysis of renal failure patients at The Moncton Hospital.

There were 13,167 patients admitted to the hospital during 1976 with 1,823 births recorded. There were 180,809 visits to the outpatient department including 3,256 day surgery patients. All services showed an increase over 1975 with the following statistics recorded: electrocardiography—17,586; electroencephalography—2,004; and electro-myelograms—359; gastrointestinal unit—865; occupational therapy—12,982; physiotherapy—31,078; radioisotope—3,863; and radiology 69,607. The new Chemotherapy Clinic recorded 289 visits with the visits to other clinics as follows: Arthritis—561; Cardiology—129; Diabetes—182; Diet Counselling—238;

Hyperlipoproteinemia—87; Obesity—165 with—382 weight checks; Orthopaedic—95; Paediatric—150 and Radio-therapy—1,427.

In January 1977 a new face appeared on the administrative scene. Douglas Apt was appointed assistant administrator. Prior to this he had been employed in the Mental Health Division of the Department of Health. In addition to supervising his share of hospital departments, he acted as co-ordinator of the hospital's various construction and renovation projects. Most of the construction projects and renovations were still only in the planning stages, however, with no permission from government having yet been received to proceed. In May, William Kilpatrick, the executive director of the hospital, was elected president-elect of the Canadian Hospital Association. At the annual meeting of the New Brunswick Hospital Association the former executive director, Dr. Austin Clarke, was honoured with a life membership.

In addition to its failure to provide any good news on construction projects, the government remained stingy in providing funds for the capital equipment budget. Fortunately, the Friends of the Moncton Hospital and many local organizations were able to help fill in the gap. The Friends purchased a Hall air drill for the Department of Orthopaedics at a cost of $3,300 and a Holter electrocardiocorder for the Department of Internal Medicine at a cost of $3,200. The DOKK's purchased a pulse width monitor. The Moncton Gyrettes donated an IMV module for MA-1 Respirator for respiratory technology. The Moncton Rotary Club presented furnishings and

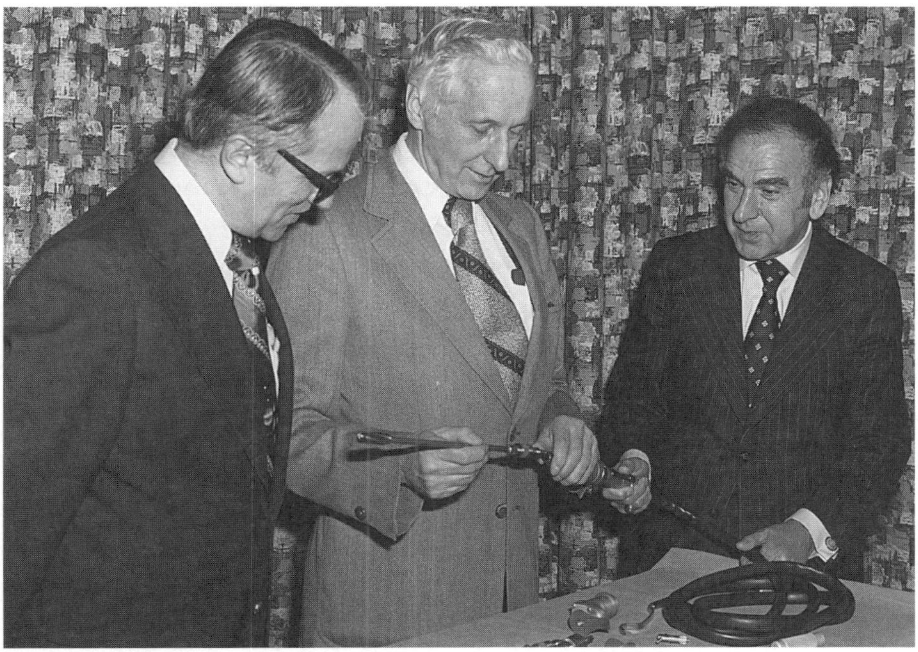

Dr. O.J. White (centre) demonstrating new power equipment to Mr. Reuben Cohen (right) and Mr. John Ward (left) who presented the equipment to the Orthopaedic Department on behalf of The Friends of the Moncton Hospital.

equipment for the rehabilitation unit lounge/dining room and the Co-operative Centre of Moncton donated a 19-inch colour TV for psychiatry. The New Brunswick Division of the Canadian Cancer Society donated $5,000 for the purchase of a diagnostic colposcope. The Hon. C.H. Blakeny Chapter of the IODE donated lymphangiography equipment and the Fort Cumberland Chapter of the IODE donated toys to the Dr. E.W. Ewart Play Therapy Unit and a cheque to the speech pathology unit to buy books and pamphlets for a lending library for patients and families on a variety of speech disorders, their nature, prevention and treatment. The Soroptomist Club of Moncton donated to the hospital one male and one female artificial larynx. The largest donation came from the Nurses' Hospital Auxiliary, which donated $61,670 for the purchase of ultrasound diagnostic equipment as well as the necessary funds for the purchase of the closed circuit TV system. Under the direction of Irene Crawford, the volunteers continued to provide many manpower hours of service to the hospital with teen volunteers alone working over 1000 hours. In addition, the proceeds from the coffee cart netted a profit of $700 which was donated to the hospital.

Prior to 1977, the spiritual needs of patients had been met by their own clergy but this presented problems for those patients from outside the Moncton area and in emergency situations. In 1977, the pastoral care staff was organized in an effort to provide a better forum for communication between community clergy and hospital staff. The organization structure approximated that of the medical staff and the preamble to the by-laws, rules and regulations stated:

> Recognizing that spiritual needs of patients in the hospital are best met by the clergy, and that to do this most effectively clergy must organize subject to the authority of the Board of Trustees, members of the clergy extending their ministry to the Hospital hereby organize themselves in conformity with the by-laws, rules and regulations hereinafter recorded.

The Hospital Pastoral Care Committee was composed of the executive of the pastoral care staff and hospital representatives with the first president being the Rev. Ronald Maund. The committee met bi-monthly with a general clergy staff meeting held annually. The hospital was now able to provide around-the-clock availability of one Roman Catholic chaplain and one Protestant chaplain, who carried pocket pagers and responded immediately to any call from nursing staff on behalf of patients or relatives. After intervening in the immediate crisis, the chaplain would notify the clergyman of the patient's faith.

The medical staff saw several departures during the year. Dr. Allan Lorimer resigned as director of the Moncton Regional Laboratory and Dr. Alfred Bastarache resumed directorship of the laboratory once again. Dr. Michael Robertson sailed across the Atlantic Ocean to Scotland and Dr. Renald Simard returned to Ottawa. New additions to the staff were Dr.

Robin Walker to the Department of Paediatrics, Dr. Douglas Baird to the Department of Radiology, Dr. Glen Brodie to the Department of Obstetrics and Gynaecology, Dr. Ronald Garston to the Department of Urology, and Dr. Daniel Zwicker to the Department of General Practice.

Dr. Alan Lorimer was appointed to the position of director of the Regional Laboratory in late 1976, to succeed Dr. Hudson, and was appointed to the medical staff by the Board of Trustees on January 6, 1977. He was born in Scotland on May 6, 1926, received his MB, ChB from Aberdeen University in 1949, and interned at Stracathro Hospital, Aberdeen, from 1949 to 1950. He began a residency in pathology at St. Joseph's Hospital, Fort Wayne, Indiana, in 1953, and then returned to the British Isles where he became senior health officer in pathology at Manchester Regional Hospital Board from 1954 to 1957. He was a lecturer in pathology at Aberdeen University from 1957 to 1959 and assistant pathologist at Salford Royal Hospital, England, from 1959 to 1960. He came to Canada and was pathologist at the Victoria Public Hospital in Fredericton from 1973 to 1975. He obtained his FRCP(C) in Pathology in 1972. In 1975 he served as pathologist at Soldiers Memorial Hospital in Campbellton and then moved on to Grace Hospital, Winnipeg, in 1976, before coming to Moncton. Before the year was out, he had also departed from Moncton.

The need for a neonatology unit at The Moncton Hospital had been established in 1975, and in 1977, the hospital was successful in recruiting Dr. Robin Walker to come to Moncton and to set up a neonatology division in the pediatric department. Robin was born on March 19, 1949, in Wilmslow,

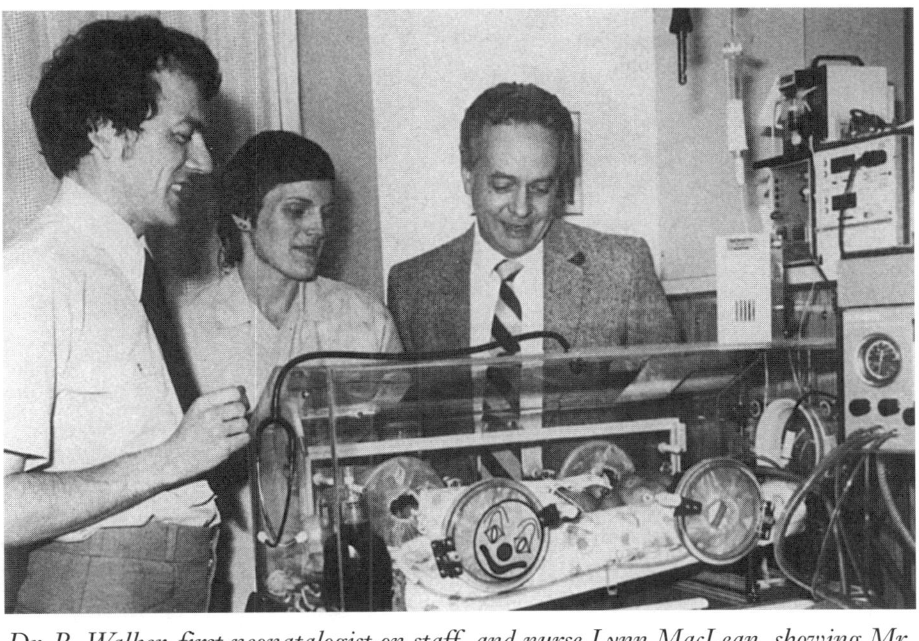

Dr. R. Walker, first neonatalogist on staff, and nurse Lynn MacLean, showing Mr. Ralph Black a ventilator presented by the Friends of the Moncton Hospital.

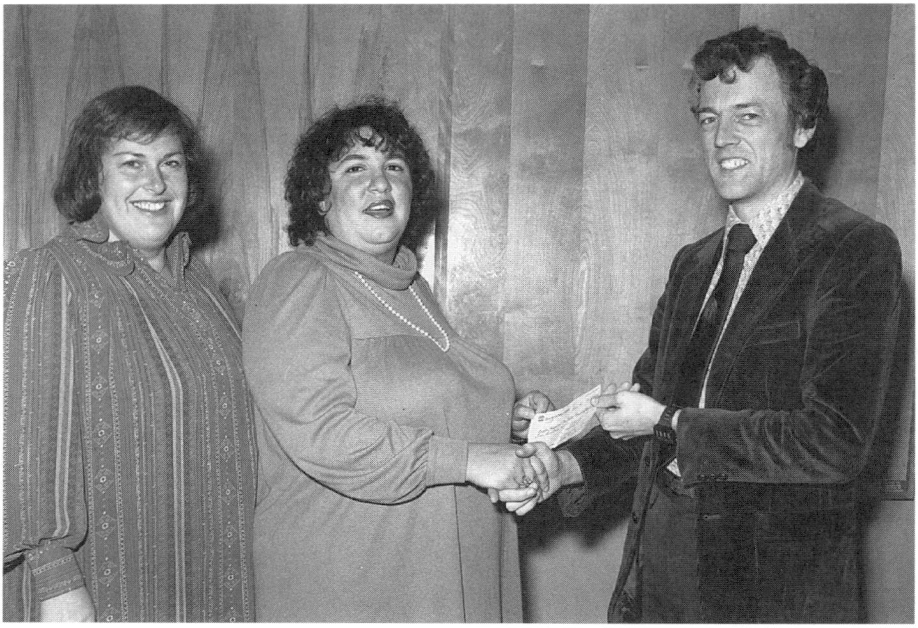

Presentation being made to Robin Walker, the hospital's first neonatologist, by Sharon Rubin (left) and Gail Zuckerman (centre) on behalf of the Sisterhood of Tiferes Israel Synagogue.

England, and after taking premedical at Kings School, Macclesfield, England, he received his MB, CM at the University of Manchester in 1971. He interned at Crumpsall Hospital and Victoria Memorial Jewish Hospital in the North-East Manchester Hospital Group from 1971 to 1972. He started his pediatric residency in England at Booth Hal Children's Hospital, Manchester, from 1972 to 1973 and then came to Canada, serving a pediatric and neonatology residency at The Grace Maternity and the Isaak Walton Killam Hospital from 1973 to 1977 and receiving his FRCP(C) in Paediatrics in 1977. He proved a wise choice to start the neonatology unit and with his dedication to the hospital and community, he built up a Neonatology Intensive Care and Regional Perinatal Service second to none in Atlantic Canada. It seemed that every month he would have his picture in the paper because, through his efforts, a service club would be donating equipment to the Neonatology Unit. His fame spread, and in June 1986, he was lured to head up a neonatology unit in Kingston at Queen's University. In 1991, he moved on to the Children's Hospital of Eastern Ontario in Ottawa.

Douglas Gale Baird was born on December 18, 1942, at Thurso, Scotland, but spent his childhood in Fredericton where his father was a doctor. He received a BA from the University of New Brunswick, in 1964 and an MD from Dalhousie in 1969 after interning at the Victoria General Hospital from 1968 to 1969. He then went into general practice in Fredericton from 1969 to 1972 before embarking on a radiology residency at Health Sciences Centre in Winnipeg from 1972 to 1976 obtaining his FRCP(C) in Radiology in 1976. Following this he remained in Winnipeg for a year at Saint Boniface General Hospital and became a lecturer in radiology at the University of Manitoba. He has remained on the radiology staff of The Moncton Hospital since 1977.

Glen Brodie was born in Glace Bay on July 16, 1943, received a BA from the University of New Brunswick in 1963 and an MD from Dalhousie in 1968 and interned at The Victoria General Hospital from 1967 to 1968. He established a general practice in Albert and was appointed to the courtesy staff of The Moncton Hospital. He left in 1973 and took a residency in obstetrics and gynaecology in the Dalhousie University program from 1973 to 1977 and obtained his FRCS(C) in obstetrics and gynaecology in 1977. He then returned to Moncton where, with a constant smile, he has provided exemplary service to The Moncton Hospital ever since. With the hospital having an active program for Dalhousie interns in obstetrics he has taken a keen interest in his teaching role and has been a clinical instructor in the Department of Obstetrics and Gynaecology at Dalhousie since 1980. In 1992 he was appointed chairman of the Obstetric and Gynaecology Section of the Medical Council of Canada.

Ronald Garston was born in Ottawa on July 13, 1947, and took his pre-medical and medical education at the University of Ottawa, receiving his MD in 1971. He interned at the Ottawa Civic Hospital from 1971 to 1972 and did postgraduate training in urology at the teaching hospitals of the University of Ottawa from 1972 to 1977, receiving his FRCS(C) in Urology in 1977.

Dr. Daniel Zwicker was born on Grand Manan, New Brunswick, on August 25, 1948, and received a BA from the University of New Brunswick in 1970 and an MD from Dalhousie in 1975. From 1975 to 1976 he served a rotating internship at the Victoria General, Isaac Walton Killam, Camp Hill, and Saint John General hospitals. He then entered general practice in Middleton, Nova Scotia, from 1976 to 1977. He joined the staff of the Moncton Medical Clinic in 1977 but left Moncton in November 1979, to set up practice again in a smaller community in Nova Scotia.

In 1978 the hospital changed its reporting of statistics and its year end to correspond with the fiscal year running from April 1 to March 31. Admissions to the hospital in the 1977-1978 fiscal year totalled 13,521, besides 1,776 newborns; 9,997 operations were performed in the surgical suite including 3,519 day surgery patients. The following services were provided: electrocardiograms—17,470; electroencephalograms—1,950; gastrointestinal unit procedures—976; nuclear medicine procedures—4,020; radiological examinations—69,117; ultrasound examinations—598; respiratory therapy treatments—6,925; speech pathology—1,346 and social services 1,980. There were 5,343 visits to the various outpatient clinics: Arthritis—698; Cardiology (Pediatric)—139; Chemotherapy—2,193; Diabetes—95; Diet Counselling—264; Hyperproteinemia—82; Obesity—124; Obesity weight checks—395; Orthopaedic (Pediatric)—80 and Radiotherapy—1,170.

In 1978, the cost per patient day of operating The Moncton Hospital was

$121.27 and was the lowest in the province. The cost at the Dr. Georges-L. Dumont was about $130, Saint Joseph's in Saint John was about $155 and the Saint John General about $165. With the funds allotted to it the hospital ran a deficit of $1,200,000, which the government picked up but without promise of a more equitable distribution of funds to hospitals. It was apparent that efficiency did not pay off, and in times of restraint, there was very little fat to cut from the budget.

In 1977, Agnew Peckham & Associates had been authorized to carry out a Functional Program and this was completed in April 1978. Still no word was forthcoming to proceed with the project. Instead, because five years had elapsed since the preparation of the Master Program and at least three years for the original cost estimates, Architects Four and Agnew, Peckham & Associates were appointed to

1. revise the Master Plan;
2. create a schedule for construction which would permit the continued operation of the hospital through the program; and
3. prepare a revised cost estimate for the project.

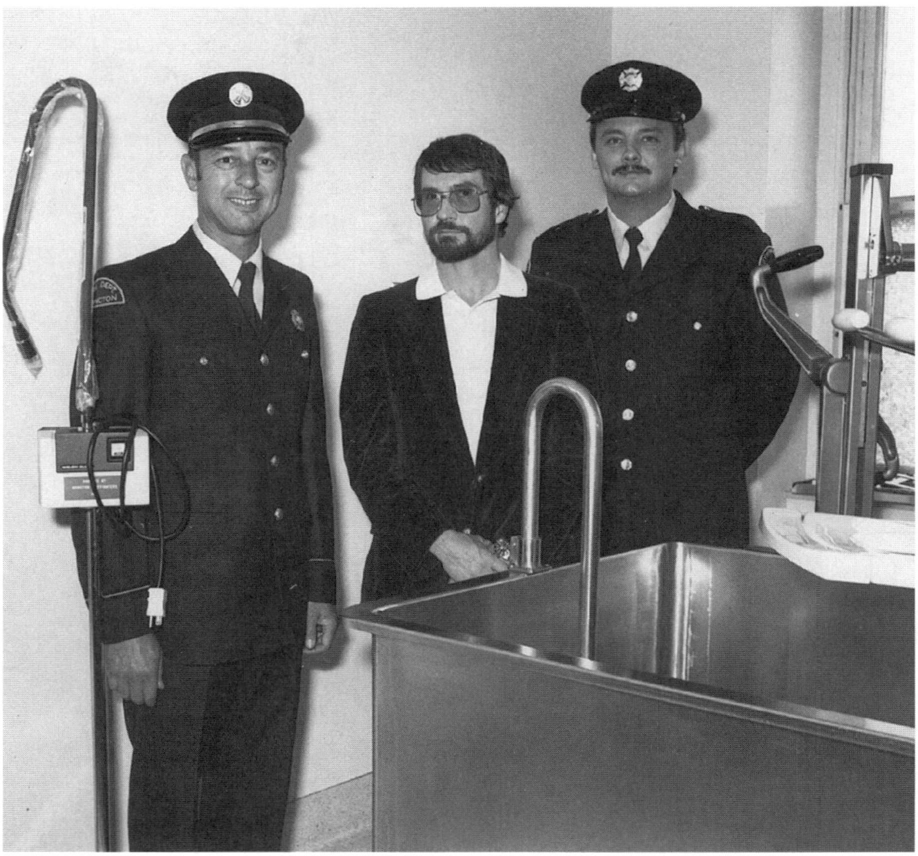

Moncton Firefighters Association making a presentation to the Burn Unit. From Left to right: Mr. Paul Cormier, Dr. Douglas Inglis, and Mr. Skip Williston.

Perhaps there was at last a glimpse of light at the end of the planning tunnel. And news was not all that bad as some projects did receive government approval. Plans for an eight-bed Coronary Intensive Care Unit and an intermediate care unit were made and a temporary unit was constructed on 1 Joyce so that the necessary construction could be carried out on 3 Joyce. In March 1978 the hospital received permission to proceed with the renovations to The Moncton Hospital laundry at a cost of $800,000. Plans called for the construction of a penthouse over the existing laundry, thereby permitting soiled laundry to be loaded from this new penthouse into new washers. In addition to the new washers, a new 400-pound tumbler and 148-inch iron were to be located in the existing laundry. Major renovations to the existing laundry layout allowed a much improved working environment, and also enabled the laundry to operate on a one shift five-day work week. At a cost of $90,000, a computerized environmental control system was installed with the up side that it would save $50,000 a year in oil and electricity costs.

On May 5 the hospital's Burn Treatment Unit was officially opened on the 6 Joyce wing with an eight-bed unit. The major portion of the funds to construct and equip this unit were supplied by Local 999 of the Moncton Firefighters Association.

In April 1978 the hospital instigated a program to prepare nurses to meet existing and future needs of hospitals' operating room staffing requirements

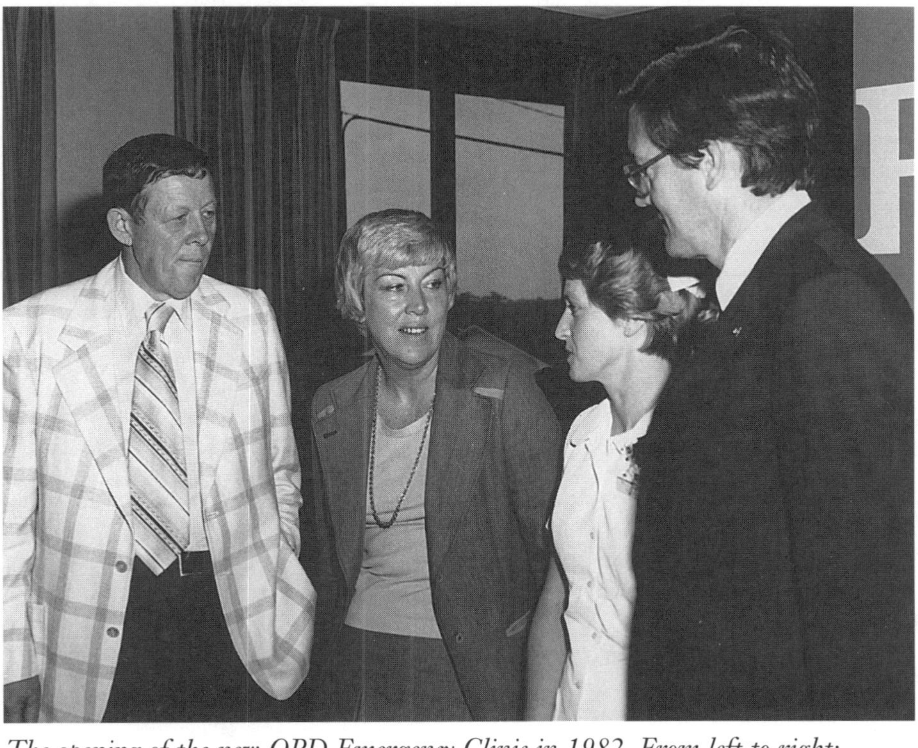

The opening of the new OPD Emergency Clinic in 1982. From left to right: Harvey Hicks, Hon. Brenda Robertson, Joan Allain R.N., and Robert MacQuade.

in the province. The program continued over the next four years with 42 graduates. Thirty-eight students came from New Brunswick and four from Nova Scotia. The Moncton Hospital sponsored twelve students.

Because of the marked lack of space in the existing outpatient department, new space totalling 4,500 square feet was acquired in the Professional Arts Building adjacent to the hospital. This area was designed for Paediatric, Orthopaedic, Radiotherapy, Chemotherapy, Arthritis and Diabetic clinics and was officially opened by the provincial minister of health, the Honourable Brenda Robertson. In addition, the Outpatient Blood Specimen Collection and GI Units were relocated to this area. A Diabetic Day Care was instituted to enlarge the scope of the Diabetic Clinic and a new Colposcopy Clinic was opened in August 1978.

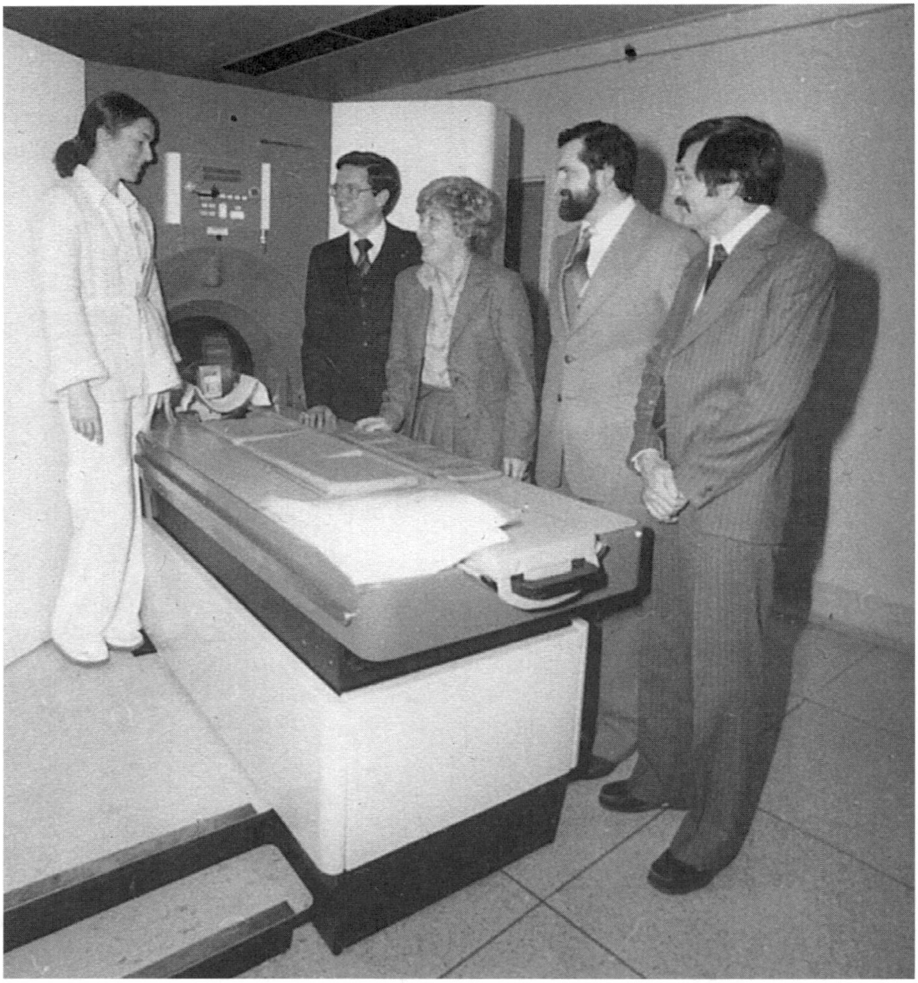

A new CT Scanner was obtained for the hospital in 1986. From left to right: Joanne Fraser, R.T., Mr. R. MacQuade, Hon. Brenda Robertson, Mr. David MacIvor, R.T., and Dr. Louis Gaudet.

The biggest new piece of equipment obtained by the hospital was the new CAT scanner. The provincial government provided $357,000 toward the cost with an additional amount of $52,000 supplied by the Friends of the Moncton Hospital Foundation. The Nurses' Hospital Auxiliary again provided a number of pieces of equipment including a shower chair, a commode chair and a Halter Patient Lift. In accordance with the times, more parents were staying overnight with their children in hospital and the Dr. John Clarence Webster Chapter of the IODE presented two bed chairs to be used by parents staying with their children.

Executive Director Bill Kilpatrick was elected president of the Canadian Hospital Association during its annual meeting. Once again The Moncton Hospital received three-year accreditation this year.

In 1978 Lionel Savoie celebrated his 25th anniversary working at The Moncton Hospital. Although there have been many dedicated employees of the hospital with twenty-five years of service, Lionel typified the dedicated hospital employee. I came in close contact with Lionel every week as he was the plaster room orderly. Except when he had to go out on ambulance call, he would work in the clinic taking his breaks or dinner hour only when it would not interfere with the smooth working of the clinic. As a child in a large family, he had to leave school at a young age and could tell stories of working in the woods when he was twelve. He continued working hard all his life and after a day's work at the hospital he would often go home at night and work at a second job doing painting. During the hunting season, he and his cohort in the plaster room, Walter Steeves, would arrange their sick days well in advance so that the plaster room would be covered when they called in sick. Lionel also served as interpreter for us unilingual Anglophones in the fracture room. Certainly most of the patients we dealt with understood his French, but I became very aware of his non-Parisian French one day when he started the interpretation to my patient with "commusca feel." Lionel had a reputation for being able to hold his liquor and, although never drinking on duty, there were Mondays when I am certain he was a little hung over. One day, one of the porters in the X-ray Department came in with a Colles fracture and later at a cast change Lionel said that he didn't think the fellow held his liquor very well becoming drunk on only a dozen beer. A delightful story about the same porter was related by Dr. Stewart when he was chief of radiology. He had to berate the employee after receiving a complaint from one of the local Baptist clergymen. The porter had gone to the patient's room to bring him to the X-ray department for an examination and the patient was being visited by his clergy. The clergyman stated that the patient would be ready to go after they had had a short prayer. After interrupting the clergyman's prayer a second time, when the prayer had lasted several minutes, the porter said, "Let's go. Did you come here to get your body or your soul fixed?"

New additions to the staff in 1978 were Dr. R.A. Trifts to the Department of Internal Medicine, Dr. Ivan H. Gibson and Dr. Wai-Leung Ying to the Department of Pathology, Dr. M.G. Forsythe to the Department of

Orthopaedics, Dr. Ian Curry to the Department of Surgery and Dr. John Meagher, Dr. Katherine Cox and Dr. William Fitch to the Department of General Practice.

Bob Trifts was born at Youngs Cove, New Brunswick, on December 2, 1943, and received a BA from the University of New Brunswick before proceeding to Dalhousie where he earned his MD in 1971. He interned at the Victoria General Hospital from 1971 to 1972 and after a year of internal medicine residency at the National Defence Medical Centre in Ottawa from 1973 to 1974, he finished his training in internal medicine and cardiology at The Health Sciences Centre in Winnipeg from 1974 to 1978. He received his FRCP(C) in 1977. He has been a faithful member of the medical staff since, serving as Chief of Medicine and a term as president of the medical staff in 1991 and 1992.

Dr. Ivan H. Gibson was a short-term addition to the staff of the pathology department, being appointed in 1978 and resigning in 1980. He was born on August 25, 1946, in Northern Ireland, and after premedical education at Bedford, England, he attended Belfast University, receiving MB, BCh, BOA degrees in 1970. He interned at Lurgan Valley and Lisburn Hospitals in Northern Ireland from 1970 to 1971, and then studied pathology at Royal Victoria and City Hospitals in Belfast from 1971 to 1976 with a further year at the Victoria General Hospital from 1976 to 1977. He received his MRC Pathology in England and his FRCP(C) in 1976 and his LMCC in 1978. After serving six months at the Sudbury General Hospital, he joined the staff of the Moncton Regional Laboratory.

Dr. Wei-Leung Ying has been a valuable addition to the pathology department, making Moncton his home for the past seventeen years. He was born on January 30, 1944, in Ninpo, China, and took premedical and medical education at the National Defence Medical Centre, Taiwan, receiving his MB degree in 1969. He then immigrated to North America and served internships at the Bronx Lebanon Medical Centre, Bronx, New York, from 1970 to 1971 and at Saint Joseph's Hospital, Toronto, from 1971 to 1972. He studied pathology at McGill at the Montreal General from 1972 to 1973, the Royal Victoria from 1973 to 1975, and the Reddy Memorial Hospital Centre from 1975 to 1976. He also took a year of internal medicine at the Ottawa General, Ottawa Civic and the National Defence Medical Centre from 1976 to 1977. He received his LMCC in 1972 and became certified by the American Board of Pathology in Clinical and Anatomical Pathology in 1977. In addition, he was qualified by the American Board of Pathology in Haematology in 1985.

M.G. Forsythe was born in Kentville, Nova Scotia, on March 18, 1945, and received a BA from Acadia in 1966 and his MD from Dalhousie in 1971, after serving in the Dalhousie rotating internship program from 1970 to 1971 at the Victoria General, St.John's General, the Grace Maternity and the Izaak Walton Killam Hospitals. After joining the Canadian Armed Forces, he served in Chatham, New Brunswick, from 1971 to 1973. From 1973 to 1974, he did a residency in surgery at the Canadian Armed Forces Hospital at Stadacona and then pursued a residency in orthopaedics at the Victoria General Hospital, from 1974 to 1977, followed by a year of fellowship in spine surgery at the University of Pennsylvania Hospital from 1977 to 1978. He received his FRCS(C) in orthopaedics in 1978, his American Boards in Orthopaedics in 1981 and his Fellowship in the American College of Surgeons in 1984. He has served the orthopaedic department in an exemplary fashion since joining the staff although he had to curtail his activities in recent years due to heart problems. He has served as chief of orthopaedics and on various hospital committees and is now serving as a program management director.

An addition to the Department of General Surgery was Dr. G. Ian Curry who specialized in plastic surgery, which had not yet become a separate department. He was born in Nigeria on August 29, 1943, but was an Irish citizen and received his education in Ireland. He took premedical education at Royal Belfast Academical Institute and then his medical education at Queen's University, Belfast, receiving the degree of MB, BCh in 1969. He interned at the Belfast City Hospital from 1969 to 1970 and then served as a resident in surgery at the same hospital from 1970 to 1971. Following his immigration to Canada, he did a residency in surgery at the Ottawa Civic Hospital in 1973 and at McMaster University from 1973 to 1975. This was followed by a residency in plastic surgery at the University of Western Ontario from 1976 to 1978 and he received his FRCS(C) in Plastic Surgery in 1978 and his LMCC in 1980. Although he had a dour personality, he was a superb surgeon, and expected perfection not only from those around him but from himself, as well. He performed the first limb reattachment in New Brunswick on October 29, 1982, when a young man, eighteen years old, had his hand amputated by a hydraulic woodsplitter. The reattachment was successful and was the subject of a feature article in the *Moncton Transcript* of November 25, 1982. Ill health forced Dr. Curry to go off the call schedule and join the senior active staff in 1990, and he resigned from the staff in June, 1993, joining the honorary staff. Following his retirement he pursued his interest in art and painting before succumbing to his illness in 1995.

John Meagher was born in Tipperary, Ireland, on June 8, 1946. He took his premedical and medical education at the National University of Ireland and received MB, BCh, BAO degrees in 1970. He immigrated to Canada and interned at Miseracordia Hospital, Edmonton, Alberta from 1970 to 1971 and received his LMCC. He entered practice at Mayer Fort General Hospital and then West Coast General Hospital in Port Alberni, British Columbia from 1972 to 1976. After a two year stint at Victoria Hospital, Castries, St. Lucia from 1976 to 1978, he returned to Canada and came to Moncton, taking over the practice of Dr. Heinz Scholtz who departed for the west coast. In 1987, he closed his office and became a full time emergency room physician. He became certified in ATLS in 1987 and ACLS in 1988.

Dr. Katherine Cox and Dr. William Fitch both came to Moncton to join the Lakeside (Riverview) Medical Clinic. Katherine Cox disappeared within a year, but Bill Fitch has remained a stalwart of the Department of General Practice. Katherine Cox was born in Truro, Nova Scotia, on March 30, 1952, and received her BSc in 1972 and her MD from Dalhousie in 1976. She then served a rotating internship in the Dalhousie program and one of her rotations included The Moncton Hospital. She served a year of residency in pediatrics at the Saint John General Hospital before coming to Moncton.

Bill Fitch was born in Moncton on August 26, 1953, the son of Dr. Ralph Fitch. He took his premedical education at Acadia University, received his MD from Dalhousie in 1977 and then served a year of rotating internship in the Dalhousie program. Since joining the staff he has served as Chief of the Department of General Practice but his most noted achievement has been the time he has spent as Chairman of the Audit Committee.

There were only 52 more admissions in 1978 than in 1977, but the average length of stay had increased from 11.6 to 12.7 days. In addition, there were 1,620 newborns admitted; 10,255 operations were performed including 4,610 day surgery patients. Most services showed just a slight increase in the number of patients with the following figures recorded: audiograms—1,061; electrocardiograms—18,342; electroencephalograms -1,915; gastrointestinal procedures—1,187; nuclear medicine procedures—4,166; radiological examinations—73,334; shock treatments—718; speech pathology—1,828; social services—1,828; ultrasound examinations—1,580. Besides 66,746 patients seen in the emergency department, there were 6,570 clinic visits as follows: Arthritis—960; Chemotherapy—2,386; Colposcopy (opened August 1978)—213; Diabetic Day Care (opened August 1978)—740; Diet Counselling—233; Hyperproteimenia—99, Obesity—166; Obesity Weight Checks—590; and Radiotherapy—1,183.

In 1979 the administration and board of trustees had to again wrestle with the problem of inadequate funding. As in previous years, the provincial government applied the same across-the-board increase to all hospitals, irrespective of existing operating costs or efficiency. The six percent increase was considerably below the amount required to meet negotiated salary increases and the other effects of inflation. By mid-year, the hospital found itself about $1.2 million short in its budget and for the first time in its history, the hospital found it necessary to lay off staff. In order to determine the areas to be cut, the hospital established a committee of representatives of the Medical Staff, Board of Trustees, and Administration and this committee reviewed every line and every dollar in the budget. As a result of this review, most departments received serious cuts in their operating capacity and 40 positions were eliminated. One casualty of the cutbacks was the closure of the Psychiatric Day Hospital.

This review, however, resulted in saving only about half of the budget shortage and it was felt necessary to close two nursing units in order to balance the budget. With the resulting publicity that would result from bed closures, the Minister of Health stepped in and commissioned a study of the hospital's use of available funds and appointed as consultants, to do so, the firm of Touche Ross & Co., in the fall of 1979. The terms of reference were to: (a) determine the adequacy of funding for The Moncton Hospital and (b) assist both the Department of Health and the hospital with the development of a common understanding of the system, and appreciation of each other's problems, and a joint approach to problem solving.

The consultants prepared their report and this was received in the spring of 1980, with the generally favourable following conclusions reached:

1. cost reduction and containment are highly evident in the hospital and relatively few opportunities exist for further significant cost savings;
2. The Moncton Hospital appears very cost effective when compared statistically to other hospitals in New Brunswick and with selected "peer" hospitals in Canada;
3. present financial information control systems and procedures at the hospital are inadequate to ensure effective control of expenditures on an ongoing basis;
4. the average length of stay (of inpatients) of The Moncton Hospital is significantly higher than the Canadian norm; and
5. a major opportunity for further cost savings at The Moncton Hospital is in the reduction of the average length of stay.

To address the critical areas of the report in items three, four, and five, the Board of Trustees, on receiving the report in 1980, took action to augment the inventory systems which would provide the additional recommended information and to do a complete review and revision of the internal financial reporting systems. A Joint Task Force from the medical staff, the board of trustees and the administration was established to look at the "length of stay" problem. With the consultant's report in hand, agreement was reached with the provincial government to renegotiate the hospital's budget.

On May 21, 1979, a Department of Health Program of User Fees was implemented. The fees applied to users of hospital outpatient facilities and included a formula for a fixed fee for each inpatient stay in hospital. Its main intention was to have patients seek treatment in the doctor's office for minor ailments rather than relying on more expensive hospital facilities. Because of political pressure, and the fact that user fees were against the Canada Health Act, the provincial government was forced to cancel user fees on March 25, 1980. During the period that user fees were in, the number of visits to the outpatient department fell by 9,055 compared to the corresponding period in the previous year. The revenue generated amounted to $288,307 with $25,697 remaining outstanding at the cessation of the program.

Despite budgetary problems, all was not at a standstill at the hospital. A new eight-bed Coronary Intensive Care Unit was constructed on 3 Joyce, as well as the intermediate care unit in the balance of 3 Joyce, and the east end of 3 Parlee. The total project cost, including new equipment, was $980,000. In addition to the improvements in coronary care, day surgery facilities were expanded and the respiratory technology department received much needed improvements.

The Day Surgery Unit was remodelled and was now capable of handling as many as twenty minor surgical cases daily. Special grants of $1.3 million by the Department of Health allowed the Radiology Department to re-equip its chest radiography room, an X-ray room for special procedures, and to install a CT scanner.

A new Speech and Hearing Service evolved with the addition of an audiologist to work with the existing speech therapist, and to carry out the hearing testing service.

The growing complexity of technological equipment resulted in the establishment of a Clinical Engineering Service. This was a joint venture with the Dr. Georges-L. Dumont Hospital and other hospitals in the region and was headed up by an engineer, Dr. Monique Frieze. With it the hospital gained the ability to improve its evaluation of proposed and new medical equipment and to raise the level of electrical safety enjoyed by the patients.

With the arrival of Dr. Robin Walker, neonatologist, in the spring of 1979, a brief was presented to the Department of Health, with Dr. Walker pointing out that perinatal morbidity was high in New Brunswick, as well as cerebral palsy and that regionalisation of perinatal care has proven benefits in reducing perinatal mortality. It was also pointed out that the Special Care Nursery was crowded and poorly equipped. The brief fell on receptive ears and the Department of Health provided funding in the amount of $81,000 to expand and properly equip the unit and $92,000 was approved to provide the required nursing coverage. Since the project was completed in December 1979, The Moncton Hospital has been able to serve as a referral centre for high risk babies from the eastern part of New Brunswick.

As 1979 was the International Year of the Child, numerous gifts were received by the neonatal unit as well as the pediatric unit and a good deal of the credit goes to Dr. Walker in publicizing the need in the community. Oxygen analysers were donated by Kentucky Fried Chicken and the Kinette Club of Moncton, apnea monitors from the Westmorland and the Fort Cumberland Chapters of the IODE, and Heart Rate monitors were received from Mrs. Christine Harper, Charlene Short, Miss Pre-Teen Majorette of New Brunswick, and the Hon. C.H. Blakeny Chapter, IODE. The Moncton Lionettes provided a parents' lounge for the Special Care Nursery and the lounge was furnished by the B'nai Brith Moncton Lodge No. 3069. Gifts to the Paediatric Unit included a wheelchair with IV holder from the Fort Monckton Chapter, IODE, a heart rate monitor from the Kiwanis Club of Moncton and Wonder Wall Murals from the Fort Cumberland Chapter, IODE, a child's walker from the Harrisville Women's Institute United Protestant Church Women's Group, a junior wheelchair and two car seats from the Meadowvale Women's Institute, a Christmas gift of four television sets from the CN Shops Employees, a rowcar from the Air Traffic Controllers' Association, and a child's stroller from the Riverview Girl Guide Company.

Although it was the International Year of the Child, donations to other departments of the hospital also continued. The Firefighters continued to support the Burn Unit and reference books were received from Local 999, Moncton Firefighters. In addition, supplies for mixing burn treatment lotions and ointments were received from the Moncton Firefighters Association Burn Unit Committee. Two colour television sets were provided by the Riverview Professional Firefighters Association. The Moncton Gyrettes provided an oxygen blender and the Pythian Sisters Tidal Wave Temple No. 16

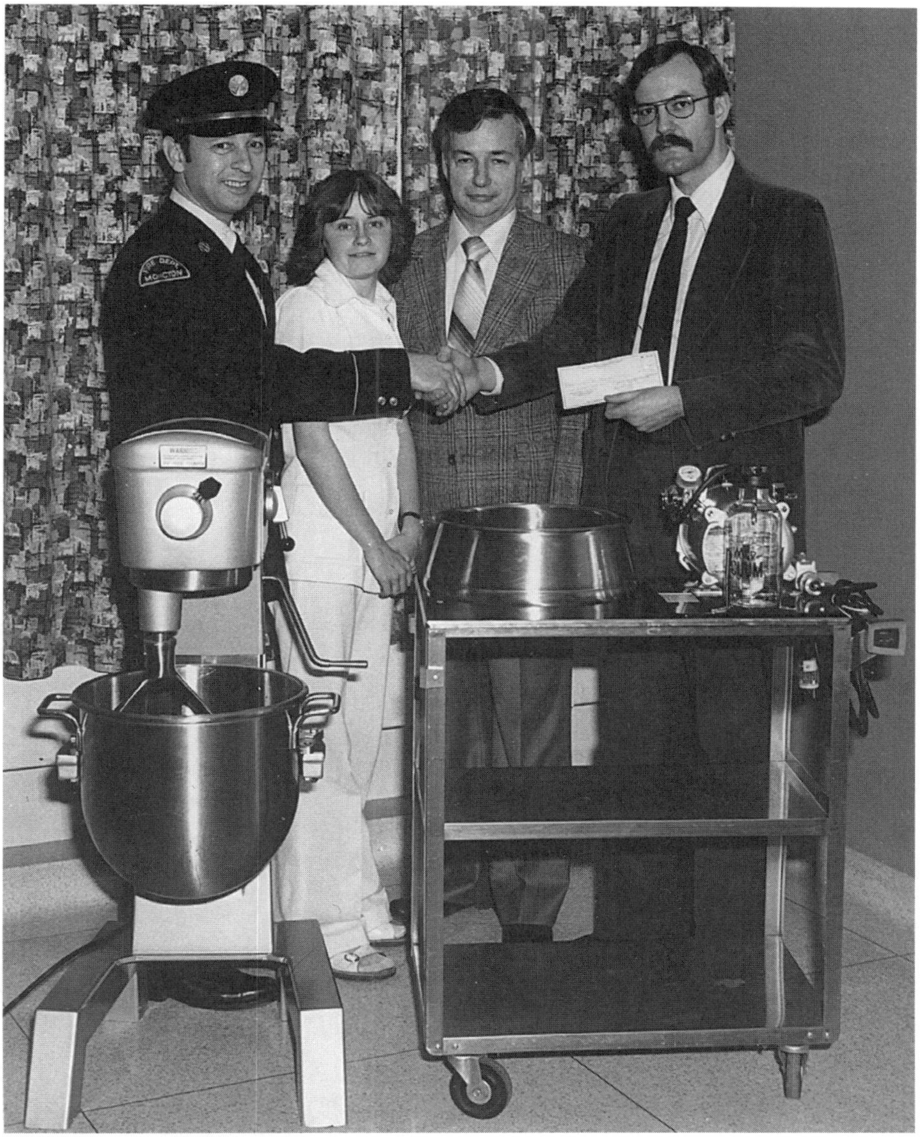

The Moncton Fire Department presents a mixing machine to the Burn Unit in 1979. From left to right: Mr. Paul Cormier, Valerie Berry, Harry Wade, Dr. Ian Curry.

a Doppler stethoscope. The Speech and Hearing Service was the recipient of a clinical audiometer from the Elks Club of Moncton, and an auditory trainer from the Municipal Chapter, IODE. Gifts also continued to pour in from the hospital organizations: The Moncton Hospital School of Nursing Alumnae, The Moncton Hospital Volunteers, The Ladies' Hospital Auxiliary, the Nurses' Hospital Auxiliary and the Friends of the Moncton Hospital. Significant among these gifts was the provision of a colonoscope and furnishing of the OPD waiting room by the Friends and financing of a cottage at Bateman's Mills by The Moncton Hospital School of Nursing Alumnae to replace the cottage at Shediac Cape which had been destroyed by fire. Contributions ranging from alternating pressure mattresses, geriatric chairs and oil paintings were also received from various individuals but, unfortunately, space does not allow them to be listed.

During the year, the medical staff, as well as the hospital staff and community were saddened by the death of Dr. Austin Clarke, executive director of The Moncton Hospital from 1955 to 1970. Also, the death occurred of Mrs. Doris Ricker, who had been secretary to the medical staff and a "housemother" to the interns and newer members of the medical staff for many years.

New additions to the medical staff in 1979 were: Dr. Gilbert Quarty, Dr. Roger Roberge, Dr. S.A. Malmud, Dr. William Harper and Dr. Thomas

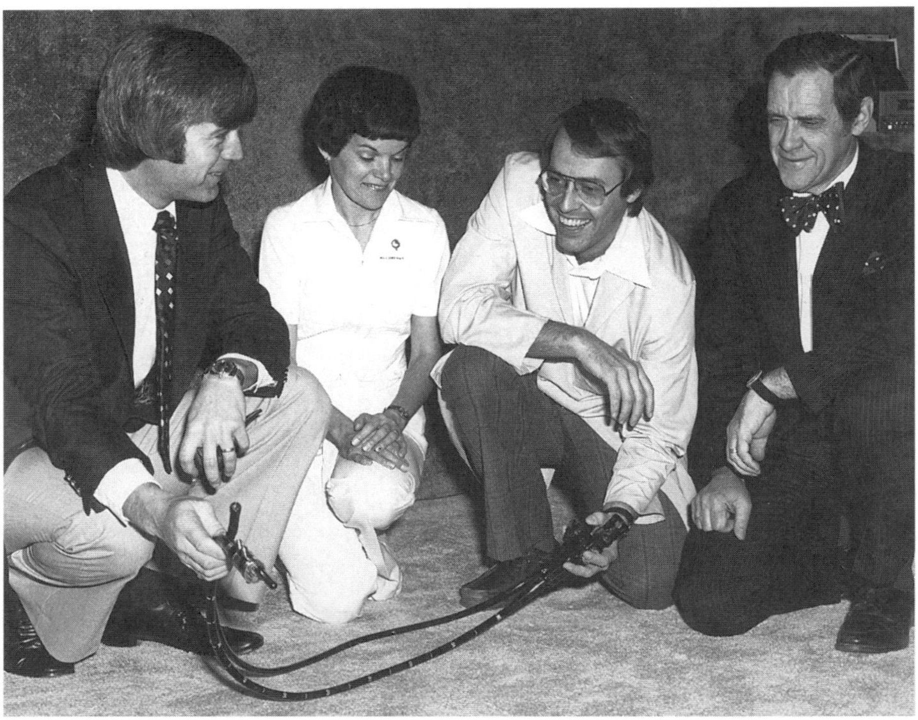

Dr. Peter Lightfoot displays the new Colonoscope presented by The Friends of the Moncton Hospital. From left to right: Mr. Douglas Apt, Carolyn Lewis, R.N., Dr. Lightfoot, and Mr. Ralph Belyea.

Laughlin. The last two joined the Moncton Medical Clinic.

With the departure of Dr. Jones, the Department of Neurological Sciences was fortunate to be able to recruit Dr. Gilbert Reginald Cato Quarty. He was born at Cape Coast, Ghana, on April 21, 1945. Educated in Great Britain, he took premedical education at University Tutorial College, London, and then graduated from Glasgow University with an MB, CHB degree in 1971. He interned at Southern General and Queen Mary's Hospital from 1971 to 1972. He did a residency in orthopaedics and emergency medicine at St. Leonard's Hospital, London, from 1972 to 1973, and then a year of general surgery at Saint John's General Hospital, Newfoundland from 1973 to 1974. He then ventured to Saskatchewan where he was a resident and clinical fellow in neurosurgery at University Hospital, University of Saskatchewan in Saskatoon from 1974 to 1979, receiving his FRCS(C) in Neurosurgery in 1979. His calm demeanour, rational thinking, and sense of fair play made him an excellent choice to serve a term as chairman of the OR Committee. In addition to his general knowledge and expertise in neurosurgery, he has established a reputation as an expert in chronic pain control management and serves in the Pain Clinic.

Dr. Roger Roberge came to Moncton with an established surgical reputation in New Brunswick. He was born in Grand Falls, New Brunswick, on August 26, 1939, and received a BA from College St Louis in 1960 and an MD from University of Laval in 1965. He interned at Chicoutimi General Hospital from 1964 to 1965 and did a residency in general surgery at the same institution from 1965 to 1969, receiving his certification and FRCS(C) in General Surgery in 1971. He had a general surgical practice in Campbellton from 1969 to 1979, before joining the active staff of the Dr. Georges-L. Dumont Hospital and associate staff of The Moncton Hospital. In 1980, he switched his main allegiance to The Moncton Hospital. Besides serving as chief of surgery in 1988 and 1989, he has served as president of the medical staff in 1989 and 1990. He is also an ATLS instructor. Aside from his general surgical practice he has gained a reputation for his special interest in management of cancer of the breast. He has been active in medical politics, serving as president of the New Brunswick Medical Society in 1979. He was also president of the College of Physicians and Surgeons of New Brunswick in 1978 and was the New Brunswick representative to the board of directors of the Canadian Medical Association from 1982 to 1985. Outside the medical field, he is an active golfer and skier. He is a medical consultant and instructor to the Canadian Ski Patrol, North Eastern Division. In 1977, he received a life-saving award from the Canadian Ski Patrol for a rescue in the woods in winter. In Campbellton he took an active role in the Saint John Ambulance Corps and was made a Serving Brother in the Order of Saint John of Jerusalem at a ceremony in Ottawa in November, 1976.

Dr. Syed Asad Malmud joined the psychiatric staff, bucking the trend of several previous appointments by becoming a long-serving member of the department. He was born on December 1, 1942, at Lahore, Pakistan. He attended D.J. Sirens College, Karachi, receiving an FSc degree in 1961. He attended King Edward Medical College, Lahore, University of Punjab, Karachi, receiving an MB, BS degree in 1966. He interned at Mayo and Kairns Hospitals in Lahore from 1966 to 1967. He went to Great Britain for postgraduate work, serving a residency in psychiatry at Roundway Hospital, Devizes, England, from 1967 to 1971 and then the University of Leeds from 1971 to 1972. He was certified in psychiatry by the Royal College of Psychiatrists (MRC Psych.) in 1973. On immigrating to Canada, he received his FRCP(C) in Psychiatry in 1973. After serving as a psychiatrist at Saint Joseph's Hospital in Saint John from 1974 to 1979, he moved to Moncton where he has remained as a well respected member of the staff. Besides serving as Chief of Psychiatry, he was elected as vice-president of the medical staff in 1995.

Thomas Laughlin was born on May 21, 1953 in Fredericton, New Brunswick, and received his MD from Dalhousie University in 1978. After serving a year of rotating internship in the Dalhousie program from 1978 to 1979, he joined the Moncton Medical Clinic in family practice and has become an examiner for the College of Family Physicians. An ardent outdoorsman, he enjoys fishing, hunting and canoeing, and is a supporter of Ducks Unlimited.

Bill Harper is a Moncton native born on August 18, 1953, and received a BA from Mount Allison University in 1974 and an MD from Dalhousie in 1978. After a rotating internship from 1978 to 1979 in the Dalhousie program which included a stint at The Moncton Hospital, he returned to practise in his native city at the Moncton Medical Clinic and became certified by the Canadian College of Family Practice in 1985. During his university years he served as an ambulance driver at The Moncton Hospital during his summer vacations. With a boyish appearance, not even hidden by the sprouting of a mustache, and an ever ready grin, Bill could be the *Saturday Evening Post*'s "boy next door". As a guileless youth, Bill was the master of ceremonies at one of the medical staffs' annual dinners, and before taking centre stage, asked one of his colleagues for a joke he could tell. His stag party joke was not well received by this mixed audience and an off-colour joke has ever since become known to the medical staff as a "Billy Harper."

There were 13,449 admissions to the hospital in 1979/80 fiscal year with 1,729 newborns for an average length of stay of 11.7 days, excluding newborns; 10,276 operations were performed including 3,935 day surgery patients. Services supplied during the year included the following: audiograms—1,206; electrocardiograms—16,848; electroencephalograms—1,438; gastrointestinal unit procedures—1,004; radiological examinations—71,427; nuclear medicine procedures—3,440; ultrasound examinations—2,118; shock treatments—564; social service caseload—1,422; and speech pathology—1,422. Although OPD/Emergency visits were down to 56,609 compared to 66,746 in the previous year, clinic visits were up significantly, from 6,570 the previous year to 8,560. Most of the increase was due to the Diabetic Day Care visits rising to 1,807 from 740 the previous year. The Public Health Orthopaedic Clinic was discontinued. Attendance at other clinics was as follows: Arthritis—1,105; Chemotherapy—2,409; Colposcopy—438; Diet Counselling—171; Hyperproteinemia—66; Obesity—193; with obesity weight checks—1,037; and Radiotherapy—1,334.

Chapter Ten

The Eighties—
A Time to Expand

In June 1979, the hospital revised the proposed development plan for The Moncton Hospital in co-operation with Architects Four and presented it to the provincial cabinet. In June 1980, the minister of health, Hon. Brenda Robertson, announced a $35 million-construction development plan with construction to begin in 1981, with a completion date in 1985. Wes Drodge joined the administration staff as project co-ordinator to supervise the construction and planning. It took a few years for the medical staff to teach Mr. Drodge and the architects that doctors did not work on nine-to-five schedules and that consultations with them should be held outside of office and operating room schedules if they were really interested in the doctors' input in the development plan. Nevertheless, over the six years of the construction project, most of the practical advice of the medical staff was heeded.

On July 1, 1980, the provincial government transferred the administration of the Regional Laboratory to The Moncton Hospital and, at the same time, established an independent laboratory at the Dr. Georges-L. Dumont Hospital. Until this time, lab employees were civil servants and it was agreed at the time of the transfer that no employee would suffer a loss of salary, classification, seniority, or other benefits, when the transfer took place. Approximately 80 lab staff members were welcomed to The Moncton Hospital staff on July 1, and to celebrate this event, a steak and lobster party was held at the hospital cottage at Bateman's Mills for all employees of the lab, hosted by the board and department heads of the hospital.

During the year, two members of the management staff retired. Jim McCafferty had been Comptroller and Treasurer since 1967. He was succeeded in this position by W. King. Frances Cudahy retired after 19 years of service as ECG technician and director of the department and regrettably died shortly after her retirement.

After the consultant's report from Touche Ross and Co. in 1979 had criticised the length of stay at The Moncton Hospital, a task force on length of stay was appointed and chaired by Dr. W.A. Oatway, the president of the medical staff. Within a year, the length of stay was reduced to that of the provincial level or slightly lower. This reduction in length of stay could not have been accomplished without the co-operation of almost every member of the medical staff and this result can be attributed directly to the personality, work, and leadership of Dr. Oatway.

There was a larger than normal number of resignations from the nursing staff in 1980. As a result of the consultants review of the operation of The Moncton Hospital, some additional nursing positions were recommended in June. These two factors resulted in a chronic shortage of nurses during the late fall and winter of 1980/81, forcing the closure of thirty beds (one nursing unit) in January 1981, in an effort to alleviate the situation. A temporary nurse recruiter, Marie Chisholm, was hired, and visits were made to all schools of nursing throughout the Atlantic provinces, university schools of nursing and nursing job fairs in Philadelphia and Toronto. A major newspaper and journal advertising campaign was undertaken, in addition. Increased activity in nurse re-orientation was undertaken with the help of Employment Canada to increase the return to work of former inactive nurses both on a full and part time basis. The staff of the education department, which had been reduced in the 1979 budget crisis, was now increased to three full-time employees, two of whom were assigned duties primarily in nursing inservice education. Mr. Kilpatrick admitted that making cuts to the education department in a budget crisis had been a mistake because of the continuing new developments in medicine and nursing, and declared that he would not be in favour of any cuts in the education budget in the future.

Numerous gifts were received from organizations and individuals during the year, taking up two pages in the annual report for 1980/81. The most significant pieces of new medical equipment obtained was an echocardiograph unit donated by the Hon. C.H. Blakeny Chapter, IODE, a new Image Intensifier from the Nurses' Hospital Auxiliary and a nephroscope, an electromyelographic unit and a three-channel ECG machine from the Friends of the Moncton Hospital. The Firefighters continued to support the Burn Unit with the Moncton Firefighters' Association pledging $6,000 for the purchase of needed equipment and the Riverview Firefighters' Association donating Christmas gifts of a microwave oven, colour television and three portable radios. The medical staff were not immune, with Dr. V. McLaughlin and Dr. G. Brodie donating a colposcope to the outpatient Colposcopy Clinic.

There were several additions to the medical staff in 1980: Dr. G. Donald, Dr. R.I. Morton, Dr. Douglas Keeling, Dr. James Livingston, Dr. John Park, Dr. Loanna Whitmore, Dr. Pamela Walsh and Dr. Francis Erwin to the Department of Family practice; Dr. T.W.A. Cooper to the Department of Anaesthesia; Dr. Peter Gorman to the Department of Neurological Sciences; Dr. David Silverberg to the Department of Neurological Sciences and Internal Medicine; and Dr. David Yule to Pediatrics. This year saw the renaming of the Department of General Practice to the Department of Family Practice and the Department of Ophthalmology was formed, splitting the ophthalmologists off from the Department of Otorhinolaryngology and Ophthalmology.

Greg Donald was born on April 9, 1951, in Charlottetown, Prince Edward Island. He received a BSc from Mount Allison in 1973 and an MD from Dalhousie in 1979. He then served a rotating internship in the Dalhousie program (1979-1980) and set up practice in Moncton joining the clinic. Like all members of the Moncton Medical Clinic, he has participated in Dalhousie medical education and serves as a preceptor for third and fourth year medical students. He has taken a keen interest in the extra mural hospital and has served as chairman of both the Driscoll Unit and the provincial Medical Advisory Committees of the Extra Mural Hospital.

Richard Morton made his entry into the world in Sussex, New Brunswick, on February 24, 1950. He obtained his BSc from the University of New Brunswick in 1972, an MD from Memorial University in 1976 and interned at St. John's General Hospital from 1976-1977. After service in the Canadian Armed Services, mostly in Lahr, West Germany, he entered practice at the Petitcodiac Health Centre joining the courtesy staff and then the active staff in 1990. Any discussion in the doctors' lounge soon reveals his right-wing political philosophy.

Douglas Keeling was born on February 6, 1953, in Saint John, New Brunswick. He attended the University of New Brunswick, receiving a BSc in 1975, and graduated from Dalhousie in 1979 with his MD. He served a rotating internship at Memorial University in Saint John's, Newfoundland, from 1979 and 1980 and did a locums at Albert, New Brunswick, from October 1980, until June 1981, when he joined the Riverview Medical Clinic. Besides his family practice, he worked shifts in the emergency department and obtained his ACLS in 1982, his ATLS in 1984 and his certification in the College of Family Practice in 1985. As a result of his work in the emergency room, he was made an honorary member of the 22nd Field Squadron of the Canadian Engineers for life-saving measures given to a young soldier in 1981. Always keen and interested in his work, he served on the National Board of Medical Examiners in 1981 and in 1985 was part of the medical team at the 1985 Canada Winter Games. In 1985 he took a leave of absence and worked in the Acadian Peninsula so that he could learn French, and from 1985 to 1987 he worked in the emergency department of the Dr. Georges-L. Dumont Hospital in addition to The Moncton Hospital. He resigned in 1987 to take postgraduate work in dermatology at the University of Ottawa, passed his American Board of Dermatology exams in 1991, and now practises in Saint John.

James Livingston, born in New Glasgow on December 12, 1952, received a BSc from Mount Allison in 1975 and an MD from Dalhousie in 1979. He served a rotating internship at The Moncton Hospital from 1979 to 1980 and then joined the staff but resigned shortly thereafter in April 1981.

John Park, born in Korea on July 3, 1954, was educated in Canada, receiving his premedical and medical training at the University of Ottawa, graduating in 1979. He did his internship in the Dalhousie rotating internship program and remained in the Maritimes to practice medicine. He was originally appointed to the courtesy staff as he began practice in Cap-Pele but joined the active staff when he moved to Moncton in 1981, at which time he assumed the practice of Dr. Tony Jong and served part-time in the Department of Emergency Medicine as well.

Loanna Whitmore was born in Moncton on February 2, 1947. After receiving a diploma in physiotherapy at Dalhousie University in 1967, she joined the staff at The Moncton Hospital. In 1973, she went to study at the University of Manitoba, from which she obtained her B PT in 1974, and then stayed on at the University of Manitoba obtaining her MD degree in 1979. She returned east to do her internship year at The Moncton Hospital from 1979 to 1980 and then joined the courtesy staff, setting up a family practice in Hillsborough. She changed from courtesy to active staff status in 1986 when she devoted her practice to working on the geriatric ward at The Moncton Hospital.

Dr. Pamela Walsh was the first member of the staff to confine her practice solely to emergency medicine, although, as yet, this was not a separate department. Pamela was born in Saint John and obtained her BSc from the University of New Brunswick in 1974 and her MD from Dalhousie in 1979. She then served an internship in the Dalhousie Integrated Program of Family Medicine from 1979 to 1980. In 1986 she received her Certification of Special Competence in Emergency Medicine from the College of Family Practice of Canada. Her knowledge and common sense approach to the practice of emergency medicine has made her one member of a team in the hospital's Department of Emergency Medicine that is second to none. From 1990 to 1992, she was a member of the New Brunswick College of Physicians and Surgeons Fitness to Practice Committee and, since 1993, has been one of the regional representatives to the College.

Frank L. Erwin was born in Montreal on October 11, 1955, and received his premedical and medical education at Dalhousie, graduating with his MD degree in 1979. He interned at Royal Columbian Hospital in New Westminster, British Columbia, from 1979 to 1980 and then joined the Moncton Medical Clinic and served part time in the emergency department. In July 1993 he resigned to undertake postgraduate work in internal medicine at Dalhousie.

Dr. Timothy Walker Argyle Cooper was born in Edgware, England, on June 7, 1947, and received his medical education at University of Saint Mary's Hospital, London, graduating in 1972 with the degrees MB, BS, MRCS, LRCP. After interning in London at St. Mary's Hospital from 1972 to 1973 and Edgware General Hospital from 1973 to 1974, he came to Canada and pursued post-graduate work in anaesthesia, first at the Victoria General Hospital in Halifax from 1975 to 1978 and then as a clinical fellow at the Royal Victoria Hospital in Montreal from 1978 to 1979, becoming certified in anaesthesia by the Quebec College of Physicians and Surgeons. The superior calibre of his work was such that he was appointed a staff anaesthetist at the Royal Victoria Hospital from 1979 to 1980. The Moncton Hospital was fortunate to recruit him to the anaesthetic staff in 1980 and unfortunate, when he left in 1990 to join the staff of the King Fahd National Guard Hospital in Riyadh, Saudi Arabia, where he went to satisfy his personal desire to travel and experience other cultures and peoples of the world. During his ten-year stay on the staff of The Moncton Hospital he joined the Pain Clinic after it was formed and was instrumental in reorganizing the Surgical Intensive Care Unit. His interest in intensive care was of great benefit to the patients but a bane to the surgeons as he would sometimes wander off to the intensive care unit between surgical cases, losing all concept of time, while the surgeon waited impatiently in the surgeon's lounge to start his next case.

Dr. Peter Gorman was born in Ottawa on July 5, 1944. After obtaining a BA from Carleton University in 1965, he received his MD from the University of Ottawa in 1969. After serving a rotating internship at the University of Toronto, he spent three years in a general surgery residency at the Ottawa Civic Hospital and then embarked on neurosurgery training at the Henry Ford Hospital in Detroit (1973-75 and 1976-77) with a year rotation to The Montreal Children's Hospital and the Montreal Neurological Institute from 1975 to 1976. Further neurosurgery training was obtained at University Hospital and Victoria Hospital, London, Ontario, from 1977 to 1979, during which time he obtained his FRCS(C) in neurosurgery. He stayed on with a fellowship in neurosurgery at University Hospital, London, from 1979 to 1980, before he was induced to throw his lot in with the Maritimes. He took to the Maritimes quite nicely and soon became an avid salmon fisherman and duck hunter. The neurosurgery department was now increased to three, although it would soon to be reduced again to a two-man department with the death of Dr. Tucker in the following year. Dr. Gorman's talents included administration and in June 1987, he was elected chief of staff for a four year period. During the centennial campaign he was tireless, speaking to numerous service clubs, promoting the Friend's campaign to raise money.

The departure of Dr. Robertson left a void in the hospital, especially with a growing Department of Neurosurgery. Dr. David Silverberg joined the staff to fill this void. David, like Dr. Gorman, was a native of Ontario, born in Toronto on August 5, 1948. He received his premedical and medical education at the University of Toronto, graduating with his MD degree in 1973. He interned at the Royal Alexander Hospital, Edmonton, Alberta, from 1973 to 1974. After a three-month stint of anaesthesia and six months of internal medicine at Royal Alexander and W.W. Cross Hospital in Edmonton, he returned to Ontario to the University of Ottawa where he studied neurology with a residency involving the Ottawa Civic, the Ottawa General and the Children's Hospital of Eastern Ontario which resulted in the awarding of a FRCP(C) in neurology in 1979. In 1983 he also was made a Fellow of the American Academy of Neurology and Psychiatry. David has remained on staff since then and has watched his department grow to include five neurologists.

David Yule was born in Glasgow on July 3, 1943, and attended the University of Glasgow, receiving his BSc in 1964 and his MB, ChB in 1967. After a rotating internship in England, he immigrated to Canada and served another rotating internship from 1969 to 1970 at Saint Anthony, Newfoundland, and a residency at Goose Bay, Labrador, from 1971 to 1972. He then entered a residency program in pediatrics at the Izaak Walton Killam Hospital from 1972 to 1976 and obtained his Fellowship in Paediatrics from the Royal College of Physicians and Surgeons of Canada in 1976. After returning to Newfoundland to practice pediatrics at Western Memorial Regional Hospital in Corner Brook from 1976 to 1980, he returned to the mainland to join the paediatric department of The Moncton Hospital.

There were 13,701 adult and children admissions in the 1980/81 fiscal year with an additional 1,614 newborns. The average length of stay was 11.5 days for adults and children and 5.7 days for newborns. There were 10,561 operations performed, of which 4,442 were day patients. All services showed some increase with the departments recording the following number of visits: audiograms—1,240; electrocardiograms—17,842; electroencephalograms—1,858; gastrointestinal unit procedures—1,010; shock treatments—641; social service caseload—1,484; speech pathology—1,713; radiological examinations—74,481; CT scans—2,359; nuclear medicine procedures—3,746 and ultrasound examinations—10,561. Outpatient clinic visits showed a marked increase to 11,916 from the previous year's total of 8,560 visits. The clinic visits were as follows: Arthritic—1,457; Chemotherapy—2,904; Colposcopy—800; Diabetic Day Care—2,068; Diet Counselling—274; Hyperlipoproteinemia—87; Obesity—194, with—1,768 obesity weight checks; and Radiotherapy—1,354.

In September 1981, the Hon. Brenda Robertson, the minister of health, approved the functional program for the development project, but it was to be January 1982, before the Minister authorized Architects Four to proceed with the planning.

As part of the provincial government's policy to increase the number of extended-care beds in hospitals, 30 acute care beds were converted to extended-care beds bringing the total of extended-care beds situated in 4-Parlee and 4-Joyce to 67.

The new angiographic suite was opened in radiology in May 1981. This latest Acromax M equipment allowed bi-plane filming, enabling rapid serial filming of the relevant anatomical area simultaneously in two planes. Adjacent to this room, a smaller room was equipped to do lymphangiography. The radiology department also obtained new ultrasound equipment.

A Pain Research Centre was established in September 1981 with the help of a grant from the Friends of the Moncton Hospital Foundation. The objective of the centre was to test the validity of using skin temperatures for the detection of the presence and exact location of pain. The total operation of the centre was governed by a steering Committee, the members of which were Dr. A. Haché, Dr. C.E. Doyle, Dr. M.G. Forsythe, Dr. W.A. Oatway,

Ruth Duffy, Y. Poussart and Dr. V. McLaughlin. As with similar research projects in other centres, the results of the research showed that skin temperatures were an unreliable guide in the evaluation of pain.

A Poison Control Centre was established in the outpatient department with four major functions:

1. information and data bank;
2. education services;
3. statistical compliance; and
4. follow-up programs.

The information data bank and the educational service were directed towards both the general public and health personnel. All accidental poisonings in children were followed up and the physicians of all intentional overdose patients were notified to ensure adequate post emergency support.

Dr. John Acres was welcomed as the first respirologist on the staff and in the fall of 1981 a fully equipped bronchocospy suite was put into operation. A Chest Clinic was established in November as well, and a flexible bronchoscope was supplied by the Nurses' Hospital Auxiliary.

Size carries with it problems, of course, and the hospital experienced its share in dealing with the increasing numbers of staff, patients and visitors to the hospital. A sign of the times was the introduction of pay parking to try and solve congestion around the hospital. A satellite cafeteria was opened on the first floor of the nurses' residence to relieve crowding in the main cafeteria. The neighbours about the hospital had frequent complaints of soot coming from the hospital's smoke stack and as a result, the incinerator was rebuilt to reduce the pollution. A heat reclaim unit was also installed so that burning garbage helped to supply some heat to the hospital.

Bill Kilpatrick continued to distinguish himself by being elected to the House of Delegates of the American Hospital Association and, of course, this could not help but spread the name of The Moncton Hospital.

The Volunteer Service continued to supply valuable service to the hospital, contributing 8,661 hours of service with 2,432 supplied by teenagers. There were now 20 volunteers with over 1,000 hours of service and 5 with over 1,500 hours. In January 1981 a new program for volunteers was initiated in the nursery for newborn babies who needed to be confined to hospital for a variety of reasons and whose parents were far away. Volunteers have the time to give the babies extra attention and cuddling while the babies respond to the stimulation of being held and talked to. Officially, the program was called the "Surrogate Grandmother Program," but unofficially it was called the "Cuddling Corps."

By 1981 the hospital was becoming a tertiary care institution with increase in the number of patients undergoing major vascular surgery and major lung surgery. By this time it also served the eastern half of the province as the major referral centre for neurosurgery, neonatology, major trauma and burns. On average, 27 percent of patients came from areas served by other hospitals outside of the Moncton and surrounding area. In certain specialties the figures were much higher with over 70 percent of neonatology, 60 percent of thoracic surgery and neurosurgery and 40 percent of orthopaedics and plastic surgery and burns coming from outside the region. Nineteen percent of patients claimed French as their mother tongue. With the reputation as an up-and-coming medical centre, it was beginning to get easier to attract doctors to join the staff and 1981 was no exception to this trend, with nine new members appointed to the active staff as well as Dr. John Carson to the courtesy staff in radiation oncology.

Dr. Ross Murphy was born on March 20, 1944, and received a BSc from

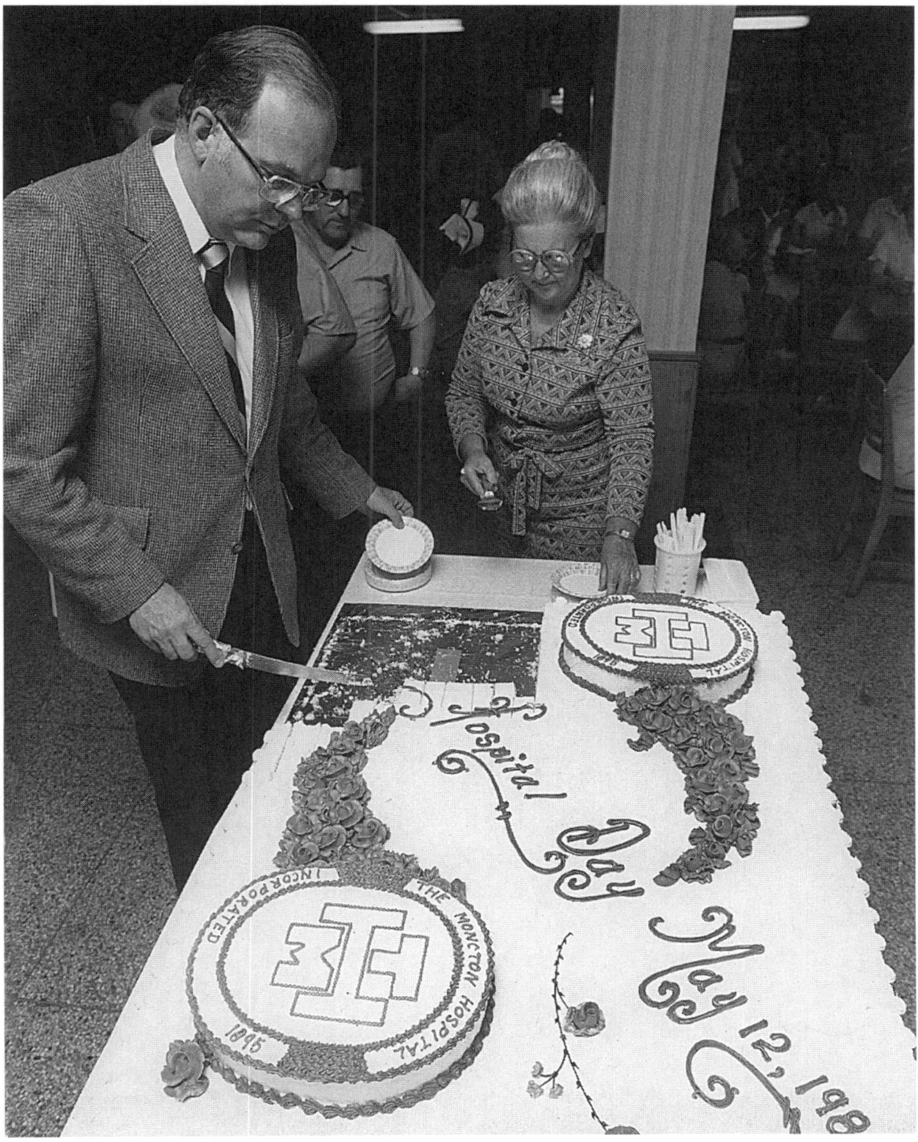

Hospital Day, 1981. Mr. Bill Kilpatrick and Mrs. Katherine Wright serve cake.

McGill in 1967 and an MD from the University of Western Ontario in 1975. He served a surgical internship at the University of Toronto from 1975 to 1976 and continued on in the Toronto Post Graduate Program in surgery from 1976 to 1980, receiving his FRCS(C) in general surgery in 1980. After another year as Ewart Angus Fellow in the Surgical Intensive Care Unit of the Wellesley Hospital, he came to Moncton. Since his appointment, he has served as chief of the Department of Surgery and was elected vice-president of the medical staff in 1993, resigning this post in 1994. He also served as president of the New Brunswick Surgical Society in 1990.

The Department of Radiology was renamed the Department of Medical Imaging in order to reflect the introduction, during the past ten years, of the many new procedures, besides X-rays, that had become part of the radiologist's armamentarium. These included such procedures as invasive angiography, ultrasound, CT scans, and radioisotope scans. With the expansion of the department's work, another radiologist was added to the staff. Dr. Frank E. Fowlie received his BSc from Dalhousie in 1972 and his MD in 1976. After interning at the Victoria General Hospital from 1976 to 1977, he remained at the same institution to study radiology from 1977 to 1980 and received his FRCP(C) in radiology in 1980, as well as a diploma from the American Board of Radiology. He served as chief of the Department of Medical Imaging from 1991 to 1994, and his attendance at the Medical Advisory Committee meetings assured a lengthy discussion on any matter involving his department.

Dr. Sajida Hussain attended Osmania University for her premedical and medical education, receiving her MB, BS in 1966. After coming to Canada she interned at the Reddy Memorial Hospital in Montreal from 1971 to 1972, studied pathology at McGill from 1972 to 1976 serving at the Montreal General (1972-73), St. Mary's (1973-74), Royal Victoria (1974-75) and Jewish General (1975-76). She received her LMCC in 1977 and was certified in pathology by the Corporation professionnelle des médecins du Québec in 1978. From 1978 to 1981 she served as pathologist on the staff of l'Hôtel Dieu de Edmundston before coming to Moncton in 1981. She resigned from the staff in June 1983.

An addition to the Department of Obstetrics and Gynaecology was Dr. Hani Albert Akoury, who was born in Egypt on May 17,1949. He obtained an MB, ChB degree from Alexandria University, Alexandria, Egypt, in 1973 and interned at Alexandria University Hospital and St. Charles Borramee Hospital, Lebanon, from 1974 to 1975. He came to Canada and, after serving an internship and then a year of residency in general surgery at the University of Sherbrooke, he entered the Dalhousie residency program in obstetrics and gynaecology from 1978 to 1981. In 1981, he obtained his specialist certificate from the Corporation professionelle des médicins du Québec (CSPQ) and then his FRCS(C) from the Royal College in 1982. From 1984 to 1987, he served as chief of Obstetrics and Gynaecology. He also served as chairman of a subcommittee of the New Brunswick Medical Society for the formation of the provincial perinatal form. Always interested in introducing new techniques, he performed tubal reanastamosis for the first time in The Moncton Hospital. He was also instrumental in setting up a urodynamics laboratory. His interest in research, however, resulted in his leaving the hospital in 1992 to pursue an academic career.

Internal medicine was now becoming oriented toward subspecialization and Dr. John C. Acres joined the staff as the first respirologist. He was born in Nova Scotia on January 28, 1946, and received his premedical and medical training at Dalhousie graduating with his MD degree in 1970 after serving a rotating internship in the Dalhousie program from 1969 to 1970. From 1970 to 1976 he did general practice in Musquodoboit Harbour and then returned to the Victoria General in Halifax from 1976 to 1979 for a residency in internal medicine. He subsequently proceeded to the Health Sciences Centre in Winnipeg for training in respirology from 1979 to 1980 and spent a year as a fellow of the Manitoba Lung Association at St. Boniface Hospital, Winnipeg in respirology and sleep apnea from 1980 to 1981. He received his FRCP(C) in 1980 and a Certificate of Special Competence in Respiratory Medicine in 1981. Since his appointment, John has enlivened departmental meetings and likes to play the role of the devil's advocate. His presence in the doctors' lounge will help liven up discussion since he likes to take a doom and gloom attitude to the stock market and world events and greets every downturn in the market with glee. His main interest outside medicine is in military history and air shows.

Robert A. Forbes was born in Moncton and attended the University of New Brunswick from which he received a BSc in 1976, and then travelled on to Dalhousie University where he received his MD in 1980. After serving a rotating internship in the Dalhousie program, he set up a family practice at the Riverview Medical Clinic.

Since emergency medicine was still not recognized as a separate department, three new physicians were added to the Department of Family Practice in 1981, although they would confine their practice solely to emergency medicine: Dr. James Goulding and Dr. Peter O'Hanley, both sons of physicians, and Dr. John Whelan.

James F. Goulding was born in Halifax on August 30, 1956, and received a BSc from Dalhousie and his MD from Dalhousie in 1980 being awarded the Dr. C.B. Stewart Gold Medal. From 1980-81, he interned at Victoria General Hospital in Victoria, British Columbia He played a large role in organizing the Department of Emergency Medicine and was its first chief. He received a certificate of competence in emergency medicine from the Canadian College of Family Practice in 1987 and a diploma from the American Board of Emergency Medicine in 1988. He resigned from the staff in May 1989, to continue emergency medical practice in British Columbia.

Peter O'Hanley, born in Charlottetown on November 3, 1954, remains a prominent member of the Department of Emergency Medicine. He received a BSc from St. Francis Xavier University in 1976 and an MD from Dalhousie in 1980. After interning, he joined the Department of Family

Practice but confined his work to emergency medicine. He obtained his ACLS in 1981 and in 1982, obtained his ATLS as well as becoming an instructor in ACLS. In 1991, he passed a course in Paediatric Advanced Life Support. In 1986 he received a Certificate of Special Competence in Emergency Medicine from the College of Family Physicians of Canada. From 1986 to 1991 he served as chief of the Department of Emergency Medicine and since 1993 has been director of the Emergency Department, The Moncton Hospital. In 1993 he was appointed by the minister of health, Dr. Russell King, to be chairman of the Regional Ambulance Planning Committee for Health Region 1.

John F. Whelan was born on April 28, 1956, and, after taking premed at Dalhousie University, he travelled to Newfoundland where he received his MD from Memorial University in 1980. He returned to Halifax where he served a rotating internship in the Dalhousie program and on completion of his internship, joined the staff of the Moncton Medical Clinic and The Moncton Hospital, serving as an emergency room physician until 1986 when he returned to the Victoria General Hospital for a residency in radiology.

Another addition to the courtesy staff in 1981 was Dr. John Carson. He played a prominent role in the hospital, however, as he served as consultant in radiation oncology. Dr. Carson graduated from the University of New Brunswick with a BSc in 1971 and an MD from Dalhousie in 1973. He interned at the Victoria General Hospital from 1972 to 1973. After serving as a general practitioner in St. Stephen from 1973 to 1976, he served a residency in internal medicine at the Victoria General Hospital from 1976 to 1978 and then a residency in radiation oncology at the Princess Margaret Hospital from 1978 to 1981, receiving his FRCP in Radiation Oncology in 1981. He joined the staff of the Saint John Regional Hospital and served as consultant to The Moncton Hospital until the opening of the Radiation Oncology Centre at the Dr. Georges-L. Dumont Hospital in 1993.

Statistics for 1981 reveal 13,471 adult and child admissions in addition to 9,162 newborns; 10,452 operations were performed, including 4,336 day surgery patients; 18,906 electrocardiograms and 1,910 electroencephalograms were done and 1,910 gastrointestinal unit procedures performed; 925 shock treatments were given. Speech pathology saw 1,678 patients and the social service looked after 1,593 cases. The Department of Medical Imaging had a busy year with 77,859 radiological examinations, 2,579 CT Scans, 4,246 nuclear medicine procedures and 3,164 ultrasound examinations. There were 12,370 visits to the outpatient clinics as follows: Arthritic—1,766; Chemotherapy—2,823; Colposcopy—979; Diabetic Day Care—2,239; Diet Counselling—422; Hyperlipoproteinemia—92; Obesity—226 with Obesity Weight Checks—2,493; Radiotherapy—1,427; and Chest—263.

If Canadians followed the example of the Chinese in giving a name to each year then The Moncton Hospital would call 1982 "the year of abortion." The Canadian government in 1969 brought in a revision to the criminal code legalizing abortion under certain guidelines. As a result, each hospital set up

Therapeutic Abortion Committees. In 1974, the board of trustees established a policy that The Moncton Hospital would only accept applications for therapeutic abortions for patients residing in hospital Region I, defined as the counties of Westmorland, Albert and Kent and the Sussex area of Kings County. Under the criminal code guidelines, pregnancy could be terminated if a woman's continued pregnancy could endanger her life or health. By 1979, the Canadian abortion rate varied from a low of 1.7 per 1,000 women in Prince Edward Island to a high of 21.1 per 1,000 in British Columbia. In New Brunswick, the rate was 2.8 per 1,000 women. However, the rate varied in the province and of 449 abortions performed in New Brunswick, 318 of them were performed at The Moncton Hospital. It became obvious that the Abortion Committee took a liberal interpretation of the guidelines taking the definition of the World Health Organization which interpreted a mother's health to include her physical, mental and social well being. The Roman Catholic Church and fundamental Baptists decried the practice of abortion and The Moncton Hospital became the target of the protest movement led by David Little, president of the New Brunswick Right to Life Association and Peter Ryan, executive director of the foundation.

There was a time set aside each week in the operation room schedule for abortion procedures. A well organized protest march would take place each week at this time with protesters marching in front of the hospital carrying anti-abortion placards. Attempts at not booking therapeutic abortions at a specific time or day of the week proved fruitless as the organizing committee obviously had an inside informant and knew whenever an abortion was to take place and the march would take place at the scheduled time of the abortion. The protest movement reached the zenith of bad taste when it took its campaign to a personal level and marched in front of the home of Dr. Robert Caddick. On Mother's Day, May 9, 1982, the protest reached its climax when a protest march of 200 protesters ended up at The Moncton Hospital claiming that this facility and the Everett Chalmers Hospital performed 80 percent of all the abortion in New Brunswick. This proved to be the straw that broke the camel's back.

On June 22, 1982, the headline in the *Moncton Transcript* was "Britain cheers new Heir." Also prominent on the front page was the announcement that there was to be a six month moratorium on abortions at The Moncton Hospital. This decision was made by all the gynecologists on staff but Dr. Robert Caddick became their main spokesman. In the *Transcript* of June 23, 1982, Dr. Caddick cited the lack of support from pro-abortionists as the major reason for the decision of The Moncton Hospital to discontinue abortions.

The anti-abortionists kept up their protest movement, however, and in December, intensified their public campaign as the end of the moratorium approached. An editorial in the *Moncton Transcript* on December 10, 1982, called for more decorum in the debate as the Right to Life Association was now calling physicians murderers, and the hospital, an abattoir. In an effort to forestall any decision to resume abortions, the Right to Life Association, on December 22, 1982, published an 18-page supplement to the *Times* and the *Transcript* as well as other newspapers in the province. This supplement contained a 33,000 name petition with the proclamation, "We the undersigned hereby proclaim our absolute respect for all human life, from the first moment of conception until natural death. We choose life." Among the signatures were 119 physicians of whom fifteen were on the staff of The Moncton Hospital. Despite these continued efforts of the Right to Life Association, Dr. Caddick, at a news conference on December 28, 1982, announced that the suspension was being lifted with the strong support of the medical staff and the Society of Obstetricians and Gynecologists of Canada. Immediately, the decision was denounced by Archbishop Donat Chiasson and by David Little, but applauded by a spokesman for the New Brunswick Advisory Council on the Status of Women. The abortion controversy received national attention with an article titled, "The doctors defy anti-abortion tide," in *Macleans* magazine on January 10, 1983. In a speech to law students at the University of New Brunswick on January 27, 1983, Gordon Fairweather, chief commissioner of the Human Rights Commission of Canada commended the group of Moncton doctors for standing firm against tough opposition from anti-abortionists.

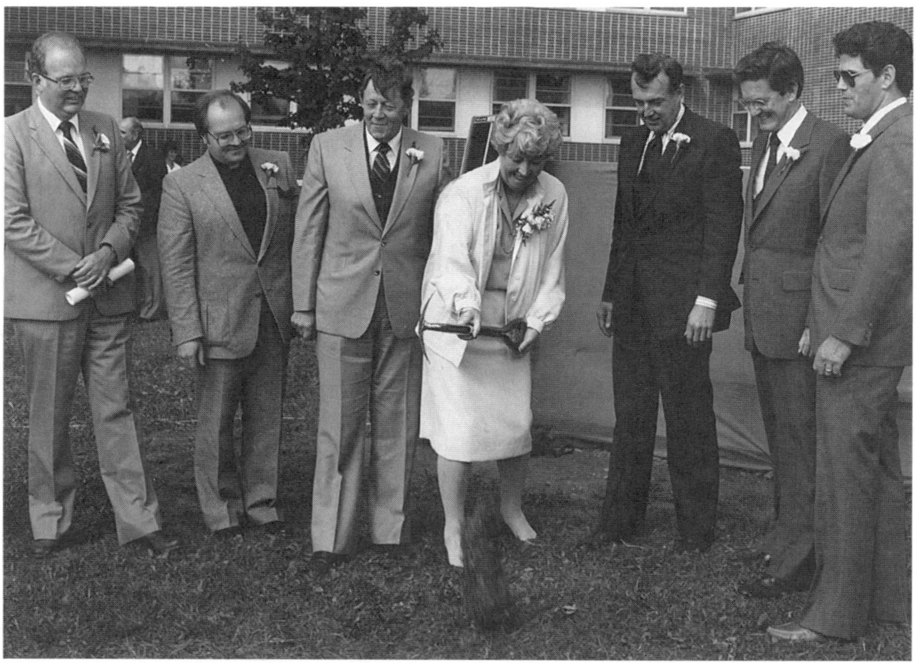

Sod-turning for the new South Tower in 1982. From left to right: Mr. William Kilpatrick, Executive Director; Rev. Ronald Maund, Pastoral Care; Mr. Harvey Hicks, Chairman of the Building Committee; Hon. Brenda Robertson, Minister of Health; Hon. Richard Hatfield, Premier of New Brunswick; Mr. Robert MacQuade, Chairman of the Board; and Dr. David Hiltz, President of the Medical Staff.

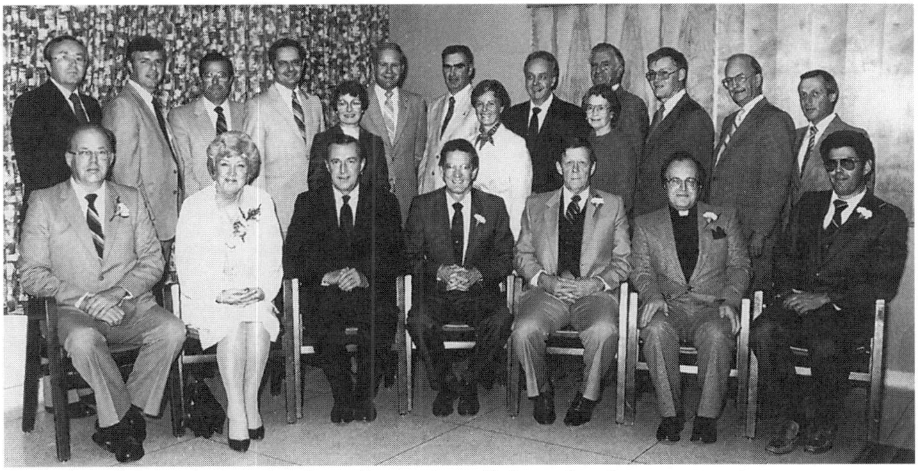

Board and participants in the sod-turning of the redevelopment project.

In all the controversy, the pro-abortion adherents stressed that abortion was not to be considered a method of birth control and that the abortion rate could be lowered by better sex education and birth control methods.

In January 1982 the minister of health, the Hon. Brenda Robertson, authorized Architects Four to proceed with the architectural plans for the Redevelopment Project. On March 1, 1982, she held a press conference to confirm The Moncton Hospital's Redevelopment Project at an estimated cost of $50.4 million (1981 dollars). The first sod was turned by the Honourable Richard Hatfield, the Premier of New Brunswick, on September 24, 1982. This was followed by the demolition of the 1A Isolation Wing and the evacuation of the property between the existing patient wings. As a result of the construction project, 32 beds were closed, never to be seen again. Once again the Department of Psychiatry was moved from the main hospital area while construction proceeded. Renovations were made to the former nurses' residence to house the In-patient Psychiatric Service. Temporary space was constructed on the Seventh Floor to house the Physiotherapy Department. Also shunted off to the nurses' residence was the Department of Social Services.

The beginning of new construction and the relocation of some departments did not mean that everything remained at a standstill. In March 1982, the new Medical/Surgical Intensive Care Unit with its increased capacity from five to twelve beds was opened on 5-Joyce. The new Intensive Care Unit was equipped with up-to-date features for patient care, including new monitors, critical-care beds, improved lighting and adequate electrical, vacuum and medical gas outlets. A group of co-ordinators was established for the unit, with a call schedule which included one internist, one general surgeon and one anaesthetist on call to the unit each day.

The Chest Clinic, opened in November 1981, was moved in the spring of 1982 to new premises on the second floor of the Professional Arts Building. In April, the Moncton TB Clinic located on Collishaw Street was transferred to The Moncton Hospital and Mrs. Bourque, RN, Miss S. Craig,

RT, and Dr. Retfalvi joined the staff. Dr. John C. Acres, director of the clinic, along with Mrs. R. Cole, RN, Co-ordinator, was responsible for developing a pulmonary rehabilitation program for those with chronic obstructive lung disease. The Nurses' Hospital Auxiliary provided two oxygen concentrators for home use by patients attending the Chest Clinic, a course in neonatology care for a respiratory technologist, and the previous year, had provided a flexible bronchoscope and four apnea monitors. The Moncton Gyro Club, with their long-standing interest in respiratory disease, donated through Gyro Charities, some equipment to the Chest Clinic as well as an ear oximeter for respiratory care.

In 1982, the untimely death occurred of Myrna Sherrard, director of nursing since December 1974. Mrs. Wright once again assumed the position of director of nursing in addition to her other administrative duties until a successor could be named. In January, death also claimed the life of a former board chairman, Howard Grayston. Retirements saw the departure of Joseph Lombard after 32 years of service, which included serving as laundry manager since 1954, and of Irene Crawford, the first director of volunteers. What started out as a part-time position was now a full-time one and included coordination of all the hospital related voluntary activities. Ruth Duffy was elected as the New Brunswick Director of the Canadian College of Health Service Executives.

When Dr. Oatway resigned from his part-time position as medical director in 1971, there was no one left in administration with a medical background. This was rectified in 1982 with the appointment of Dr. Ginette Gagné-Koch as medical director. Ginette was born in Quebec and received a BA with Honours in Sciences from the University of Montreal in 1963 and her MD from the University of Montreal in 1967. Her professional career started out as a clinician in Public Health Services for the Province of Quebec (1968-69), and as a clinician in alcoholism and other drug addictions for Domremy-Montreal from (1970-73). She then entered the administration field full time serving as director of Rehabilitation Services and director of Professional Services, Domremy-Montreal, from 1973 to 1977, followed by the position of Administrative Consultant to the Executive Director and board of trustees, Domremy-Montreal, from 1977 to 1978. She then ventured to western Canada and, after an internship in Calgary from 1979-80, she became assistant executive director of Medical Services, Holy Cross Hospital, Calgary, Alberta. The east coast of Canada proved irresistible, however, and when The Moncton Hospital advertised for a medical director, she gladly came back east and accepted the post and challenge when it was offered to her. She has continued her climb up the administration ladder, being appointed the president of The Moncton Hospital in October 1991, when Mr. Kilpatrick resigned.

One development in 1982 meant that female patients would no longer have to be concerned with how to care for their hair while in hospital. On

March 31, the Curly Corner hairdressing shop was opened for the patients—a project of the Nurses' Hospital Auxiliary.

In 1981 the end came to the independent intern program and 1982 saw the completion of the first year of affiliation with Dalhousie University. Negotiations were completed to expand the program to include internal medicine and general surgery during 1983/84.

In April 1982 the extramural hospital concept was introduced to the Moncton area with two units: the Driscoll Unit, to serve the anglophone population and the Blanche Bourgeois Unit to serve the Francophone population. The main contact person at The Moncton Hospital became Marie Brown who, in addition to her cheery attitude, became famous for her green outfits on Saint Patrick's Day each year. With the extra mural plan in effect, many patients were able to be discharged early and be cared for at home. It has especially been a welcome relief to those terminally ill who are able to remain at home in relative comfort in their final days.

During 1982 the board funded, from its own resources, a special study on the relative level of sickness of our inpatients and how to develop a system of assigning the nursing staff in the most effective way. In general, the study showed that the previous nursing staffing patterns were not significantly out of line but that the Grasp System was here to stay as a system for assigning nurses from shift to shift on the basis of the needs of the patients.

In 1977, the first annual campaign by the Friends of the Moncton Hospital Foundation was held, but with a limited target audience. In view of the ever more pressing needs for funds to augment government approved budgets, in 1982 the Friends of the Moncton Hospital Foundation embarked on a community-wide annual campaign to raise funds. Over 45,000 flyers were mailed to local residences and individuals and the response was quite gratifying with $40,000 raised, compared to $13,000 the previous year, although the total net revenue of the Friends from all sources had been showing a healthy growth each year since its inception. With the funds received in 1982, the Friends were able to purchase several ventilators, including a portable one.

The sudden death of Dr. Tucker created a void in the Department of Neurosurgery. The death of Dr. L.A. Goodridge, a pioneer in Ear, Nose and Throat Surgery, also occurred during the year. New members to the staff in 1982 included Dr. Amar Pal to Otorhinolaryngology, Dr. David Parton to Neurological Sciences, Dr. L.B. Eidus to Pathology, Dr. Preston Smith to Family Practice and Dr. Andar A. Retfalvi to the courtesy staff as a result of transferring the TB Chest Clinic to The Moncton Hospital.

Amarnath Pal was born in India and took his premedical and medical training at Calcutta University, receiving his MB, BS in 1963. He travelled to England where he received his FRCS(Eng) in General Surgery in 1971. On coming to Canada, he served a rotating internship at Dalhousie from 1977 to 1978 and an EENT residency at Dalhousie from 1978 to 1981, receiving his FRCS(C) in 1981. He was appointed to the staff in February 1982.

David Parton provided the hospital with a second neurologist. Receiving a BSc in 1973 and an MD in 1977 from the University of Ottawa, he served a rotating internship at Memorial University from 1977 to 1978. This was followed by a residency in neurology at Dalhousie from 1978 to 1981 and a Fellowship in Clinical EEG at Dalhousie from July 1981-December 1981. He received his FRCS(C) in Neurology in 1981. After a six-year stay in Moncton, he departed for British Columbia in August 1987.

Leslie Bence Eidus was born in Budapest, Hungary, on June 27, 1950, but became a Canadian citizen and was educated in Canada. He received his Bachelor of Applied Science (Electrical Engineering) from the University of Ottawa in 1971 and his MD from the same institution in 1977. He served a surgical internship at Wellesley Hospital in Toronto from 1977 to 1978 and a residency in pathology at the University of Toronto at Princess Margaret Hospital (1978-79), St. Michael's Hospital (1979-80), Toronto General (1980-81) and the Hospital for Sick Children and Sunnybrook Hospital (1981-82). He received his FRCP(C) in Anatomical Pathology in 1981. Like so many others appointed to the pathology staff, his stay was short, departing for greener fields in 1984. While in Moncton he participated in teaching a histology course at the Université de Moncton, where he was known as a very popular lecturer who could hold the students' attention.

Preston A. Smith was born in Charlottetown on June 30, 1957. After starting out on a BSc in engineering at the University of New Brunswick in 1975, he switched to premed at Dalhousie in 1976 and continued on to receive his MD with Honours and the Dr. C.B. Stewart Gold Medal in 1981. After serving a rotating internship in the Dalhousie program from 1981 to 1982, he joined the Moncton Medical Clinic in family practice. He became certified by the College of Family Physicians of Canada in May 1992, receiving the Irwin W. Bean Award given to the eligible candidate in actual practice, who achieved the highest marks in the 1991 certification examinations in family practice. Since joining the staff he has shown leadership in both the professional and administrative side of medicine. He served as medical director of the Reproductive Health Clinic at The Moncton Hospital (1984-June 1990). He was chief of Family Practice from 1988 to 1991. He was president of the Moncton and District Medical Society from 1990 to 1991 and has served on the Economic Committee of the New Brunswick Medical Society. He also served as a board member of Family Services, Moncton, from 1983 to 1986. In June 1991, he was elected to the position of chief of staff, succeeding Dr. Peter Gorman, but resigned in September 1992, when he was appointed vice-president Medical Affairs Region 1 Hospital Corporation (South East). He took this job on a part-time basis until he could get someone to take over his family practice. Because of PRAC (Professional Resource Advisory Committee, the government's committee designed to limit the number and location of physicians in New Brunswick) he was unsuccessful in getting someone to take over his practice and he resigned his position as vice-president in 1995 to return full time to family practice. In 1988 and in 1992, he attended the Physicians Management Institute of the Canadian Medical Association. One of his most noteworthy duties as vice-president had been as chairman of the Program Management Steering Committee.

Andor A. Retfalvi, born in Budapest on November 15, 1913, graduated from the Royal Hungarian Elizabeth University Medical School, Pecs, Hungary, in 1938. He interned at Royal Hungarian University Medical School, receiving his MD degree in 1939. After further training, he was certified a specialist in tuberculosis disease in Budapest, Hungary, in 1943. After the Second World War, he served as chief doctor at a tuberculosis hospital for Hungarian refugees in the US zone of occupied Germany from 1945 to 1948. In 1951, he immigrated to Canada and was appointed Assistant Medical Superintendent of Saint Joseph's Sanatorium, Saint-Basile, New Brunswick. He received his LMCC in 1956 and was made a Fellow of the American College of Chest Physicians in 1959. He was appointed to the TB Chest Clinic in Moncton and when it moved to The Moncton Hospital in April 1982, he was appointed to the courtesy staff. He retired on May 1, 1987, and his duties at the clinic were taken over by Dr. Acres.

There were 12,987 adult and children admissions in 1982/83 fiscal year with 1,593 newborns in addition; 9,980 operations were performed in the surgical suite including 4,189 day surgery patients. Services provided included: audiograms—2,162; electrocardiograms—18,514; electroencephalograms—2,844; gastrointestinal unit procedures—1,745; social service caseload—1,166; speech pathology—3,904; radiological examinations—79,586; nuclear medicine procedures—4,236; ultrasound examinations—3,418; and CT scans—4,189. There were 64,394 emergency visits to the outpatient department exclusive of 13,143 visits to the various clinics as follows: Arthritic—1,750; Chemotherapy—3,025; Colposcopy—1,242; Diabetic Day Care—2,674; Diet Counselling—384; Hyperlipoproteinemia—110; Obesity—275 with obesity weight checks—2,825; Radiotherapy—149; and Chest—2,191.

In 1983 Mr. MacQuade stepped down as board chairman to be replaced by Ralph Black, who would carry the reins through the construction project. Evidence that the project was really underway could be seen by the rising steel frame on the south side of the hospital. In addition to the start of the new tower, three new boilers were installed. The assistant secretary to the board, Dorothy Flemming, who also served as secretary to the executive director, retired after 28 years of service to the hospital and was replaced by Marlene MacLeod, who continues to serve in this position. Not long after assuming the chairmanship, Mr. Black became the centre of discontent among staff and the citizens when in September 1983, the board adopted the policy that the hospital would provide bilingual services in certain specified departments which, in this region, are found only at The Moncton Hospital. This included neurosurgery, neonatology and the ambulance service, with the ambulance drivers presenting the most vocal dissent.

In July 1983, the provincial government reintroduced user fees for O.P.D. Services and this resulted in a ten percent reduction in the number of patients seen in the outpatient and emergency departments. Again, user fees did not last long because the Federal Government threatened to apply the letter of the law and withhold funds equal to the amount of user fees obtained.

A highlight of 1983 was the presentation of a brief concerning cancer services in Moncton to the Hon. Charles G. Gallagher, minister of health and welfare, in Fredericton on July 21. The Woods-Gordon Report on Cancer Services in New Brunswick (October 1982) and the Tertiary Care Advisory Committees' report based on it (January 1983) recommended the establishment of a second radiooncology centre in New Brunswick. The brief was generally supportive of the recommendations of the Woods-Gordon Report, but felt that it would be a mistake to establish radiation therapy services in Moncton other than at, or adjoining, The Moncton Hospital. Attending the meeting in Fredericton were representatives from the board: Ralph Black, David Deware, Fred Gaudet, Harvey Hicks, C. Morris, and Robert Radford; Administration: Ruth Duffy, Dr. Ginette Gagné-Koch and William Kilpatrick; Medical Staff: Dr. J.T. Edgett, Dr. J. Gagnon, Dr. O. Messenger, Dr. D.I. MacLellan, Dr. James Noonan, Dr. W.A. Oatway and Dr. Sheldon Rubin. Although a well thought-out brief, it failed to impress the minister and the government, as the decision was made to establish the unit at the Dr. Georges-L. Dumont Hospital.

With rising health care costs, the cry in the 1990s seems to be that we are spending too much money on treating disease and that the emphasis should be on its prevention. Although not a disease, head injuries and multiple trauma as a result of motor vehicle accidents constitute a major source of expense to the health care system. Yet preventative measures are often met with great resistance by the public. The use of seat belts is a case in point. For many years it was known that seat belts would cut down the number of serious injuries in motor vehicle accidents, yet people would not comply. It was only after the provincial government instituted compulsory seatbelt legislation in November 1983, that the number of serious head injuries admitted to the Neurosurgery Intensive Care showed a decline.

In September 1981, a pain research project was started and this evolved into a pain clinic for the treatment of chronic pain. Budget restrictions in 1983 forced its closure, however, since it had been funded by non-governmental sources and the board did not feel that it could continue to divert money from other patient care needs.

An innovation from the Volunteer Service in 1983, was the establishment in October of the Post-Operative Information Service. Every day from 9 am to 4 pm, volunteers would staff a lounge where families could wait while their loved ones were undergoing surgery and be kept informed of their progress, as well as meet with surgeons after the surgery.

Under the guidance of Dr. Hani Akoury, a urodynamics laboratory was set up for the investigation of urinary flow problems in women. A new vascular laboratory for non-invasive investigation of peripheral vascular disease was opened under the direction of Dr. F.G. Murphy and was located in the Professional Arts Building.

The hospital would be in a sorry state if it were not for the help of outside organizations in providing much needed new and replacement equipment. The Friends of the Moncton Hospital Foundation contributed substantially with the purchase of a monitor-defibrillator for a second crash cart in the emergency department for cardiac arrests ($9,295); an upper and lower limb passive motion orthopaedic equipment ($4,495); a teaching arm for the bronchoscope, which enables interns to view a part of the lung while the surgeon is carrying out a procedure ($2,700); a K-Thermia unit to bring very high or low body temperatures back to normal ($7,150); and an incubator for the Nursery at ($11,800). In addition, numerous donations were made by church groups, service organizations and individuals throughout the year. One interesting contribution was a freezer for kosher foods by the Sisterhood of Tiferes Israel Synagogue.

There were two losses by death to the medical staff in 1983, with the sudden death of Dr. S.A. Hopper and that of Dr. Loyola LeBlanc who died in an automobile accident. There were several new additions to the staff during the year: Dr. Ogundimu to the Department of Neurosurgery, Dr. Alatishe to the Department of Psychiatry, Dr. John C. Crompton to the Department of Anaesthesia, Dr. Enrique Silva and Dr. Lewis Abbott to the Department of Pathology, Dr. Efram Barrera to the Department of Internal Medicine, Dr. Ernest McKenzie to the Department of Medical Imaging and Drs. Mary Ann Carlos, Stephanie Casey, James MacKillop, Eva Eros, Michael Camphyn, and Patrick Phelan to the Department of Family Practice.

Fad e Gbola Ogundimu was born in Nigeria and received his MB, BS degree from the University of Ibadan in Nigeria in 1974. After a year of internship in Lagos (1974-75), he served a two-year residency in general surgery at the University of Ibadan and then came to Canada for training in neurosurgery at Dalhousie University (1978-82), receiving his FRCS(C) in Neurosurgery in 1982 as well as his American Boards. Dr. Tucker had died in September 1982, leaving a void in the Neurosurgery Department. As a result, Dr. Ogundimu, who had planned on returning to Nigeria in twelve to eighteen months after his wife had finished postgraduate work in Canada, joined Dr. Quarty and Dr. Gorman in the department in May 1983, after satisfying the Immigration board that there was no Canadian available for the position and being registered under Section 26(1) of the Medical Act. By December 1985, his temporary work permit had run out and he had to leave the staff.

Moses Adeoye Alatishe was also from Nigeria, born on March 9, 1942, and, after receiving his premedical training at Ijebu Muslim College, he journeyed to Russia for his medical training at the Leningrad State Medical Institute of Pediatrics, graduating in 1970 with his MD degree. He then returned to Nigeria where he interned at the Lagos General Hospital and the Lagos Island Maternity Hospital from 1970 to 1971. He came to Canada for psychiatric training at the University of Saskatchewan, Saskatoon, from 1973 to 1977, including a fellowship year from 1975 to 1976 on mental retardation for which he received an MSc in 1976. From 1977 to 1978 he was senior psychiatrist at the Weyburn Psychiatric Centre and then returned to Nigeria to work as a psychiatrist for the federal government of Nigeria (1978-79), after which he returned to the Weyburn Psychiatric Centre. He received his FRCP(C) in Psychiatry in 1980. He worked at Swift Current Union Hospital, Swift Current, Saskatchewan (1980-82), and then in 1982 became program director of the William F. Roberts Hospital School in Saint John. He moved to Moncton in 1983, where he has continued to serve as a valuable member of the psychiatric staff. His main interest has been in child psychiatry and he is now director of the Child and Adolescent Psychiatric Program. He also serves as a member of the board of the Canadian Mental Health Association.

John Crompton was born in England on February 6, 1952, and received his MB, BS, MRCS(Eng), LRCP(London), in 1976 from Saint Mary's Hospital, London. In 1977 he served an internship at St. Helier Cevshalton Hospital, London, followed by six months' work in emergency medicine. He then came to Newfoundland and Labrador where he did nine months of general practice before beginning a pediatric residency at the Janeway in Saint John's from 1978 to 1979. He decided that pediatrics was not his calling and went to Halifax where he served a residency in anaesthesia, including time in internal medicine and intensive care (1978-82), receiving his FRCP(C) in 1982. His proficiency in anaesthesia was well recognized at this stage and he was appointed an assistant anaesthetist at the Victoria General Hospital on completion of his residency. Fortunately, his fellow countryman, Tim Cooper, was able to persuade him to throw his lot in with the anaesthetic group in Moncton. His technical skill and steady composure in the operating room makes any surgeon happy to have him on his case even if the nurses have to do a little picking up after him. His tardiness in cleaning out his hospital mailbox once resulted in it encroaching on Doug Crawshaw's space, until finally one day Doug gathered up all John's mail, encased it in plaster and delivered it to him in the OR. Soon after joining the staff he showed an interest in pain management and with Dr. J.S. Wright, served in setting up the Pain Clinic in 1985. Many a patient can attest to his skills in performing blocks for pain relief. In activities outside medicine he is an accomplished pilot who flies his own plane.

Enrique Silva was born in Uruguay and received his MD from the University of the Republic, Uruguay, in 1968. He practised family medicine in his homeland in Mercedes, from 1968 to 1974 and then served a residency in anatomical pathology at the University of the Republic from 1974 to 1975. He came to Canada in 1975 to complete a residency in anatomical pathology and microbiology at the University of Western Ontario from 1975 to 1981. He was certified by the American Board of Anatomical Pathology in 1979 and received his FRCP(C) in Pathology in 1980. He was appointed pathologist at the Carleton Memorial Hospital in 1981 and came to Moncton in 1983. After a four-year stint he left to become a pathologist at the Pembroke Civic Hospital in Ontario.

Lewis Abbott was born on Prince Edward Island on December 20, 1940, and obtained a BSc from Acadia in 1962 and an MSc in microbiology from Dalhousie in 1964. Setting higher goals, he enrolled in Dalhousie Medical School and obtained his MD in 1971 after serving a rotating internship at Dalhousie (1970-71). After serving as a medical officer at the Canadian Forces Base in Halifax (1971-73), he did family practice in Montague, Prince Edward Island, from 1973 to 1979. Seeing the important place that infectious diseases occupied in medical practice, he returned to his first love, microbiology, and entered on a residency program at the Victoria General Hospital in microbiology from 1979 to 1983. The recent death of John Casey, longtime microbiologist at The Moncton Hospital, had created an opening for this position in the laboratory and Lewis accepted the call after the government agreed to accept and pay for a physician in this position. This was welcomed by the medical staff as now instead of just sitting in the laboratory, the medical microbiologist would be able to assist the treating physician by becoming more involved in the treatment of complicated infections. He obtained his FRCP(C) in medical microbiology in 1986. Dr. Abbott was well liked by his colleagues who were sad to see him resign on September 15, 1988, to return to his native province.

Efram Barrera was born on December 12, 1926, in LaGuaira, Venezuela, and received his MD from Venezuela Central University in 1950. He interned at the Traumatology Institute in Caracas (1950-51) and the Caracas Emergency Hospital (1951-53). He then took training in rehabilitation medicine at Caracas Vargas Hospital and Caracas Emergency Hospital from 1953 to 1954, with an additional two years at the Rehabilitation Institute in Montreal from 1954 to 1956 and became certified in rehabilitation medicine by the Royal College of Physicians and Surgeons of Canada in 1956. From 1956 to 1982 he served as chief of service, Physical Medicine and Rehabilitation, National Centre of Rehabilitation of the Social Security in Caracas. On the recommendation of Dr. Gustave Gingras, he was appointed director of the Rehabilitation Unit in June 1983, as this position had remained vacant since the departure of Dr. Simard in 1977. Although very pleasant and active in his church community, Dr. Barrara did not enjoy the confidence of the nurses and medical staff in his approach to running the rehabilitation unit and he resigned on December 31, 1987.

Ernest MacKenzie was born in Corner Brook, Newfoundland, on April 25, 1948, and graduated with his MD degree from Memorial University in 1974. He served a rotating internship at the Ottawa Civic Hospital from 1974 to 1975. After serving a family practice in Come-by-Chance from 1975 to 1977, he did a residency in radiology at Saint John's General Hospital (1977-81), with another year in nuclear medicine at the University of Alberta from 1981-82. He received his FRCP(C) in diagnostic radiology in 1981. In March 1982, he returned to his home town as a radiologist at the Western Memorial

Hospital in Corner Brook, Newfoundland but moved to the mainland and Moncton, in June 1983, remaining on the staff of The Moncton Hospital for only four years.

Mary Ann Carlos, born on December 11, 1956, obtained her BSc in 1978 and her MD in 1982 from Dalhousie. Following a rotating internship in the Dalhousie program (1982-83), she set up a family practice at the Petitcodiac Health Clinic.

Jeanne Stephanie Casey, the daughter of John Casey, a long-time microbiologist at The Moncton Hospital, was born in Moncton on April 26, 1956. After receiving a BSc from St. Francis Xavier University in 1978, she entered Dalhousie Medical School, obtaining her MD degree in 1982. After a rotating internship in the Dal program from 1982-83, she also joined the Petitcodiac Health Clinic but only remained for one year before moving to Bedford, Nova Scotia, in 1984.

Another one-year appointment to the medical staff was Dr. James MacKillop, who joined the Moncton Medical Clinic to replace Dr. Gary Chesser while he was on a one-year sabbatical. James received a BSc from Acadia in 1976, and then went to Dalhousie University to obtain a BEd in 1977 and then an MD in 1981. He served an internship and residency program in family medicine at Dalhousie (1981-83) and received his certification in family practice. On completing his locums, he moved to Sydney, Nova Scotia.

Michael Camphyn was born on December 9, 1947, and received his MD degree from the University of Louvain, Belgium, in 1972. He interned in Namur, Belgium, from 1972 to 1973 and served a residency in internal medicine in Jolinot and Louvain, Belgium, from 1975 to 1976. From 1976 to 1982 he had a tendency to wander, serving, at various times, a general practice in Brussels and also in Saudi Arabia. In 1982 he came to Canada and served a rotating internship at St. Coeur, Ste. Justine and Notre Dame hospitals in Montreal from 1982 to 1983, receiving his LMCC. He set up a general practice in Salisbury in 1983, but his life ended tragically with a drug overdose in June 1985.

Eva Eros was born in England on July 1, 1949. After premedical education at University College, London, she received her medical education at University College Hospital, being awarded her MB, BS in 1972. She interned at Edgware General Hospital, London, and Nottingham General Hospital, Nottingham, England (1972-73). She served as senior house officer at Nottingham City Hospital, Saint James Seacoast Hospital and Nottingham Children's Hospital (1973-75) and received a diploma in child health from the Royal College of Physicians, London, and the Royal College of Surgeons, England. She came to Canada and did a family practice at Kincardine, Ontario (1975-76) and at London, Ontario (1976-77). She served as an emergency room physician at St. Joseph's Hospital, Saint John (1977-78) and at the Halifax Infirmary (1978-79). From 1980 to 1982 she served as a physician at the Dalhousie University Health Service. She moved to Moncton in 1982 with her husband, Dr. Amar Pal, and subsequently opened up a family practice in Riverview.

Patrick Phelan was born on August 23, 1951, and before medicine, embarked on an engineering career, receiving his BSc in engineering from the University of New Brunswick in 1974. He abandoned engineering and received his MD from Memorial University in 1981. He entered the family practice program at McGill at the Jewish General Hospital (1981-83). Besides his family practice, he served emergency room shifts and obtained his ACLS in 1983 and his ATLS in 1985. His compassionate nature made him an excellent choice to become director of the Palliative Care Unit of the hospital when it was established in 1988. He also serves on the provincial Palliative Care Association. Besides his interest in computers, he played the trumpet, with the Thomists while at the University of New Brunswick, and now plays with The Moncton Hospital Jazz Band ("The Greens"), when they make their infrequent appearances at medical functions.

David Symington was born in Metz, France, on April 4, 1957, and received his MD from the University of Alberta in 1982. After a rotating internship at Victoria Hospital, London, Ontario (1982-83), he began a family practice at the Albert County Hospital and was appointed to the courtesy staff. He was subsequently appointed to the active staff in 1984 when he began working part-time shifts in the outpatient department. He resigned in October 1985, but served a locums in the emergency department in October 1986.

Statistics for the 1983/84 fiscal year, remain about the same as the previous year, except that the average percentage of occupancy of active treatment beds rose to 90.76 percent from 83.4 percent the previous year. This can be explained by the bed closures associated with the redevelopment project. There were 13,117 adult and children admissions with 1,612 newborns; 10,328 operations were performed in the surgical suite, including 4,505 day surgery patients. Services provided included: audiograms—2,660; electrocardiograms—18,811; electroencephalograms—2,163; gastrointestinal unit procedures—1,843; social service caseload—857; speech pathology attendance—3,148; radiological examinations—79,022; CT scans—3,140; nuclear medicine procedures—4,367; and ultrasound examinations—3,537.

There was good news from the provincial government when the premier and the Minister of Health confirmed in writing the government's intention to complete the whole of the redevelopment project, including the renovations, in 1991. I guess that the key word here is "intention" as, of course, by the time the South Tower was completed there was no money to proceed with Phase II. Phase I was proceeding on schedule but it did result in the loss of 30 beds and another 85 rooms facing the new construction became windowless rooms. Another bright spot was the new Provincial Department of Health Policy to provide for orderly replacement of so-called high-tech equipment. Our 20-year-old electroencephalography equipment was able to be replaced with two 16-channel units incorporating the latest technology for the production of clinical information on brain function. Sophisticated computerized equipment was also obtained for the haematology laboratory, eliminating the time consuming method of doing manual cell counts.

To establish better rapport with the government and to make our concerns known to it, a breakfast meeting was held at the Hotel Beausejour on November 5, 1984, between the medical staff and our local representatives of the legislature. Representing the medical staff were: Dr. J.T. Edgett, Dr. D.I. MacLellan, Dr. K.J. Deware, Dr. C.E. Doyle, Dr. P.D. Lightfoot, Dr. J.S. Noonan, Dr. P. Gorman, Dr. F.G. Murphy and Dr. W.A. Oatway. The invited attendants were the Hon. Mabel Deware, the Hon. Brenda Robertson, the Honorable William Harmer and the Hon. Malcolm MacLeod. Dennis Cochrane, MP was unable to attend, but sent his assistant, Mrs. Murray. The staff outlined treatment problems at The Moncton Hospital as they related to the health care of Greater Moncton and all eastern New Brunswick and showed that the solutions depended on the early completion of the new South Tower stage of the hospital's redevelopment program.

After serving as operating room supervisor for 32 years, Aline Forsythe retired and was honoured at a dinner held at the Hotel Beausejour on September 5, 1984. She was born in Sussex and graduated in the class of 1948 from The Moncton Hospital School of Nursing. She completed a six-month course in operating room technique at the Winnipeg General Hospital in 1953, the Nursing Unit Administration Extension Program sponsored by the Canadian Nursing and Hospital Associations in 1962, and was awarded the Silver Jubilee Medal in 1977. She also served as the first president of The Moncton Hospital Nurses' Union. A strict disciplinarian, she ran a tight ship, treating doctors and nurses alike. The only time I saw her stumped was when she walked into the operating room one day and one of the nurses had a paper bag stuck over her head. Mrs. Forsythe asked when we would be ready for the next case and completely ignored the embarrassed nurse. One day in the locker room, the same nurse, unaware that Mrs. Forsythe was present, was relating to her fellow nurses how she thought she would have her bunions fixed one summer, and her gallbladder removed the next, but when she said she didn't know what she would plan for the summer after that, Mrs. Forsythe's voice was suddenly heard, saying that she would probably be looking for a new job.

Diagnostic services in the cardiology department were enhanced with the purchase of a Holter Monitor System at a cost of $113,000. The credit for this goes to the Nurses' Hospital Auxiliary, which provided the funds raised mainly through their operation of the gift shop. In addition, the auxiliary helped the Department of Thoracic Surgery with the purchase of a bronchoscope for $11,000, instruments for the use with the mediastinascope at a cost of $2,000 and ten biopsy forceps totalling $4,000. They also contributed $1,500 for mobile pharmacy carts. The Friends of the Moncton Hospital Foundation was raising increasing amounts of money with their annual financial appeal and in 1984, collected over $60,000. In the process, they were becoming the second largest contributor of non-governmental funds to the hospital. In 1984, the foundation contributed $6,050 for a mobile cart specially equipped for examining and treating patients with ear, nose and throat problems, $11,000 for a cardiac and respiratory monitor and $3,850 for an apnea monitor to save babies from sudden death syndrome.

New staff appointed in 1984 included Dr. Paul Dubois, Dr. Warren Davidson, Dr. S.B. Zimmer, and Dr. Michael Peters. Dr. D.J. Doiron and Dr. J.T. Trofmick were appointed to the courtesy staff on their appointment to the Albert County Hospital. Except for Dr. Peters, none of the additions to the Department of Family Practice in 1984, would have any long-term commitment to the community.

Dr. Paul Dubois added strength to the Department of Surgery, with his training in thoracic surgery enabling the department to have two qualified thoracic surgeons on staff. Paul, the son of a physician, was born in Ontario, on March 6, 1952, received his BSc in 1972 and his MD cum laude from the University of Ottawa in 1976. After interning at the Ottawa General Hospital (1976-77), he served as a resident in general surgery at the Ottawa General Hospital (1977-82), including the position of chief Administrative Resident (1981-82). His training in general surgery was followed by service as chief resident in the Department of Thoracic surgery at the University of Toronto (1982-83) and as a clinical fellow in the Division of Cardiac Surgery at the Ottawa Cardiac Institute from July-December 1983. He received his FRCS(C) in 1981 and a certificate of special competence in thoracic surgery in 1983. He was also certified by the American Board of Surgery in 1982. He served as an attending surgeon at the Ottawa General Hospital (1983-84) but, fortunately for New Brunswickers, he ventured east and began practice in association with Dr. Messenger in October 1984. Dr. Messenger took a three-month sabbatical to study in England at that time, but within a year, illness forced him to abandon his surgical practice and Dr. Dubois had to assume the position as the only thoracic surgeon in the city, a role which he has played to the utmost benefit to the citizens and physicians of New Brunswick. In addition to his surgical skills, he has the distinct advantage of being able to offer his services in both official languages. In 1986, he introduced the use of the YAG Laser in Endoscopic Laser Therapy and was one of the first to introduce Endoscopic Cholecystectomy to The Moncton Hospital in 1991. Since 1987, he has served as chairman of the Laser Safety Committee and from 1990 to 1992, he served as chief of surgery and chairman of the OR Committee. His pastimes include skiing, windsurfing, and "surfing" the internet on his computer.

The hospital had two wards devoted to chronic care at this time. Most of the patients in these wards were elderly and attended to by their family doctor but the general attitude was that these were patients that were either awaiting transfer to a nursing home or were in such a state that they would remain in hospital until their deaths. The hospital felt that more use could be made of these chronic care beds and Dr. Warren Davidson arrived on the scene on August 1, 1984, as the Director of the Extended Care Unit and, of course, brought with him new ideas in the treatment of these geriatric patients. Fully 25 percent of the admissions to The Moncton Hospital were over the age of 65 and these patients occupied 40 percent of the beds. On arrival, Warren immediately developed a Moncton Hospital Geriatric Program, the goal of which was to restore individuals to their maximum level of functioning, to return them to their own homes and to co-ordinate the available community services to ensure that they could maintain their autonomy and well-being. Dr. Loanna Whitmore and Dr. Sylvia Argouarch soon joined Dr. Davidson to build an interdisciplinary team including specialised nursing, physiotherapy, occupational therapy, social service, discharge planning and pastoral care staff. Several features of the program included:

1. consultation, assessment and rehabilitation services provided throughout southern New Brunswick to both French and English communities and province-wide public and professional education in geriatric medicine and interdisciplinary care;
2. the team organized and maintained family support programs;
3. an intermittent readmission program through which patients, often with Alzheimer's disease, could be regularly admitted for one week to provide much needed relief for family members who were providing this care at home; and
4. family conferences held during critical periods in patient management or prior to discharge to discuss the patient's diagnosis, functional problems, medications and care needs.

Warren Davidson was born in Selkirk, Manitoba, on October 9, 1945, and received a BSc from the University of Manitoba in 1969 and an MD from the University of Calgary in 1974. He did a straight internship in internal medicine at the Winnipeg Health Sciences Centre (1974-75) and a residency in internal medicine (1975-79), including a clinical fellowship in geriatric medicine (1977-78) and a year off to serve as an emergency medical officer at St. Boniface General Hospital (1976-77). After serving as a staff geriatrician at the Winnipeg Health Sciences Centre and Deer Lodge Hospital from 1979 to 1980, he went to England where he was senior registrar and honorary lecturer in geriatric medicine at St. George's University, London, England. In 1981, he returned to Winnipeg and served as clinical director, Geriatric Assessment and Rehabilitation Unit at the Health Sciences Centre until 1983. Since coming to Moncton, he has played a prominent role in geriatric care, province-wide. He has been chairman of the Subcommittee on Health Care of the Elderly, Health Care Committee of the New Brunswick Medical Society since 1986. He has been president of the New Brunswick Gerontology Association since 1988. As well, he has served as a member of the board of Directors of the Alzheimer's Society of New Brunswick and as a member of the Medical Advisory Committee of the New Brunswick Extra Mural Hospital, Driscoll Unit. Since 1989 he has been a member of the Provincial Design Committee, Single Entry Project, Department of Health and Social Services. This project has helped make it much easier to transfer patients to nursing homes, thereby freeing up active treatment beds in the hospital. Since 1987 he has served on the Product Selection Committee, Prescription Drug Program, Department of Health and Community Services. With the collaboration of professors from McMaster University, he made a study of the overuse and abuse of drugs in the elderly in New Brunswick for which he has gained a Canada-wide recognition with his findings, not only generating much heat after being published in the *Canadian Medical Journal*, but also in the national press, principally in the *Globe and Mail*. Warren also demonstrated his social consciousness when, as a reserve officer in the Canadian navy, he served on a team to provide medical aid to the refugees in the Rwandan civil war in October 1994.

Stephen Zimmer was born on September 7, 1955, and educated at Queen's University, receiving a BSc in 1978 and an MD in 1983. After an internship in family medicine at Dalhousie from 1983 to 1984, he joined Dr. Eva Eros in the practice of family medicine but resigned from the staff in 1985 to take postgraduate work in internal medicine at Dalhousie.

Michael Peters was born on July 16, 1955, in Prince Edward Island. He received a BSc from the University of Prince Edward Island in 1977 and an MD from Dalhousie in 1982. He interned in the Dalhousie rotating internship program (1982-83). In April 1984, he began a family practice in Moncton.

Timothy Trofimuk, born on January 6, 1958, received his BSc in 1978 and his MD from the University of Alberta in 1982. After an internship in the family medicine program at Dalhousie (1982-84), he remained in the Maritimes and began a family practice in Albert, but returned to Alberta in September 1985.

Daniel Doiron received a BSc from the University of New Brunswick in 1979 and an MD from Memorial University in 1983. He served in the Dalhousie rotating internship program from 1983 to 1984 and then set up family practice in Albert while also serving part-time in the Emergency Room. He obtained his ACLS in 1983 and his ATLS in 1984. In 1986 he resigned to pursue a residency in psychiatry.

Statistics in 1984/85 showed 13,588 adult and child admissions and 1,640 new-born. 10,646 operations were performed in the surgical suite, including 4,651 day patients. The number of services provided included the following: audiograms—2,280; electrocardiograms—19,902; electroencephalograms—2,113; gastrointestinal unit procedures—1,953; social service caseload—990; speech pathology attendance—4,463; radiological examinations—82,158; CT Scans—3,939; nuclear medicine procedures—4,842. Clinic visits totalled—13,592.

It became popular in the 1980s for every company and organization to develop a mission statement and The Moncton Hospital was no exception. The long-range planning committee felt that a clear comprehensive role statement was needed before the committee could re-examine the direction in which the hospital was going and formulate a long-range plan. When completed, its role statement began with the mission statement:

> **Mission and Philosophy of The Moncton Hospital**
> The mission of The Moncton Hospital is to achieve excellence in providing and promoting health services that improve the quality of life for the population we serve. We believe in the importance of:
> - Concern, compassion and individualized care for our patients.
> - Commitment to competence and progressive standards of excellence in all that we do.
> - A climate fostering personal satisfaction and co-operation amongst all who work in support of this mission.

Some new services were developed in 1985, including the Department of Emergency Medicine, the Pain Clinic, a Pastoral Care Co-ordinator, a Donations Co-ordinator and Materials Management.

For a few years, there had been doctors on the staff who confined their practice to emergency medicine but who were still attached to the Department of Family Practice. In 1985 the Department of Emergency Medicine was formed with four full-time staff members: Dr. J.F. Goulding, Dr. C.B. Levesque, Dr. P.H. O'Hanley and Dr. Pamela Walsh. Naturally, four persons could not staff the emergency room on a twenty-four-hour, seven days a week basis and it was necessary to have part-time staff to fill in the gaps. Those appointed part-time included: Dr. D.J. Doiron, Dr. D.N. Keeling, Dr. R.J. Leger, Dr. J.M. Meagher, Dr. J. Park, Dr. P.J. Phelan, Dr. L.M. Smith and Dr. P.A., Smith. Two of these, Dr. J.M. Meagher and Dr. Luella Smith, would eventually devote their practice to full time emergency room medicine. In addition, other members of the family practice staff were given courtesy staff privileges so that they could work occasional shifts in the emergency room rotations. The emergency room and the outpatient department were still in one location on the ground floor of the Parlee Wing. In anticipation of the move to the new patient tower in late 1986, when these two departments would become physically separated, the outpatient department was divided into an emergency department and an ambulatory care department.

A Pain Research Clinic had been established in 1981 and its role had eventually evolved to include some treatment of chronic pain before it was disbanded in 1983 due to budget cuts. The need for such a clinic, however, was still apparent and in the spring of 1985, with the financial support of the Worker's Compensation Board, a pain clinic was re-established in the Professional Arts Building under the direction of Dr. J.S. Wright and Dr. John Crompton, with a physiotherapist and a psychologist on staff to round out the clinic personnel. In future years more anaesthetists would be added to the staff, including Dr. Tim Cooper, Dr. Ken Porter and Dr. Kent Monteith.

One of the recommendations of the last accreditation survey in 1984 had been the establishment of a Pastoral Care Department. The clergy had been

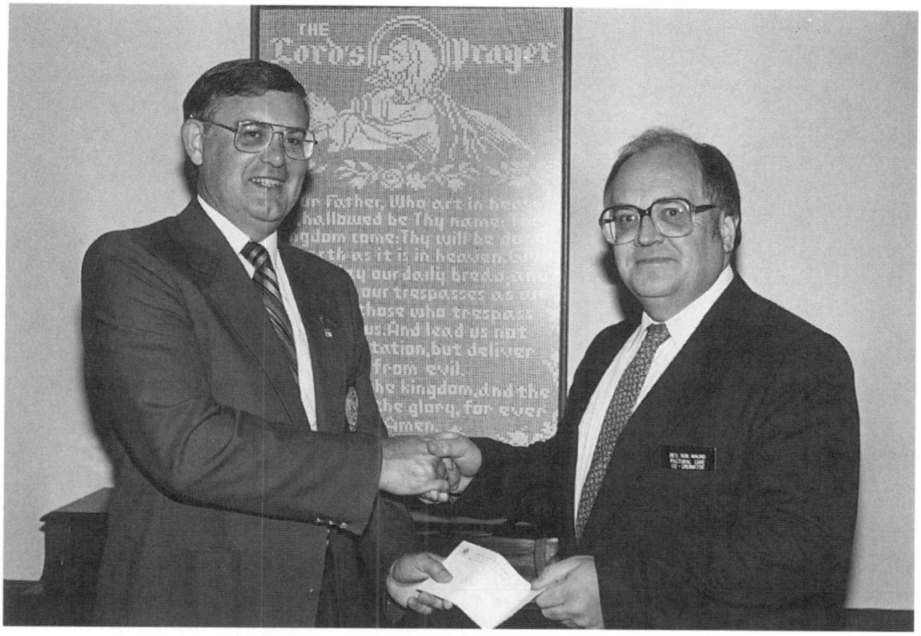

The Pastoral Care Department was formed in 1986. There was a presentation of GIC to the Pastoral Care Department by Bill Field, Moncton Kiwanis Club in 1988 to Rev. Robert Maund.

previously organized with an on call system for the hospital but a formal department was now set up with a full time Pastoral Care Co-ordinator. The Rev. Ronald Maund was appointed to this position and continues to occupy the post to this day. An Interfaith Chapel was created in the former nurses' residence and was dedicated to the memory of Myrna Sherrard in September 1986. The School of Nursing Alumnae funded the furnishings for the entire Pastoral Care Department, including the chapel. The chapel was subsequently moved to the hospital proper on completion of the new South Tower.

Although the largest donations to the hospital came from the Nurses' Hospital Auxiliary and the Friends of the Moncton Hospital, there were literally hundreds of individuals and organizations that wished to participate in helping to better the lot of those citizens who needed treatment in the hospital. Much new and replacement equipment was needed that could not be bought with the limited funds supplied by government. Many individuals and organizations had funds ranging from $100 to $5,000, to donate and liked to see something tangible for their money rather than having it dumped into the general pool. The hospital, however, could only use so many wheelchairs and TV sets, and so a part-time donations co-ordinator was appointed in the fall of 1985 to show these individuals and organizations where their money could be put to the best use.

Another new department which was formed was the Material Management Department which amalgamated stores, central sterile supply, print shop and distribution into one department, providing a more effective co-ordination of these related functions. Ms. Donna McIntyre became the head of this new department.

In the fall of 1985 the volunteers took on a new look when the pink smocks which had been used for years were replaced by crisp, crested blue and white pinstriped lab coats. Men now were participating in the volunteer service as well as women. In December 1985, Ann Cunningham became the first volunteer to contribute 5,000 hours of service, followed soon after by Georgina Allen. Translated into 40-hour work weeks this represents almost two and one-half years of service. In 1985-86 the combined efforts of adult and student volunteers totalled 21,981 hours.

There were several new additions to the staff in 1985: Dr. Sheila Mackem, Dr. Gilles E. Brisson, Dr. William So, Dr. Janet Fultz, Dr. John Steeves, Dr. Christopher Levesque, Dr. Kenneth Mitton, Dr. James G. Stewart, Dr. Francis Anthony and Dr. Hans Korritz.

Sheila Mackem was born in Ireland on September 21, 1955, and received MB, BCh, BAO degrees from University College, Dublin, National University of Ireland in 1979. After a rotating internship at Mater Hospital, Dublin, from 1979 to 1980, she did a residency in internal medicine at General Hospital, Letterkenny, Ireland (1980-81). On embarking on a pediatric career, she came to Canada and served a residency at the Hospital for Sick Children in Toronto (1981-83), followed by two years at the Izaak Walton Killam Hospital (1983-85), receiving her FRCP(C) in Paediatrics in 1985. She proved a very capable pediatrician and served as chief of pediatrics in 1987 and 1988. In June 1989, she left to specialize in neuropediatrics and the neurosurgeons at The Moncton Hospital looked forward to her returning to the staff. On completion of this training, however, she returned to her native Ireland.

Dr. Gilles E. Brisson received his MD, CM from McGill in 1949 and from 1949 to 1950 served a rotating internship at the Montreal General Hospital. From 1950 to 1956 he was a resident in general surgery at the Centre Hôpital de l'Université de Sherbrooke and he practised general surgery at the Montreal General Hospital (1956-68). He then deserted surgery and took a residency in pathology at Centre Hospital (1968-71) and the Montreal General (1971-73), receiving his FRCS(C) in Pathology in 1972 and certification in pathology from the College of Physicians and Surgeons of Quebec in 1975. After serving as Director of Cytology at the Victoria General Hospital from 1973 to 1984, he came to Moncton to do a locums in the pathology department for six months but remained on staff until 1989.

William So was born on August 7, 1981, and received a BSc from McGill in 1971 and an MD from the University of Toronto in 1975. He interned at the Toronto General (1975-76) and served a residency in neurosurgery at the University of Toronto (1976-81), followed by two years at the University of Ottawa (1981-82). He became certified by the American Board of Neurological Surgery in 1980 and received his FRCS(C) in Neurosurgery in

1982. He served as a fellow in neurosurgery at the Ottawa General (1982-83) and as a fellow at University of Cornell Medical Centre (1984-85). He proved a competent neurosurgeon but affairs of the heart ruled when he resigned in June 1988 to join his wife, whose career path took her to the United States.

Dr. Janet Fultz has the distinction of being the first female surgeon on the staff of The Moncton Hospital. She was born on December 1, 1953, and received her BSc from the University of Guelph in 1977 and her MD from Queen's in 1978. After a surgical internship at the Wellesley Hospital, Toronto, she did a residency in plastic surgery at the University of Manitoba Teaching Hospitals (1979-84) receiving her FRCS(C) in Plastic Surgery in 1983. After a six-month fellowship in craniofacial surgery in France with Dr. Marchac at Collège Français de Chirgurgie Plastique Reconstruction & Esthétique, she came to Moncton. With her arrival, Plastic Surgery now became a separate department. Other than hiking and travelling, her recreational activities include bicycling. This activity put her at the scene of the Cormier Village hayride disaster where she helped triage and gave first aid to the unfortunate victims of this accident.

John Steeves, the son of Dr. Lea Steeves who has had a distinguished career as a cardiologist and as an educator at Dalhousie University Medical School, was born on December 12, 1949. He received his BSc from Mount Allison University and his MD from Dalhousie in 1974. After a rotating internship in the Dalhousie program (1974-75), he did general practice in New Glasgow from 1975-80. He entered the residency program in orthopaedics at Dalhousie in 1980 and on completing it in 1984, he received his FRCS(C). From January to July 1985, he served a fellowship at St. Michael's Hospital in Toronto before joining the orthopaedic department at The Moncton Hospital. Besides serving in the orthopaedic department, he served as In-Training Medical Education Co-ordinator for four years before handing over the reins to Dr. Dubois in December 1993. He resumed the position again in 1995.

Dr. Chris Levesque was born on December 14, 1950, in Saint John, New Brunswick, and seemed to be destined for a brilliant career in law before switching to medicine. He received a BSc degree from the University of New Brunswick in 1972, an LlB degree from the University of New Brunswick in 1975 and then a LlM from the London School of Economics in 1976. Forsaking law, he obtained a B.Med.Sc. degree from Memorial University in 1979 and an MD from the same institution in 1982. After a rotating internship at the Ottawa Civic Hospital (1982-83), he was on the staff on the Charlotte County Hospital in St. Stephen before coming to Moncton to serve as an emergency room physician. He received his ACLS in 1981, his ATLS in 1988 and his pediatric ALS in 1991.

Kenneth Mitton was born on May 22, 1958, and received his MD from Dalhousie in 1983. After serving in the Dalhousie family medicine internship and residency program (1983-85) he became certified in family practice by the College of Family Practice. He joined the Riverview Medical Clinic in family practice. In 1995 he served on the Region 1 Ad Hoc Medical Manpower (Primary Care) Planning Committee.

James G. Stewart was born in Moncton on March 16, 1959, the son of a Moncton optometrist. He was educated at Dalhousie University, receiving his BSc in 1980 and his MD in 1984 and interned in the Dalhousie rotating internship program from 1984 to 1985. He began a family practice in Albert in 1985 and was appointed to the courtesy staff but then transferred to the active staff in 1988 when he moved his practice to Moncton.

Francis Anthony was born on August 10, 1934, and received an MB, BS degree from S.N. Medical College, Agra University, India, in 1962. He went to Great Britain and after interning, received training in general surgery and urology. In 1967 he was made a Fellow of the Royal College London in General Surgery and in 1974 a LRCP/MRCS in Urology. He then immigrated to Canada and practised general surgery in Saskatchewan from 1978 to 1981. He left his surgical practice and served as chief resident in urology at Dalhousie from 1982 to 1984 to get his Canadian qualifications and was rewarded with his FRCS(C) in Urology in 1983. He joined the active staff of the Dr. Georges-L. Dumont Hospital and the courtesy staff of The Moncton Hospital in 1985, but because of the common call schedule, is a frequent visitor to The Moncton Hospital.

Hans R. Koritz was born in Uddenalla, Sweden, on February 15, 1946. He took his medical education in Switzerland, receiving a Certificat d'Études Médicale from the University of Zurich in 1976. After practising family medicine in Norway (1977-78) he came to Canada and served a rotating internship at The Moncton Hospital in 1978-79. He took one year of internal medicine at Dalhousie (1979-80) and then a year of family medicine at University of Western Ontario (1980-81), followed by a residency in anaesthesia at the same institution (1981-83). He did not complete his anaesthetic training, however, and started general practice in Sackville from 1983 to 1985. After some disagreement with the Sackville Hospital he moved to Dorchester and was appointed to the active staff of The Moncton Hospital but left Dorchester in September 1987.

In 1985-86 there were 13,786 adult and child admissions and 1,581 newborns. 10,827 operations were performed in the surgical suite, of which 5,019 were day surgery patients. Services provided included: audiograms—1,885; electrocardiograms—21,336; electroencephalograms—21,336; gastrointestinal unit procedures—2,179; social service cases—1,159; speech pathology—4,361; radiological examinations—87,774; CT scans—4,319; nuclear medicine procedures—4, 657; and ultrasound examinations—3,763. Visits to the various clinics were as follows: Arthritis—2,453; Chemotherapy—3,804; Chest—606; TB—866; Colposcopy—1,311; Diabetic Day Care—3,125; Diet Counselling—601; Multiple sclerosis—31; Pain—249; Reproductive Health—2,626; Urodynamics—390; Weight Checks—1,007; and Diagnostic—1,748.

By the end of 1986, the South Tower was about 70 percent completed but no word was forthcoming from government on plans for Phase II—the construction of North West and North East Towers. Some preliminary planning of space requirements and floor plan layouts for the existing space designated for renovations, was being carried out.

The search for a new vice-president in charge of nursing ended with the selection of Carroll Ann O'Leary for the post. Katherine Wright resumed other administrative duties before retiring in 1988.

The most significant purchase of equipment in 1986 was a new CT Scanner to replace the out-of-date model. Compared to the old scanner, the new one was able to produce a far superior image resolution. Shorter exposure times, increased computer capacity and an extensive array of software programs now made it possible to obtain a high diagnostic yield from CT scanning of all body organs and systems. With the success of the 1985 Annual Appeal, the Friends were able to donate $96,000 to purchase a special operating microscope and the hospital's first carbon dioxide laser. In addition, the Friends made it possible for the hospital to acquire state-of-the-art echocardiography equipment. The Friend's annual campaigns were now centred on a particular annual need for the hospital after consultation with the medical staff. The Nurses' Hospital Auxiliary also continued to make equipment purchases in response to direct requests from physicians. To demonstrate their dedication to health care, however, the Auxiliary gave up one source of funds by discontinuing the sale of tobacco products in their hospital gift shop. The volunteer department launched its first fundraising project in 1986 when it opened "The Pantry", a bakery cart which offered freshly baked goods. The proceeds from this business would go to the Ladies' Hospital Auxiliary.

In February of 1986, The Moncton Hospital submitted a Proposal for the Establishment of a Comprehensive Cardiovascular Program at The Moncton Hospital to the Hon. Nancy Clark-Teed, the minister of health. This proposal supported the need for a Cardiac Surgery Unit in New Brunswick. In February 1985, the hospital undertook to carry out a study on the feasibility of instituting a comprehensive cardiovascular program at The Moncton Hospital. This study was carried out in two phases. Phase 1 was contracted out to Education Health Environment Ltd.(EHE), Ottawa, as consultants and confirmed the volume of patients which could be expected at a centre in the province. Phase 2 was carried out by Agnew Peckham and Associates and detailed the cost and other implications of providing this service at The Moncton Hospital. External consultants included Dr. Murphy and Dr. Chandler from the Cardiac Unit, Victoria General Hospital, Halifax, and Dr. Jablowsky from Department of Cardiology, University Hospital, London, Ont. The proposal emphasized that The Moncton Hospital was the best centre in the province to meet the criteria for the establishment of a Cardiac Surgical Unit. The proposal was not accepted by government and the Cardiac Surgery Unit for the Province ended up in the city of Saint John. Members of the medical staff providing input into the proposal were: Dr. Robert Trifts, Dr. David Douglas, Dr. Kim Deware, Dr. Robert Dysart, Dr.

Paul Dubois and Dr. Fred Murphy, as well as members of the executive of the medical staff.

During the year the hospital increased its use of computers with the installation of a new patient information system, including a central patient index and systems for the emergency and medical imaging departments. Future plans to include laboratory, pharmacy and nursing stations remained unfulfilled until 1996 and 1997. Concurrent with the installation of the new patient information system was the full computerization of the hospital's financial information systems including: general ledger, accounts payable, inventory, purchasing, payroll, personnel and management reporting.

New members of the staff in 1986 included Dr. Bruce Bender, Dr. Roddy Canning, Dr. Michael McGonigle, Dr. Colin Nath, Dr. Kenneth Porter, Dr. Jennifer Huntsman, Dr. Bruce Fraser, Dr. Kevin Black, Dr. Sylvie Argouarch, Dr. Christine Telfer, Dr. Alan Munroe, Dr. Ross Leighton, Dr. Margaret Leighton and Dr. Margaret Stevens.

Bruce Bender was born in Philadelphia on October 16, 1949, and received a BSc from the University of Michigan in 1971 and an MD from the same institution in 1975. After interning at the University of Virginia and starting a pathology residency there, he shifted to the University of Pittsburgh in 1977 and became certified in anatomical and clinical pathology by the American Board of Pathology in 1979. From 1979 to 1981 he was an assistant professor of pathology at the University of Pittsburgh and in 1981 he became head of chemistry and anatomical pathology at Faber Health Centre, Monroeville, Pennsylvania, remaining an assistant professor at the University of Pittsburgh. He was interested in research and had 19 publications to his credit when he came to Moncton to become director of the laboratory at The Moncton Hospital. This position was gradually requiring more administrative work as the lab now had over 100 employees and a budget of $4.6 million. In his quiet unassuming manner, Bruce soon took charge, introducing additional personnel, new equipment and revised methods in the lab. He served as chairman of the Utilization Committee for several years. He took his administration duties to heart and enrolled in a course of administration medicine at the University of Michigan and received his Masters Degree in Administrative Medicine in May 1990. In 1981 he became a Diplomate of the American Board of Medical Management. This extra education proved the hospital's undoing, however, as he resigned in March 1991, to accept a position as vice-president of Medical Affairs at Sacred Heart Hospital in Allentown, Pennsylvania.

In July 1986, Dr. Robin Walker left for Kingston, Ont. Although the pediatricians continued to provide neonatal care, this was a tertiary service and it was important to have a pediatrician with special skills in neonatology to run the program. The hospital was fortunate to obtain the services of Dr. Roderick Canning in December 1986. Roddy was born in Galway, Ireland, on August 8, 1953, and received his medical education at National University of Ireland, University College, Galway, Ireland, obtaining the degree MB,

BCh, BAO in 1977. After a surgical internship at the Regional Hospital, Galway, and a medical internship at the General Hospital, Sligo (1977-78), he served as a medical house officer at these hospitals from 1978-79 and then as pediatric house officer at the General Hospital, Castlebar, and the Regional Hospital, Galway, from 1980 to 1981. He then came to Canada and served as a pediatric resident at the Hospital for Sick Children in Toronto from 1981 to 1983, followed by an appointment as chief resident in pediatrics at Queen's University in Kingston (1983-84). He obtained his LMCC in 1982 and his FRCP(C) in pediatrics in 1984. His expertise in neonatology came with a two-year stint as a neonatal fellow at Mount Sinai Hospital in Toronto from 1984 to 1986. Besides his interest in paediatrics he has been involved in the New Brunswick Medical Society, being appointed to the board of Directors in 1990 and elected as its president in 1994.

Michael J. McGonigal received his premedical education at St. Malachy's College, graduating in 1963 and then graduated from medical school at Queen's University, Belfast, Northern Ireland, in 1969 with the degree MB, BCh. After a rotating internship at Moter Hospital, Belfast (1969-70), he did a residency in internal medicine (1970-73) at Royal Victoria Hospital, Belfast City Hospital and Belfast Fever Hospital. From 1974 to 1975 he was senior resident in the Department of Metabolic Medicine, Royal Victoria Hospital, Belfast, and from 1975 to 1977, a research fellow at Royal Victoria Hospital. He came to Canada and spent a year as a research fellow in the Department of Endocrinology at Victoria General Hospital, London, Ontario, from 1976-77. He had become a member of the Royal College of Physicians (UK) in 1972 and received his LMCC in 1972 and his FRCP(C) in 1976. He joined the staff of the Department of Internal Medicine as chief of endocrinology at the Saint John Regional Hospital in 1978 and remained there until he moved to Moncton to assume the position as the first endocrinologist on staff. As a member of the Department of Internal Medicine, he felt unsure in caring for patients in the Coronary Intensive Care Unit and in 1988 was relieved of the burden of taking call. He felt he lacked support among the staff in establishing his specialty and he resigned in October 1990, and went to Saudi Arabia.

Colin Nath was born in Trinidad on September 11, 1955, and received his premedical education at St. Mary College, graduating in 1972. He graduated from the University of the West Indies with an MB, BS degree in 1978. He interned at Port of Spain General Hospital (1978-79) and undertook an additional year at Foothills Hospital, Calgary, from 1979 to 1980. He then remained at the Foothills Hospital, taking a residency in internal medicine from 1980 to 1983 and receiving his FRCP(C) in 1983. From 1983 to 1985 he had a fellowship in cardiology at the Foothills Hospital and the University of Calgary resulting in his receiving his certification in cardiology in 1985. He joined the staff of The Moncton Hospital where his pleasant manner and abilities were recognized and appreciated. On coming to Moncton, he had training in cardiac catherization and had envisioned that the hospital might become the cardiac surgery centre for the province. When this did not happen, he resigned in May 1987 so that he could find another centre that could use his special skills.

Kenneth Porter was born in Plaster Rock, New Brunswick, on January 10, 1953, and received his BSc from the University of New Brunswick before travelling to Newfoundland where he obtained his MD degree in 1980. He interned in family medicine at the General Hospital in Saint John's (1980-81) and, after a one-year paediatric residency at the Janeway (1981-82), he returned to a family practice residency (1982-83), receiving certification by the College of Family Practice in 1983. He then switched to a residency in anaesthesia (1983-85) and became certified and received his FRCP(C) in Anaesthesia in 1985. While on the anaesthetic staff he became interested in pain management and joined the pain clinic. In 1990 he passed examinations by the Acupuncture Foundation of Canada and in 1992 he opened his private Harrisville Pain Clinic. On July 1, 1995, he resigned from the anaesthetic staff to devote his full time to his pain clinic.

Jennifer Clare Huntsman, the wife of Dr. Ken Porter, was born on October 18, 1957, and received her BMed Sciences from Memorial in 1979 and her MD in 1981. She did an internship and residency in family medicine at Memorial (1981-83), receiving certification in family medicine from the College of Family Practice. After a further year of residency in anaesthesia (1983-84), she worked as a casualty officer at the Janeway Child Health Centre in Saint John's (1985-86), after which she came to Moncton with her husband and joined the part-time emergency room staff.

Douglas Bruce Fraser was born in Minnedosa, Manitoba, and received a BSc from Brandon College in 1965 and an MD from the University of Manitoba in 1969. He served a rotating internship in the Dalhousie program (1969-70) and then returned west to do general practice at Wilkie, Saskatchewan, from 1970 to 1971. He then served at the Student Health Centre, University of Saskatchewan before proceeding to a residency in psychiatry at the University of Saskatchewan from 1972 to 1974. He completed his psychiatric training at the Kingston General in 1974-75 and the Regional Psychiatric Hospital in Kingston in 1975-76, obtaining certification from Royal College of Physicians and Surgeons of Canada in psychiatry in 1976. From 1976 to 1979 he was senior psychiatrist at Moose Jaw Union Hospital. This was followed by private practice of psychiatry in Moose Jaw from 1979-86 before his decision to come to Moncton. He received his FRCS(C) in 1986. He is a long-term survivor of kidney transplantation, having undergone a transplant in 1974.

Kevin Black was born in Northern Ireland on August 30, 1953, and took his premedical and medical education at Queen's University, Belfast, receiving the degrees of MB, BCh, BAO in 1978. He interned at Erne Hospital, Enniskillen, and Waveney Hospital, Ballymena, from 1979 to 1980. After stints as house officer in casualty, surgery, obstetrics and gynaecology and internal medicine (1980-82), he immigrated to Canada and did family practice (1982-86) at Shoal Lake and Strathclair Health Centre. On coming to

New Brunswick he started practice in Salisbury but soon moved to Moncton. In August 1989, he gave up his family practice to work full time as an emergency room physician. He obtained his ACLS in 1984 and his ATLS in 1985.

Sylvie Argouarch was born in France on July 18, 1957. She received her undergraduate BacC from Lycée de Kerrshe, Brest, France, in 1975 and her medical degree in 1982 from the University of West Brittany, Brest, France. After a residency in pediatrics in France in 1982-83, she came to Canada and served a rotating internship at Dalhousie in 1984-85 and then a medical internship in 1985-86, and received her LMCC in 1986. She joined the Department of Family Practice but worked in the geriatric unit that had been set up by Dr. Davidson. In 1989, she left to pursue a residency in psychiatry at the Victoria General in 1989-92, and became certified in psychiatry in 1992. After working at the Nova Scotia Hospital in 1992-93, she was appointed to the psychiatric staff of The Moncton Hospital in December 1993. In November 1994, she took a year's leave of absence to obtain a fellowship in geriatric psychiatry.

Christine Telfer was born on December 18, 1956, and received a BSc in Medical Science in 1978 and an MD from the University of Alberta in 1980. She was introduced to the Maritimes when she served a rotating internship at Dalhousie University in 1981-82. She remained in the Maritimes for the next four years, doing locums in Oromocto, Kentville, Wolfville, Chatham and Bathurst, except for 1985, when she spent a year in Cambodia. She came to Moncton to do a locums for Dr. John Meagher in September 1986, but stayed on and started her own family practice and stopped her wanderings when she married Dennis Livingston, a music teacher in Moncton.

Alan Munroe was born in Moncton on June 4, 1958, and received his MD from Dalhousie in 1984. He did the intern and family practice residency at Dalhousie (1984-86). He first came back to his home town to do a locums for Dr. John Meagher but then stayed on, setting up his own family practice in Moncton.

Ross Leighton was born on December 15, 1954, the son of Dr. Claude Leighton. He received a BSc from Acadia in 1975 and an MD from Dalhousie in 1979. After a rotating internship at the Victoria General Hospital in 1979-80, he entered the orthopaedic residency program at Dalhousie from 1980 to 1984, receiving his FRCS(C) in 1984. From 1984 to 1985, he did a further year of fellowship in trauma and arthroplasty at St. Michael's Hospital in Toronto. From July to December 1985, he was a fellow in trauma and research at University of Davis, Davis, California. He joined the orthopaedic staff in January 1986 and after a successful practice in Moncton, resigned in October 1991, to take up a position at the Victoria General Hospital in Halifax.

It seemed that every male physician coming to Moncton lately was accompanied by a physician wife who also joined the staff, and Ross' arrival did not prove to be an exception. Margaret MacRae Leighton (Peggy) was born in Halifax on December 26, 1953, the daughter of a physician. She received her premedical and medical education at Dalhousie, obtaining her MD in 1977. After a rotating internship in the Dalhousie program in 1977-78, she had a large family practice in Halifax until she moved to Moncton with Ross and set up a family practice. She has since returned to Halifax with Ross and re-established her family practice there.

Dr. Margaret Stevens, the wife of Dr. Eric Stevens, who is on the ophthalmology staff, joined the family practice staff in 1986 with privileges limited to participation in the Reproductive Health Clinic. She was born in the United Kingdom on December 8, 1936, and graduated from Edinburgh University in 1960 with the MB, ChB degree. She interned at Bangour General Hospital, Scotland, Royal Hospital for Sick Children, Edinburgh, and Dufenline and West Fife Hospital (1960-62). She then did a residency in obstetrics and gynaecology at Bangour General Hospital (1962-64), Elsie Inglis Maternity Hospital, Edinburgh, in 1964-65, and Newcastle General Hospital in 1965-66. On coming to Canada she obtained her LMCC in 1971 and worked part-time doing office gynaecology in the offices of Dr. McLaughlin, Dr. Caddick, Dr. Pugh and Dr. Brodie. In 1992, she was appointed to the sexual assault team.

Statistics for 1986-87 showed a slight increase for most services over 1985-86. There were 14,386 adult and child admissions with 1,551 newborn. Operations performed numbered 10,824 including 4,975 day patients. Services provided were: audiograms—1,555; electrocardiograms—22,977; electroencephalograms—2,252; gastrointestinal unit procedures—2,052; social service caseload -1,420; speech pathology attendance—3,413; radiological examinations—90,495; CT Scans—4,639; nuclear medicine procedures—4,784; and ultrasound examinations—4,065. 72,994 visits were made to the OPD/Emergency department exclusive of G.I. Unit and Clinics. Clinic visits numbered 20,996 as follows: Arthritic—2,530; Chemotherapy—3,383; Chest—912; TB—567; Colposcopy—1,067; Diabetic Day Care—3,715; Diagnostic—1,422; Diet Counselling—740; Multiple Sclerosis—54; Pain—3,389; Reproductive Health—2,823; Urodynamics—388 and weight checks—1,002.

In the fall of 1987, the Liberal Party under Frank McKenna totally decimated the previous Conservative government of Richard Hatfield taking all fifty-eight seats in the legislature. With a change in government, there was naturally some trepidation in the hospital over the redevelopment project, as it seems that when each new government comes to power it immediately finds the books worse than they ever imagined and begins to talk of cutbacks and inability to fulfil their election promises. Nevertheless, the new government promised to complete the remainder of the project in the least possible time. With expenses of $52,739,086, the hospital was able to show a surplus of $193,805 before depreciation in 1987. This was possible because of an increase in the base budget of $871,554 and increased payments by Hospital Services to offset new labour agreements, particularly with nurses.

A program initiated in 1987 by the Employee Recognition Committee was the awarding of pins to those employed by the hospital for varying periods of time. At a special ceremony to launch the program over 1,000 pins were awarded. Three employees—Mary LeBlanc, switchboard, Désiré Saulnier, housekeeping, and Katherine Wright, administration, each received pins, recognizing 35 years of service. In common with many organizations, the hospital recognized that happy employees make for efficient workers and an Employee Assistance Program was established as a joint project of the hospital and the four unions which represented the employees. Recognizing that employees with difficulties caused by physical or emotional illness, financial, marital, or family problems, alcohol or drug abuse, legal problems and other concerns, have an opportunity for recovery or improvement when help is provided at an early stage, the program promised increased confidential assistance to the employees and did not replace any community based programs.

The 1987 annual appeal of the Friends of the Moncton Hospital was focused on the laboratory and over $100,000 was raised to supply advanced laboratory equipment which was able to analyse thousands of blood tests previously sent to other hospitals. This year, the Friends established an Education Fund as a result of memorials received at the time of the deaths of Dr. A.M. Clarke and Myrna Sherrard, along with a bequest from the estate of Harold Tait. The interest from this fund would be set aside to support staff members wishing to further their education.

The Moncton Hospital Ladies' Auxiliary donated $14,000 to the hospital for the purchase of equipment, with the major purchase being an Impedance Audiometer for the Speech and Hearing Department at a cost of $9,000. In the meantime, the School of Nursing Alumnae extended the operation of their coffee shop to 24 hours and with their funds, more computer equipment and furniture was provided to the Nursing Office. Funds were provided to purchase nursing texts for the nursing units and The Moncton Hospital Health Sciences Library. The Alumnae's project "Lifeline" was also the beneficiary of their largesse with an additional 15 units made available to the public.

The volunteers continued to supply stellar service to the hospital and in the fall of 1987 introduced a new program, "The Oncology Volunteer Program." A Terry Fox grant allowed the hiring of a co-ordinator, Barbara Joudry, to develop and supervise the program. Oncology volunteers were specially trained to help cancer patients cope with living through their illness and to provide support to patients and their families.

A trial operation of a Child and Adolescent Psychiatry Unit was carried out in 1987 and it was envisioned that if the assessment were favourable, a permanent unit would be established to provide a much needed service to south-eastern New Brunswick.

With an increasing number of AIDS patients requiring hospital services, the Medical Advisory Committee formed a special committee to examine these problems and to ensure the co-ordination of all elements of the hospital organization for the benefit of patients and those caring for them.

Despite the hospital's by-laws which required that the chief of staff be appointed for a two-year term with an option of another two-year term, Dr. C.E. Doyle had held this position since 1975. He retired in June 1987, to be replaced by Dr. Peter Gorman.

The hospital again continued to attract new members to its staff with several additions during the year. Dr. Ann Canning (née Cunningham) finished her training in pediatrics and joined her husband, Roddy, on the pediatric staff. Born in Ireland, like her husband, she received her MB, BCh, BAO from the National University of Ireland in 1977. From 1977 to 1978 she did a medical internship at Merlin Park Hospital, Galway, Ireland, and a surgical internship at the General Hospital, Mayo, Ireland. From 1978 to 1981 she served a year each in obstetrics and gynaecology, ENT, psychiatry and anaesthesia at various hospitals in Ireland before coming to Canada for training in pediatrics. She did a pediatric residency at the Hospital for Sick Children in Toronto in 1982-83 and from 1984 to 1987 with the 1983-84 year at the Kingston General Hospital. Her last year at the Hospital for Sick Children was spent as a Fellow in Pediatric Gastroenterology. She received her FRCP(C) in 1987.

Monique B. Harize received her BA from the University of Toulouse College of Sciences, Toulouse, France, in 1955 and her MD from the University of Toulouse Medical School in 1962. She did a residency in medicine at University Hospital, Toulouse, from 1960 to 1962 and was certified by the Specialty Board in Serology in 1963, and in Microbiology in 1964. After family practice in Toulouse from 1964 to 1966, she moved to the USA and, after working as a microbiologist, she began a residency in pathology at Maricopa County General Hospital, Phoenix (1981-82), and the Medical College of Ohio (1983-86). This was followed by a fellowship in anatomic pathology at Children's Hospital of Los Angeles in 1987. She became a Diplomate of the American Board of Pathology in 1987. In August 1987 she joined the pathology staff but she resigned in June 1989 to return to the USA.

For some time Peter Lightfoot had been holding down the fort as the only gastroenterologist on staff and his burden was lightened in 1987 with the appointment of Dr. Franz Joseph Schweiger. Born in West Germany on December 2, 1954, he was educated in Canada, receiving a BSc from the University of Windsor in 1978 and an MD from the University of Toronto in 1982. He had a medical internship at the Toronto Western Hospital (1982-83) and began his training in internal medicine at Toronto Western Hospital in 1983-84 and the Toronto General in 1984-85. He finished his training at Queen's University with a residency in gastroenterology (1985-86) and a fellowship in gastroenterology from 1986 to 1987. He became certified in internal medicine by the American Board of Internal Medicine in 1985 and received his FRCP(C) in Internal Medicine in 1986. He also received a certificate of special competence in the subspecialty of gastroenterology from the Royal College in 1987. He has introduced many new diagnostic tools and treatments to the practice of gastroenterology in Moncton, most notably

ERCP, and he served as chief of the Department of Internal Medicine in 1993 and 1994. He was appointed director of the Gastrointestinal Unit in 1991.

The Department of Medical Imaging had been showing yearly increases in the amount of its work and in order to cope with the increased workload, Dr. Keith Costello was recruited to augment the staff. Keith was born on July 14, 1955, and received an MD degree from Memorial University in 1980. He came to the mainland and took an internship in internal medicine at the Victoria General Hospital from 1980 to 1981 and served a year as a resident in internal medicine in 1981-82. This was followed by a residency in diagnostic radiology from 1982 to 1985 and in 1986 he received his FRCP(C) in diagnostic radiology in 1986. After serving as radiologist at Central Newfoundland Regional Health Centre in Grand Falls, Newfoundland, he returned to the mainland and joined the Department of Radiology in April 1987.

The Department of Obstetrics and Gynaecology received a big boost with two new appointments in 1988. Francis MacDonald was born on October 16, 1952, and received a BSc from St. Mary's University in 1974 and an MD from Dalhousie in 1978. He served a rotating internship in the Dalhousie Program from 1978 to 1979 and from 1980 to 1984 took a residency in obstetrics and gynaecology at Dalhousie. He received his FRCS(C) in Obstetrics and Gynaecology in 1985 and practised in New Glasgow from 1985 to 1987. He only remained on the staff for two years, resigning in 1989 to go to the Charlottetown Clinic.

The other addition to the Department of Obstetrics and Gynaecology was Naheed Masood Chaudry. She was born in Rawalpindi, Pakistan, on January 8, 1951. After taking her premedical education at the University of Karachi she attended medical school at the University of Punjab, graduating in 1975 with the MB, BS degree. From 1975 to 1977 she was a house officer at Lady Dufferin Hospital in Karachi. She immigrated to Canada and passed her ECFMG exams in 1979 and after a fellowship in medical genetics she interned at The Moncton Hospital in 1981-82. She then did a residency in obstetrics and gynaecology in 1982-83 and from 1985 to 1987, taking the year 1984-85 off while she did general practice in North Bay Psychiatry Hospital. She received her certification from the Royal College in 1987 and then joined the staff of The Moncton Hospital. She resigned from the staff in 1996.

Gilles Belisle was born on July 2, 1955, and received his premedical education at St. Jerome, Quebec, and his MD from the University of Sherbrooke in 1978. After a straight surgical internship at CHUS, Sherbrooke, in 1978-79, he was a resident in internal medicine at Maisonneuve, Rosemont, Montreal (1979-80). He returned to Sherbrooke for postgraduate training in ENT from 1981 to 1983 and completed his training at Notre Dame Hospital, Montreal, from 1983 to 1984. He became certified by Corporation professionelle des médicins du Québec in 1984 and received his FRCS(C) in 1986. He first joined the courtesy staff in 1987 while on the active staff of the Dr. Georges-L. Dumont Hospital. A very talented, personable and dynamic individual, he had interests besides his profession and while practising, was taking political science at the Université de Moncton. He was serving as chief of his department in 1991 when he resigned from the staff to pursue other interests. His free spirit was demonstrated when one Christmas he decided to celebrate by decorating his house with a tree from the campus of the Université de Moncton. Unfortunately, he was caught in the act of cutting it down and had to pay the price of receiving a call from the local police.

The Department of Surgery received a boost when it was able to add a second general surgeon with training in vascular surgery to its roster. Dr. Stephen Brown was born in Charlottetown, Prince Edward Island, on December 5, 1954. He graduated from Queen's University with a BSc in 1976 and then attended Ottawa University, receiving an MD degree in 1981. After a straight surgical internship at Mount Sinai Hospital in Toronto, he underwent a general surgical residency at the University of Ottawa from 1982 to 1986, receiving his FRCS(C) in General Surgery in 1986. He then took further training in vascular surgery at the Ottawa Civic and Ottawa General Hospitals from 1986 to 1987 and received certification in vascular surgery. In 1990 he became a Fellow of the American College of Surgeons in General and Vascular Surgery.

Michael MacEachern provided the Department of Neurological Sciences with a second neurologist. He was born on October 16, 1949, in Cape Breton, and after receiving a BSc from Dalhousie in 1949, he went to the Université de Liège, Belgium, where he received his MD degree in 1980. He did a rotating internship at the Jewish General Hospital in Montreal in 1980-81, followed by a year of residency in internal medicine at the same institution in 1981-82. He went to the University of Ottawa for a neurology residency at the Ottawa General, Ottawa Civic and Children's Hospital of Eastern Ontario from 1983 to 1986 and a fellowship in neurophysiology in 1986-87. He joined the active staff of the Dr. Georges-L. Dumont Hospital and the courtesy staff of The Moncton Hospital but spends a lot of time at The Moncton Hospital as a result of his duties in the Department of Neurological Sciences. He is one of several on the staff who spend their spare time on the golf links where he reportedly is as cognizant of the rule book as he is of neuropathways.

Catherine Ann MacLean (née Plant) is the grandchild of Dr. Arthur Ross and the only grandchild of a member of the medical staff to join the staff. She was born on June 26, 1957, and was educated at Dalhousie University, receiving her BSc in Health Education in 1981 and her MD in 1985. She joined the Moncton Medical Clinic after completing the two-year family medicine program at Dalhousie and becoming certified by the College of Family Practice. Once she joined the staff, she became very active in the Department of Family Practice and on hospital committees and was a strong supporter of continuing education. She served on the Palliative Care Advisory Committee, Environmental Advisory Committee, Patient Education Committee. She served on the Family Violence Task Force and became a member of the Sexual Assault Team. She also became active in the New Brunswick Division of the College of Family Physicians, serving as Chairperson of AIDS Testing Education Committee in 1988-89 and nationally, as Chairperson of the National Advisory Committee on patient Education for the College of Family Physicians in 1990-91, and as an examiner in 1990-91. After five years in practice, she resigned to accept a full-time teaching position at Victoria Hospital, University of Western Ontario.

Sharon Northrup was born on January 1, 1959, and received a BSc from the University of New Brunswick in 1981 and an MD from Dalhousie in 1986. After a rotating internship at Dalhousie in 1986-87, she came to Moncton to do a locums for Dr. Kevin Black and decided to remain.

Dr. Daniel Landry was born on December 31, 1959, and received a BSc in 1981 and an MD from Dalhousie in 1985. After a two-year internship and residency in the family practice program at Dalhousie in 1985-87, he joined the Riverview Medical Clinic.

The statistics for 1987-88 show 14,905 adult and children admissions and 1,495 newborns. 11,020 operations were performed including 4,941 day surgery patients. Services provided were: audiograms—1,874; electrocardiograms—23,566; electroencephalograms—1,911; gastrointestinal unit procedures—2,441; social service cases—1,332; speech pathology—3,413; radiological examinations—93,729; CT Scans—6,424; nuclear medicine procedures—5,238; and ultrasound examinations—4,918. There were 22,954 clinic visits as follows: Arthritis—2,515; Chemotherapy—3,491; Chest—1,208; TB—596; Colposcopy—1,317; Diabetic Day Care—4,027; Diet Counselling—1,228; Weight Checks—1,047; Multiple Sclerosis—4; Pain—2,505; Reproductive Health—3,131; and Urodynamics—427.

After 14 years of service on the board and five years as chairman, Ralph Black retired, and his position as chairman was assumed by Robert Radford. Mr. Black steered the hospital through most of the construction of the South Tower and also through some tough years financially. When he assumed the chairmanship he was faced with the task of introducing bilingualism to the hospital and even when he retired five years after its implementation the hospital's bilingualism policy continued to be a controversial issue. As a practical matter, the policy only affected a few services such as neurosurgery, neonatal intensive care and ambulance and positions in these services were filled with bilingual staff as vacancies occurred. Out of a hospital staff of 1600, this amounted to only 51 positions.

Wrestling with inadequate budgets to look after the number of people served by The Moncton Hospital, the board took its message to the people of the greater Moncton area by launching a public awareness campaign. Representatives of the board, the medical profession and administration met and spoke to many organizations and groups throughout the greater Moncton area, but it is doubtful if this had any beneficial effect other than to gain some understanding from anyone waiting for a hospital bed. Information sessions were held with the staff in May and June to introduce them to the hospital's revised Role Statement. In addition, over 1,000 hospital staff viewed a slide-sound presentation on the activities of the hospital. Many signed their name to the Mission and Philosophy poster which was then hung on the wall of the lobby for all to see.

After many years of service to The Moncton Hospital, Katherine Wright retired during the year. On the occasion of her retirement the Friends of the Moncton Hospital received many gifts in her honour and the Friends decided to name one of the educational grants awarded each year, the Katherine Wright Bursary. Meanwhile, Mr. Kilpatrick received yet another accolade when he was presented with the George Findlay Stephens Memorial Award by the Canadian Hospital Association. This award was made "in recognition of his outstanding contribution to the health care system of Canada."

In May 1988, the Hon. Raymond Frenette, the minister of health and community services, officially opened the Haemophiliac Clinic under the directorship of Dr. Sheldon Rubin. This clinic was established in co-operation with the New Brunswick Haemophilia Society and was designed to meet the needs of haemophiliacs throughout the province.

Some changes took place in the emergency department. A triage service had been in effect during the daytime and through this system, every non-scheduled patient was assessed on arrival by a nurse and categorized as acute, urgent or non-acute. This allowed the early identification of life threatening emergencies. This triage system was now expanded to the evening hours as well. This had become especially necessary since so many patients were now using the hospital as their point of entry into the health care system and clogging the emergency room with non-emergencies that could easily be handled in their family practitioner's office. Another change in the emergency

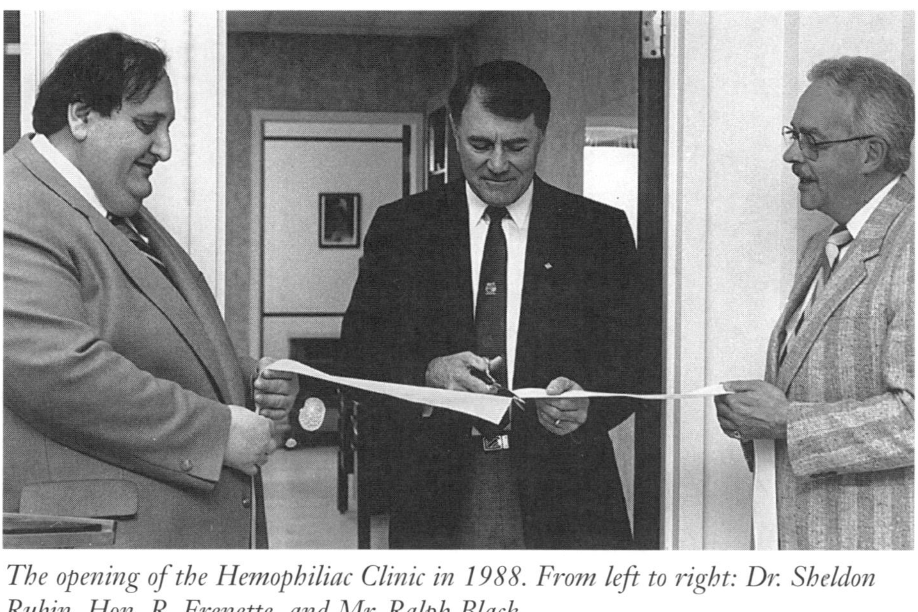

The opening of the Hemophiliac Clinic in 1988. From left to right: Dr. Sheldon Rubin, Hon. R. Frenette, and Mr. Ralph Black.

department was a major reorganization of the ambulance service. In order to further the professional development of the ambulance personnel, maintain adequate service levels, and meet the needs of the two linguistic groups in the community, the service was integrated administratively and clinically with the emergency department. This integration provided an opportunity to upgrade the training of the attendants so that all personnel now exceeded the training standards of the Department of Health and Community Services.

A morale booster to the staff this year was the presentation of "Spring Thaw." This variety show was performed at Mathieu Martin High School and included performances from many departments, including contributions from the medical staff. The evening was a great success with a sold-out house and was followed by a dance.

Any medical staff that wants to rest on its laurels and fails to look inward and review its programs and plan for the future is a dying organization. We like to feel that The Moncton Hospital is alive and well, and, although plans for a cardiac surgery unit and radiation oncology did not bear fruit, for instance, the staff remained undeterred in trying to plot its future. In 1988 the medical staff identified the need for review of our infectious diseases services. Dr. Tom Marrie, an infectious disease specialist, was brought in from Halifax for consultation and he provided a list of suggestions to improve the hospital's management of infections.

In 1988, the Friends of the Moncton Hospital embarked on two new fundraising strategies. As part of the Annual Fall Appeal, a very successful corporate appeal was launched. Forty volunteer canvassers approached businesses in the Greater Moncton Area for donations and this provided 25 percent of the total campaign funds raised that year. The second strategic thrust was the formal solicitation of the employees of The Moncton Hospital which included payroll deduction privileges. In total, the foundation raised in excess of $200,000 in 1988. The fall campaign was directed toward the Gastrointestinal Unit and raised over $150,000 to purchase much needed equipment for the Gastrointestinal Unit. The Nurses' Hospital Auxiliary provided an addition to the duodenoscope as well as funds to the emergency room for a new type of thermometer which can be used in the ear.

Departures from the medical staff in 1988 included: Dr. Willam So from neurosurgery, Dr. James Goulding from the emergency department, Dr. Gopal Nanjudan from ENT, Dr. Arthur Oatway, who retired from the Department of Anaesthesia and Dr. Arthur Armstrong, who retired to Sackville but would continue to work in the day surgery unit at the Sackville Hospital. Identification by the board of trustees of a deficiency in ophthalmology prompted the hospital to invite Dr. Raymond LeBlanc, chairman of ophthalmology at Dalhousie University, to meet with representatives of the hospital to determine the direction and needs of the future. His recommendations were helpful and the hospital sponsored one ophthalmology resident's training as a result. Despite departures from the staff, new additions made up for losses.

Dr. William So was replaced in the neurosurgery department by Dr. Antoine Salloum. Antoine was born in Lebanon on May 27, 1949, and received a BA from Jesuits College, Janhour, Lebanon, in 1966. He went to France for the first two years of his medical training at the University of Bordeaux, and then completed the third to sixth year at St. Joseph University, Beirut, Lebanon, receiving his MD degree in 1973. He then came to Canada and after serving a rotating internship at Centre Hôpital de l'Université de Sherbrooke (1973-74), he embarked on a neurosurgery residency at the same institution from 1974 to 1980, except for 1975, which was spent in pediatric neurosurgery at the Montreal Children's Hospital. He received his FRCS(C) in Neurosurgery in 1981. He returned to his native Lebanon and did private practice at St. George Hospital and Sacré Coeur Hospital, Beirut, from 1980 to 1988, except for working at Hamad General Hospital, Daha, Quatar, in 1986-87, after which he returned to Canada to join the neurosurgery staff of The Moncton Hospital. In 1992 he became a Fellow of the American College of Surgeons and in 1993 was certified in Neurosurgery by the College of Surgeons and Physicians of Quebec. He served as chief of Neurosurgery in 1992 and 1993 and at the same time served on the OR and Critical Care Committees. Besides his skills as a neurosurgeon, his quiet reasoned approach to problems assured him of the confidence of his colleagues who elected him chief of staff in December 1993.

In 1988, Dr. William Sigsworth joined the full-time staff in the new Department of Emergency Medicine. Bill was born in Halifax on May 28, 1958, and attended Dalhousie, from which he received a BSc in 1980, a BEd in 1981 and an MD in 1985. After a rotating internship at Dalhousie in 1985-86, he already had his eyes set on emergency room medicine receiving his ACLS in 1985 and ATLS in 1986. He worked in the emergency department of the Aberdeen Hospital from 1986 to 1988 and then came to Moncton. From 1989 to 1990, he took a year off to serve in the family practice residency program at Dalhousie and became certified in family practice by the Canadian College in 1990. He then returned to practise as an emergency room physician at The Moncton Hospital.

Roel Poblete was born in the Philippines on October 11, 1951, and received a BSc in Biology in 1972 from Philippine Union College and an MD from Manila Central University College of Medicine in 1976. He did a rotating internship at Manila Sanatorium Hospital in 1976-77 and then served as a rural physician in Metro Manila in 1977-78. He immigrated to Canada and served a rotating internship at Regina General Hospital in 1979-80. After a residency in pathology at Kingston General Hospital from 1980 to 1982, he did a residency in internal medicine at St. Mary's Hospital, New York, University of Rochester School of Medicine, from 1982 to 1985, becoming certified and a Diplomate of the American Board of Internal Medicine in 1985. He then did a fellowship in cardiology at the Royal Victoria Hospital in Montreal in 1985-86 and after a year of private practice in Willowdale, Ontario, in 1986-87, returned to McGill for another year of fellowship in cardiology in 1987-88. He received his FRCP(C) in internal medicine in 1986 and his certification in cardiology in 1990. After only three years on staff, he resigned in 1991, for family reasons.

It was a good year for cardiology with another addition to that department by the name of Vincent Robinson. Vincent was born in Westmoreland, Jamaica, on October 30, 1950. He took his premedical and medical training at the University of West Indies in Kingston, Jamaica, receiving his MB, BS in 1976. He interned at the Kingston Regional Hospital Board in 1976-77. After a year as an emergency room physician at the Kingston Public Hospital in 1977-78, he came to Canada for a residency in internal medicine at the Victoria General Hospital in Halifax from 1978 to 1982. He became certified by the American Board of Internal Medicine in 1981 and received his FRCP(C) in Internal Medicine in 1982. From 1982 to 1985 he had a fellowship in cardiology at Foothills Hospital and in 1984 received a specialist certificate in cardiology from the Royal College. He stayed on doing clinical research at Foothills Hospital from 1985 to 1988 before coming to Moncton bringing with him his expertise in nuclear cardiology. Although slow moving and slow talking, he always had something to offer when he did talk. When he came to Moncton he already had 15 published articles to his credit and because of his interest in research, he resigned in March 1994, to take an academic position in Augusta, Georgia.

The Department of Rehabilitation Medicine, sitting in limbo and run by a committee since the departure of Dr. Berrara, was in need of a director. The hospital was able to recruit Dr. Elliott Weiss in 1988. Elliott was born in Toronto on December 12, 1957. He received his premedical and medical education at the University of Toronto, graduating with an MD degree in 1982. After an internship at the Toronto East General Hospital in 1982-83, he entered the residency program in physical medicine and rehabilitation at the University of Toronto from 1983 to 1988 and became certified in physical medicine and rehabilitation in 1989. He was appointed the clinical director of Rehabilitation Services in October 1988. Since joining the staff, he has furthered his education by receiving an Executive MBA from St. Mary's University and as a result the hospital has to worry about losing him to an administrative post. It has not been the custom to have one-man departments and so there has never been a separate category in the staff for the Department of Physical Medicine and his initial appointment was to the Department of Family Medicine. In 1981, he was placed on the active staff in internal medicine but in 1995 more appropriately placed on the active staff of the Department of Neurological Sciences.

Elliott came to Moncton alone with his wife, Dr. Maureen Bulger, who also joined the staff. Maureen was born on November 12, 1954, and received her premedical and medical training at the University of Toronto graduating in 1979 with an MD. She interned in Montreal at the Jewish General Hospital in 1979-80 and then did locums in British Columbia and Alberta from 1980 to 1982. She did a general practice anaesthesia residency in 1982-

83 and from 1984 to 1988 did a family and anaesthesia practice at Ross Memorial Hospital, Lindsay, Ontario. Since coming to Moncton she has mainly pursued a locums practice while other family practice doctors are on holidays.

Frank Kelly was born on November 22, 1947, and received a BSc from St. Dunstan's University in 1969 and an MD from McGill in 1973.After a rotating internship at Saint Joseph's Hospital in London, Ontario, in 1973-74, he established a family practice in Inuvik, North West Territories, from 1974 to 1976. In 1977, he did a six-month residency in pediatrics at the Janeway Hospital in Saint John's, Newfoundland, and from 1978 to 1979 he did locums in family practice in Antigonish. In 1980 he received a diploma in tropical medicine and health from Liverpool, England, spending a year doing missionary work in South America. On returning to Canada, he did family practice at the Highland View Hospital in Amherst from 1981 to 1985. He then abandoned medicine to study theology at College Dominican in Ottawa from 1985 to 1987 and at the Atlantic School of Theology from 1987 to 1988. He returned to medical practice in Moncton in 1988 where he remained in family practice until 1996, although he took a sabbatical in 1991-92 to further study theology in Ottawa. His training in theology has made him an ideal person to serve on the Ethics Research Committee.

Eliva Instrum was born on November 5, 1958, and received her MD from Dalhousie in 1984. She did the two-year family medicine internship and residency at Dalhousie from 1984 to 1986 and then began serving locums in British Columbia, Ontario, Nova Scotia and New Brunswick from 1986 to 1988 after which she joined the Petitcodiac Medical Clinic. She married in 1992 and resigned from the Petitcodiac Health Clinic establishing a general practice in Moncton under her married name Eliva Morrison.

Richard Lewington was born on June 8, 1955, and received a BSc in 1978 and an MD in 1987 from the University of British Columbia. He did a rotating internship at Memorial University from 1987 to 1989 and then joined the staff while practising in Albert. He stayed less than a year, moving to Springhill, Nova Scotia, in August 1989.

The statistics for 1988-89 fiscal year show 14,245 adult and child admissions along with 1,479 newborns; 10,928 operations were performed including 4,833 day patients. Services provided included: audiograms—2,173; electrocardiograms—23,838; gastrointestinal unit procedures—2,657; social service cases—1,318; speech pathology—3,468; radiological examinations—90,795; CT Scans—7,265; nuclear medicine procedures—5,512; and ultrasound examinations—4,971. Besides 87,454 emergency visits there were 21,924 clinic visits as follows: Arthritis—2,805; Chemotherapy—4,132; Chest—1,322; TB—1,187; Colposcopy—1,847; Diabetic Day Care—2,389; Diet Counselling—1,309; Weight checks—922; Diagnostic—1,160; Eye—39; Hemophiliac—74; Multiple Sclerosis—0; Pain Clinic—1,795; Reproductive Health—2,498; and Urodynamics—446.

The decade ended on a good note with the opening of the South Tower,

16 years after its conception. Planning had begun in 1973 and construction of the project began in 1982. The final cost of the project was $97 million, including $85 million for construction costs and $12 million for new equipment. An additional 125 employees were hired to bring the hospital's total employment to 1,500. On Friday, November 24, 1989, New Brunswick's minister of health and community services, the Hon. Raymond Frenette, cut the ribbon to officially open the South Tower of The Moncton Hospital. He was assisted by the Hon. Bruce Smith, minister of supply and services, and Robert Radford, chairman of the board of trustees of The Moncton Hospital. The chairman for the ceremonies, Mr. Radford, paid special tribute to Harvey Hicks who had chaired the Building Committee of the board since planning had begun in 1973. Katherine Wright served as co-ordinator for all the celebration events. Tour guides took citizens through the new tower and refreshments were served to all the guests.

Although the new construction did not result in any new beds, the new tower included beds for 170 patients and allowed for the closing of beds in the older wings. The third, fourth and fifth floors contained patient beds. With the opening of the new patient tower the familiar names for the wards disappeared and 4 Clarke became 4600, 4 Joyce, 4400, and 4 Parlee, 4500, with the new wards in the tower named 4100 and 4200. To older physicians and employees the names Parlee, Clarke and Joyce will always be associated with these wards, although the habit will likely fade in time. One unique feature on

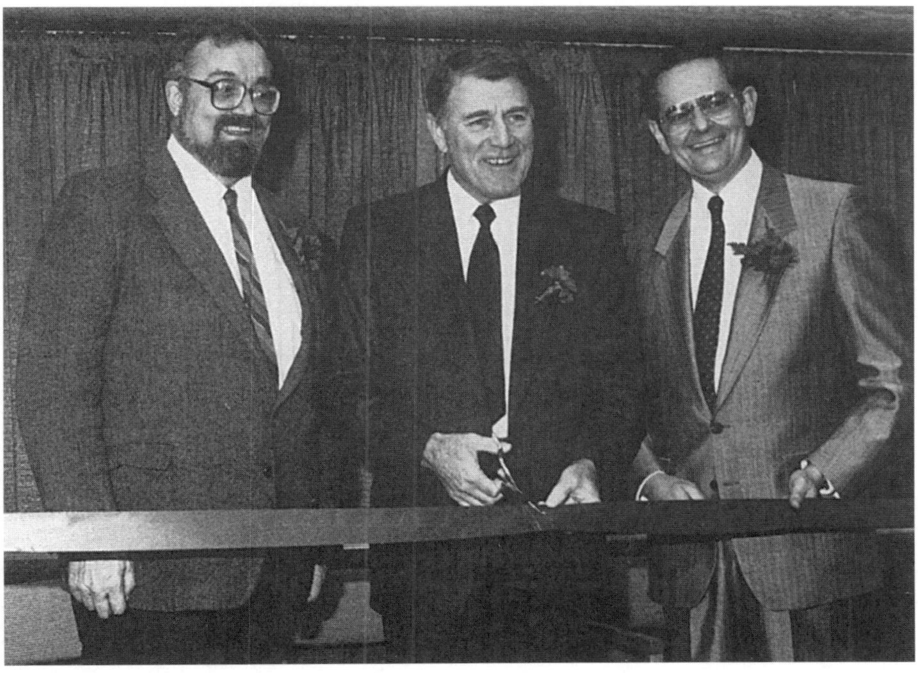

The opening of the new South Tower in 1989. From left to right: Hon. Bruce Smith, Minister of Supply and Services; Hon. Raymond Frenette, Minister of Health; and Mr. R. Radford, Chairman of the Board.

the fourth floor 4200 ward was the construction of a secure two-bed unit with an anteroom for guards for Correctional Services Canada to service sick inmates. In the new tower two thirty-four bed units for gynaecology and general surgery patients were created. Psychiatry, which had been exiled to the former nurses' residence during construction, was rewarded with a unit in the new tower. The spacious new unit provided 28 inpatient beds arranged in an apartment style pod concept which encourages patients to spend less time alone. Each pod was designed to accommodate four patients with separate sleeping areas, a common room and a bathroom with shower. There were several group rooms where sessions could be conducted in assertiveness training, anti-anxiety, self esteem and stress management. Large comfortable areas for activities and socialization were part of the design. One of the guiding design principles was that the unit should facilitate a multidisciplinary approach to caring for patients. Next to the inpatient units, facilities were constructed for a psychiatric day hospital able to accommodate 40 patients and to work closely with the inpatient unit to provide for earlier discharge and help prevent readmission.

The fifth floor of the South Tower became the new home of the Geriatric Service with seventy beds allotted for a variety of services, including patient assessment, short and long term rehabilitation, extended care and relief care. Like psychiatry, this unit was created to facilitate a multidisciplinary approach to patient care. The objective of the Geriatric Unit was to help patients maintain or regain the greatest degree of independence possible and to enjoy the best quality of life they can. All bathrooms were designed to be wheelchair accessible with equipment that facilitates independence, such as grab bars and mirrors and sinks which are at wheelchair height. Group activities could take place in a large common lounge area and patients could enjoy their meals together in a common dining room. A quiet room offered space where families may visit together or where patients may read or watch television. Treatment facilities include physiotherapy and occupational therapy rooms, the latter including a kitchen. Additional features include a laundry room where patients can do their own laundry, a small hairdressing room and a whirlpool bath. The large occupational therapy area includes space suitable for light crafts, one for heavier activities and a kitchen/dining area. The program operated by the department provided a balance of activities, including exercises, stress management, woodworking, ceramics and life skills and can meet the needs of both inpatients and day patients.

The main floor of the new tower became the nerve centre of the hospital. The new main lobby, located between the existing hospital and the new tower, featured skylights to give a bright airy appearance to those entering the hospital. Furnishings for the lobby were provided by the Nurses' Auxiliary. The coffee shop, operated by The Moncton Hospital School of Nursing Alumnae with eighty seats, was located in the lobby and the gift shop was located on the opposite side of the lobby. The bank of elevators for the Clarke wing faced the lobby and became the route to all the floors of the hospital for visitors. Just beyond the coffee shop was an entrance to a large 240-seat lecture theatre extending down into the basement where the Education Department was situated with offices and smaller lecture rooms. The theatre contained the latest in audiovisual equipment and was intended to be made available for use by hospital staff and also community groups. Up a flight of stairs and off the mezzanine overlooking the lobby, was situated the new Health Sciences Library. The School of Nursing Alumnae chose the library as their main recipient of donated funds that year.

Just off the main lobby was situated a new large Department of Medical Imaging containing 22 equipped diagnostic rooms for radiology, nuclear medicine, ultrasound and CT scanning.

The new Emergency Department, approximately four times larger than the old, was divided into three distinct functional areas:

1. a four-bed resuscitation/trauma unit with state-of-the-art equipment including X-ray units for the immediate assessment and care of patients with life threatening injuries or illnesses;
2. a 16-bed acute care section designed to serve patients who are acutely but not critically ill. It contained centralized cardiac monitoring, an isolation unit, a decontamination room for patients who have been exposed to harmful chemicals and a security room;
3. a non-acute area with 14 rooms equipped to treat problems related to eyes, ears, nose and throat illnesses or injuries and dental, pediatric, gynaecology, orthopaedic, minor surgical and general emergencies.

The department also contained three inter-related programs: the Emergency Service, Ambulance Service and Poison Control Centre. With 80,000 patients visiting the unit annually, 4,000 individuals being transported by ambulance and 1,800 consulting the Poison Control Centre, it was now one of the busiest emergency units in Canada. The Ladies' Auxiliary contributed funds to provide furnishings for the medical imaging and emergency departments, including seating for patients and furniture for the children's play area in each department.

The time to transport a patient from the emergency room to the surgical suite was vastly improved with the operating rooms now located next door to the Emergency Department. The new suite consisted of 12 operating rooms, an increase of 4 over the old facility. Four of the rooms were custom designed for cystoscopy, orthopaedic surgery and neurosurgery. All rooms contained the latest in fixed and mobile equipment and furnishings designed to accommodate current and emerging trends in surgery and anaesthesia. A sophisticated system was supposed to control temperature, humidity and medical gases, but those who work there would question how well the temperature and humidity controls work. Operating room instruments and other supplies were now made available by Materials Management staff through a case cart system. Under this system, a cart is provided for each operation which contains all of the material required by a specific surgeon for a particular case.

The suite was constructed to have its own delivery elevator for supplies from stores and processing. Additional facilities included waiting rooms and lounges, an anaesthetic office, classrooms, patient holding area and space for lab and X-ray processing. Entrance to the OR suite was restricted, with access only by a security card to the dressing rooms where OR attire must be donned before proceeding to semi-restricted and restricted areas. Located next to the operating room was a new recovery room with 20 recovery stretcher spaces. Also adjacent to the operating room was a new day surgery unit containing spaces for 22 patients at one time.

On the ground floor of the new tower, besides the education department, space was allotted to many of the auxiliary services. The new Health Records Department replaced one that was designed for a 200-bed hospital. For the first time in many years all sections of the department were united in one location. The department houses and manages the dictation system used by physicians throughout the hospital. With the new system, a doctor using his access code can listen to a dictated report from another consultant even before the typed copy becomes available. Emergency room records, which used to be filed separately, are now integrated into the inpatient chart.

Also in the basement was situated the new pharmacy, a far cry from the area set aside when the Parlee wing was built in 1953, with expansion from 1,500 to 5,500 square feet. The computerization of patient profiles and the acquisition of new medication storage and delivery carts made it possible for the pharmacy to greatly improve the hospital's drug distribution system. Both the chemotherapy and the total parental nutrition program have been newly centralized in the large modern sterile product area.

The largest area in the basement or ground floor was given over to Material Management which would provide five services to the hospital:

1. Shipping and receiving, responsible for all goods entering and leaving the hospital;
2. The stores section, warehousing supplies awaiting assembly or delivery;
3. The print shop, fulfilling the hospital's huge need for printed material;
4. The processing section, responsible for manufacturing and sterilizing the instruments and supplies required by the surgical suite and nursing units; and
5. Distribution, delivering equipment and supplies throughout the hospital.

Office space was also provided on the ground floor for the 100-member Housekeeping Department, responsible for cleaning approximately 575,000 square feet of hospital space daily. With the new tower came new equipment with labour saving devices such as automated carpet cleaners, automated floor scrubbers and high speed burnishers.

To feed the patients and staff, approximately 2,200 meals had to be prepared daily by the 104 member Food Service Department in 17.5 hours of daily operation. To meet these requirements, the whole sixth floor of the south tower was devoted to the food service with a spacious new kitchen and a 250-seat dining area. Adjacent to the dining area were provided a lounge and three spacious meeting rooms, one of which is now used for the Medical Advisory Committee meetings.

For some time, parking had been a problem at the hospital. With the building of the Blue Cross building on Main Street, the hospital, with the assistance of the provincial government, was able to purchase the vacant Blue Cross property at the corner of MacBeath Avenue and Garfield Street and, after tearing down the building on the lot, build a new parking lot. This made it possible to move virtually all staff parking from the main lot opposite the hospital leaving it available for patients and visitors. The house at the corner on the main parking lot which was previously occupied by Dr. Clarke until he retired in 1970 and then occupied as an interns' residence, was also torn down to provide more parking space.

For years the hospital had held disaster exercises and on Thanksgiving weekend, 1989, the hospital had a chance to put all its practice into good use. In Cormier Village, the Cormier Family were having a reunion and were on a hayride when a truck loaded with logs overturned onto their haywagon, resulting in thirteen deaths and more than fifty casualties. Dr. Janet Fultz, on a leisure biking expedition at the time, was one of the first doctors on the scene. Both The Moncton Hospital and the Dr. Georges-L. Dumont Hospital put their disaster plans into effect and proved equal to the task of looking after the large number of casualties.

The upgrading and expansion of the ophthalmology department was identified as a major program priority in 1989-90. In response, the Friends of the Moncton Hospital selected eye-care equipment as the focus for their annual appeal for funds. Through their superb efforts, $155,000 was raised. The Moncton Lions Club then showed their community spirit when they announced that they would donate $190,000 to completely equip the Lion Hugh T. Reardon Eye Clinic in the ambulatory care department. It is sad to have to report that while we have been provided with the equipment to do the job, the hospital has been hampered in its efforts to adequately staff the ophthalmology department by the PRAC guidelines of the provincial Department of Health.

There were 18 additions to the medical staff, although only 10 now remain on staff. There were 4 additions to the Department of Pathology: Dr. Jasim Radhi, Dr. Magdalena Kuhn, Dr. Hank Taylor and Dr. Shani Jones; Dr. Rachel Cormier to the Department of Otorhinolaryngology; Dr. Benoit Grenier to the Department of Ophthalmology; Dr. Ralph Ellis to the Department of Medical Imaging; Dr. Michael Greschner to the Department of Anaesthesia; Dr. Callum MacLeod to the Department of Paediatrics; Dr. Bruce MacDonald to the Department of Internal Medicine; Dr. John Murphy to the Department of General Surgery; Dr. Barbara Ross to the Department of Psychiatry; Dr. David Ross, Dr. Michelle Conrod, Dr. John

Li and Dr. Leona Harries to the Department of Family Practice and Dr. Ashu Ruparella to the Department of Emergency Medicine.

Jasim Radhi was born in Baghdad on July 1, 1950, and received his medical education at the University of Baghdad College of Medicine, receiving the MB, BCh degree in 1976. From 1976 to 1977 he was a house officer at Alyarmuk Teaching Hospital in Baghdad and then from 1978 to 1980 a house officer at Sadah Aldin Military Hospital. After a year in pathology at the College of Medicine at the University of Baghdad (1980-81), he went to England where he underwent further training in pathology (1982-84). From 1984 to 1987 he was a registrar in pathology at Freean Hospital, Newcastle-upon-Tyne. He came to Canada in 1987, serving as pathologist at Grenfell Regional Health Services at Saint Anthony, Newfoundland. He was appointed to the staff of The Moncton Hospital but after receiving his FRCP(C) in pathology in 1991, he left Moncton in 1992.

Magdalena Kuhn was born in Czechoslovakia on March 9, 1948, and immigrated to Canada where she received her education. She graduated in 1973 from the University of Saskatchewan with an Honours BSc in Microbiology. She then went on to receive her MD from the same institution in 1978, followed by a rotating internship at St. Paul's Hospital, Saskatoon, in 1978-79. From 1979 to 1981 she was an emergency room physician in Regina and from 1981 to 1985 she did a family practice in Regina. In 1985 she came east to the University of Western Ontario where she did a residency in microbiology from 1985 to 1989, becoming certified in microbiology in 1989 and receiving her FRCP(C) in microbiology. She then came further east to join our staff where she has been a welcome addition. Because of her previous clinical experience she brings to her work as a microbiologist a deep appreciation of the clinician's problems and moves easily out of the laboratory to give sound clinical advice in her consultations with the medical staff.

Hank Taylor was born on December 19, 1939, and received a BA degree from the University of Detroit in 1961 and an MD from Wayne State University in 1965. He did a year of rotating internship and a year of residency in internal medicine at the Kaiser Foundation Hospital in San Francisco from 1965 to 1967 and then a year in internal medicine at Henry Ford Hospital in Detroit in 1967-68 and a fellowship in haematology and clinical pathology at St. Joseph Hospital and William Beaumont Hospital in 1968-69. Following this, he served as a consultant in internal medicine in Nigeria in 1970 and toured Europe in 1971-72. On returning to the US, he finished another year as a resident in clinical pathology at William Beaumont Hospital and became certified by the American Board of Pathology in clinical pathology in 1972. He was made a Fellow of the American College of Clinical Pathology in 1982. From 1973 to 1974 he was assistant professor of clinical pathology at West Virginia University of School of Medicine. He subsequently moved to Columbia, Missouri, where he served as assistant professor, associate professor of pathology and chief of section of morphologic haematology until he was recruited by Dr. Bender to come to Moncton. He became acting chief of the Department of Pathology and interim director of the laboratory on April 24, 1991. Despite being well-liked by his colleagues and despite efforts on the part of the administration, he had difficulty with the College of Physicians and Surgeons of New Brunswick recognizing his American qualifications, and his wife, a registered nurse, also had difficulty in being registered in New Brunswick, so he regrettably resigned from the staff and returned to the United States in July 1993.

Elizabeth Shani Jones was born in Saint John, New Brunswick, on March 22, 1957, and went to Dalhousie on a Sir James Dunn Scholarship where she received a BSc in 1978. She then went on to Memorial University where she received a BMedSc in 1980 and an MD in 1982. She did a rotating internship in the Dalhousie Program in 1982-83. From 1984 to 1988 she did residency training in anatomical pathology at Dalhousie and after receiving her FRCP(C) in anatomical pathology in 1988 she joined the staff of The Moncton Hospital in February 1989.

Dr. Rachel Cormier was born on October 29, 1958, and received her MD degree from Laval University in 1982. She interned at Centre Hôpital de l'Université de Sherbrooke in 1982-83. After a year of general surgery residency at Laval University in 1983-84, she did an ENT residency at the University of Ottawa from 1984 to 1987. From January to June 1988, she did a fellowship in facial cosmetic surgery at the University of Toronto. In 1988 she received her FRCS(C) in otorhinolaryngology and head and neck surgery and became certified by the American Board of Otolaryngology. She was appointed to the associate staff in February 1989 and the courtesy staff in March 1990. She was on the active staff of the Dr. Georges-L. Dumont Hospital but a frequent visitor to The Moncton Hospital. She left Moncton in 1996 to set up practice in New York State.

Benoit Grenier was born on March 21, 1955, and received his MD from University of Montreal in 1978. After an internship in 1978-79 and an internal medicine residency from 1980 to 1982 at Sacré-Coeur Centre Hospital, Saint Eustace, he did an ophthalmology residency at the University of Montreal from 1982 to 1986 and became certified by the Quebec College and the Royal College in 1986. He did further training with a retina and vitreous fellowship at Notre Dame Hospital in 1986-87 and became a Diplomate of the American Board of Ophthalmology in 1988. Appointed to the active staff of the Dr. Georges-L Dumont Hospital, he was appointed to the courtesy staff of The Moncton Hospital, but left Moncton in July 1990.

Dr. Ralph Ellis was born on August 10, 1957, and received his BSc from the University of Prince Edward Island in 1979 and an MD from Dalhousie in 1983. He did a rotating internship in the Dalhousie program in 1983-84, followed by a residency program in radiology at Dalhousie from 1985 to 1989, becoming certified in diagnostic radiology in 1989 and then joining the medical imaging staff of The Moncton Hospital.

Dr. Michael Greschner, a Montreal native, born on July 12, 1957, took his education at McGill University, obtaining a BSc in 1979 with first class honours in physiology, an MSc in physiology in 1981 and then an MD in 1984. He started his anaesthetic training in Montreal at the Jewish General Hospital in 1984-85 but completed his training at the University of Toronto from 1985 to 1989 at various hospitals in the Toronto program such as Wellesley, Sunnybrook, St. Michael's, Toronto General, Toronto East General and the Hospital for Sick Children. He became certified in anaesthesia and received his FRCP(C) in 1989. Since joining the staff, he has served as chief of anaesthesia in 1992 and 1993.

Calum MacLeod was born on April 17, 1958, in Kirkealdy, Scotland. He received his MB, ChB from Glasgow University in 1981 and interned at the Glasgow Royal Infirmary in 1981-82. He then came to Canada and underwent pediatric training at the Hospital for Sick Children in Toronto from 1982 to 1987, except for 1983-84 when he took a year off and did a general practice at Drayton Valley, Alberta. His last year at the Sick Childrens was devoted to a clinical fellowship in respiratory medicine. He received his FRCP(C) in pediatrics in 1987 and entered private practice in Etobicoke, Ontario. He joined the pediatric staff in June 1989, but only remained a year before going to Kingston, Ontario, in October 1990.

Bruce MacDonald was born on May 4, 1934, and educated at the University of Western Ontario, receiving a BA in 1958 and an MD in 1962. He served a rotating internship at Grace Hospital in Detroit and a residency in internal medicine at the same hospital from 1963 to 1966. He then did a residency in medical oncology at Wayne State University, Detroit, Michigan, from 1966 to 1967. In 1988 he received his FRCP(C) in Internal Medicine. From 1967 to 1986 he served as an internist and medical oncologist at Metropolitan General Hospital, Grace Hospital and l'Hôtel Dieu of St. Joseph's in Windsor, Ontario, as well as senior medical oncologist at the Regional Cancer Centre in Windsor, Ontario from 1971 to 1986. In 1986 he moved to the Toronto area where he served as the medical director of palliative care and chief of staff at Providence Villa and Hospital, Scarborough, as well as consultant at Sunnybrook Hospital and Toronto Bayview Cancer Centre.

John Lawlor Murphy was born on June 7, 1957, the son of Dr. Fred Murphy. It is unusual for the son of a McGill graduate to go to Dalhousie University, but this is what John did, receiving a BSc in 1978 and an MD (cum laude) in 1982. After interning at the Ottawa Civic Hospital in 1982-83, he spent 1983-84 doing a locums in Owen Sound, Ontario, before deciding to follow in his father's footsteps and become not only a surgeon but also a vascular surgeon. From 1984 to 1988 he served as a resident in general surgery at the University of Ottawa, receiving his FRCS(C) in general surgery in 1988. He also received his American Boards. He remained in Ottawa in 1988-89, serving as a resident in vascular surgery as well as chief administrative resident. He then joined his father in practice in Moncton.

Barbara Ross was born on December 31, 1956, and received a BSc from Saint Mary's University in 1977 and an MD from Dalhousie in 1981. She served a rotating internship in the Dalhousie program from 1981 to 1982 and then did general practice in Ontario from 1982 to 1984. She did a six-month pediatric residency at Memorial University in 1983 before taking a psychiatry residency at Queen's University from 1984 to 1987. She became certified in psychiatry and received her FRCP(C) in 1987 and, after doing a psychiatry locums from 1988-89, she joined the psychiatric staff in June 1989, planning on doing child and adolescent psychiatry. In May 1991, she resigned from the staff of the hospital but continues in private practice in Moncton.

Barbara Ross's husband, David Ross, was born in Moncton on April 8, 1956. He received his BSc from Dalhousie in 1977 and his MD in 1981. He interned in the Dalhousie rotating internship program in 1981-82. He did family practice locums from 1982 to 1986 in British Columbia, Bellville and Kingston, Ontario, including stints in Dr. Ted Atkinson's office in Moncton in 1983, 1984 and 1985. From 1985 to 1989 he did a general practice at St. Mary's of the Lake Hospital and the Kingston Psychiatric Hospital before moving back to his native Moncton and establishing a family practice here.

John Li was born on August 13, 1958, and educated at Dalhousie University where he received a BSc in 1980 and an MD in 1985. After a rotating internship in the Dalhousie University program he did general practice in Nova Scotia from 1986 to 1989 before moving to Moncton and opening a family practice at the Mountain Road Medical Clinic.

Michelle Conrod was born on November 29, 1959, and also was educated at Dalhousie University, receiving a BSc and then an MD in 1987. She served in the two year Dalhousie family medicine internship and residency program from 1987 to 1989, becoming certified in family practice by the Canadian College of Family Practice and then joined the staff of the Moncton Medical Clinic, taking over the practice of Dr. Ed MacLeod.

Dr. Leona Harries was born on October 16, 1964. Educated at the University of Calgary where she received her MD in 1988, she interned at St. Thomas Hospital, Akron, Ohio, in 1988-89. She started a practice in Alma and was appointed to the staff of the Albert County Hospital and the courtesy staff of The Moncton Hospital. Like so many doctors before her, her stay in Albert was short and she departed in May 1990.

Asutosh (Ashu) Ruparelia was born on April 27, 1960, and received his BSc from Dalhousie in 1980 and his MD in 1985. From 1985 to 1987 he did the family medicine internship and residency program at Dalhousie. He obtained his ATLS in 1987 and his ACLS in 1988. From 1987 to 1988 he served in the emergency room of the Halifax Infirmary and from 1988 to 1989 in the emergency room of Health Sciences Centre, Saint John's, Newfoundland. He joined the emergency room staff of The Moncton Hospital in 1989 to serve for one year while Dr. William Sigsworth took a year's leave of absence.

For the 1989-90 year there were 14,754 adult and child admissions with 1,646 newborns; 9,993 operations were performed, including 4,434 day surgery patients. Services provided included: audiograms—1,718; electrocardiograms—24,563; gastrointestinal unit procedures—2,909; social service caseload—1,410; speech pathology—4,548; radiological examinations—89,789; CT Scans—7,440; nuclear medicine procedures—5,815 and ultrasound examinations—4,914. Besides 81,325 emergency visits there were 25,060 clinic visits as follows: Arthritis—2,858; Chemotherapy—4,537; Chest—2,445; TB—1,617; Colposcopy—2,114; Diabetic Day Care—1,282; Diet Counselling—1,501; Weight checks—1,120; Haemophiliac—160; Eye—0; Pain—1,671; Reproductive Health—1,617 and Urodynamics—346.

CHAPTER ELEVEN

THE NINTIES— ONE HUNDRED YEARS OF CARING

The 1990s bring with them a new look for the annual reports of the hospital as they begin to be produced in both official languages. While the opening of the South Tower allowed for greatly improved services to patients, there were still many deficient areas in the older parts of the hospital. The provincial government announced in response that $100,000 would be allotted in 1991-92 for planning the completion of the redevelopment of The Moncton Hospital. In the meantime, consultants were engaged to help develop measures to meet some of the most pressing needs on an interim basis, bridging the gap until the necessary redevelopment work could be completed to upgrade the aging sections of the building. Interim renovations were begun in 1990 to improve conditions in the gastrointestinal, orthopaedic and oncology clinics, diabetic day care, electrodiagnostics and the library. The renovations were to be carried out using the hospital's maintenance staff.

One area that was renovated was the old X-ray department with the opening of the Lion Hugh T. Reardon Eye Clinic. Funds for this construction and the equipment were supplied by the Moncton Lions Club and the 1989 Annual Appeal of the Friends of the Moncton Hospital.

Renovations were also undertaken to the old operating room area where an eight-bed Child/Adolescent Psychiatric Unit was opened in November 1990, with Premier Frank McKenna cutting the ribbon. He was assisted by the minister of health and community services, the Hon. Raymond Frenette, and the chairman of the board, Robert Radford. This was the first unit in the province specifically for children and adolescents, and provided a tertiary service with patients accepted from anywhere in New Brunswick.

With the completion of the South Tower, Wes Drodge moved on and became vice-president of the Oshawa General Hospital. Douglas Apt, who had been with the hospital since 1977, moved to Halifax to become vice-president of the Victoria General Hospital. His place was taken by Alan Mongraw who had previously been director of administration of the Ottawa-

Carleton Health Department. Also making a departure was Fred Rayworth. After 18 years of service and honing his skills in public relations and human resources, he moved to Saskatchewan where he joined the Saskatchewan Hospital Association as vice-president of labour relations. It was apparent by this time that running a hospital is big business and the administrative staff changed their titles to reflect its structure so that the executive director became a president and the next lower echelon became vice-presidents.

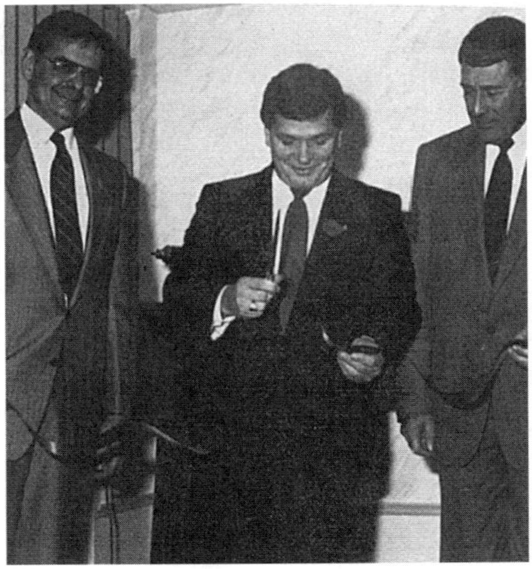

The opening of the Child/Adolescent Psychiatric Unit in 1990. From left to right: Mr. Robert Radford, Chairman of the Board; Hon. Frank McKenna, Premier of NB; and Hon. R. Frenette, Minister of Health.

An innovative service, begun in 1990, was the fitness centre, called "Stretchers," which was opened in renovated space in the basement of the former nurses' residence. The centre soon proved popular with over 500 members enrolled. It is operated on a non-profit basis by the Employees' Fitness Association and offers aerobics and karate classes as well as facilities for weight training.

The Friends of the Moncton Hospital Foundation again had a successful annual appeal and raised over $180,000 in 1990 to provide microbiology equipment for diagnosing and treating infectious diseases. Equipment purchased included a blood culture system (Bactec), automated microbiology system and CO2 incubators. The board also authorized the ordering of a $6,620 Aerosol Treatment and Sputum Induction Chamber for the treatment of HIV infected patients. As part of their fund raising, the Friends appointed a committee under the chairmanship of Les Buzzell and they undertook to sell to the public and the hospital staff a personal security alarm system called Red Alert.

Dr. Harry Rich, Dr. Austin Delaney and Dr. Gerald Allanach all retired from the staff in 1990, each having given over twenty-five years of service to the hospital. Other members of the staff with much less service, who also departed, included Dr. Michael Burslem, Dr. Calum MacLeod and Dr. Michael McGonigal. Several departments welcomed new additions with Dr. Kent Monteith and Dr. Mario Goselin joining the Department of Anaesthesia, Dr. Frederick Coop to the Department of Medical Imaging, Dr. Peter Feero to the Department of Urology, Dr. Edmond Jones to the Department of Otorhinolaryngology, Dr. Bill Thompson to the Department of Internal Medicine, Dr. Vitia Kozel and Dr. Patricia Thomas, to the

Department of Family Practice and Drs. Randall Lee and David Smozarski to the courtesy staff in family medicine while practising in Albert.

Kent Monteith was born in Moncton on August 13, 1960, and received a BSc in 1981 and an MD from Dalhousie University in 1985. He served a rotating internship at the Ottawa Civic Hospital in 1985-86, did a residency in anaesthesia from 1986 to 1990 at University of Ottawa affiliated hospitals and became certified in anaesthesia by the Royal College in 1990. Since joining the anaesthetic staff he has also worked in the Pain Clinic.

Another welcome addition to the anaesthetic staff was Dr. Mario Gosselin. He was born on August 23, 1959, and received his MD in 1983 from Université de Sherbrooke. After an internship in anaesthesia at Centre Hôpital de l'Université de Sherbrooke, he did a residency in anaesthesia at the same hospital from 1984 to 1987 with six months of pediatric anaesthesia at Hôpital Sainte-Justine, Montreal. He became certified in anaesthesia by the Corporation professionelle des médicins du Québec and received his FRCP(C) in anaesthesia in 1987. He practised anaesthesia at the Chaleur Regional Hospital from 1987 until coming to Moncton in June 1990. There must be some contagious gases in anaesthesia which induce a desire to fly as he has joined two of his other colleagues on the anaesthetic staff, Dr. A. Dobson and Dr. John Crompton, in obtaining his pilot's license.

Frederick Coop was born on March 6, 1957, in Brampton, Ontario, and received his MD from the University of Western Ontario in 1982. He served a rotating internship at St. Paul's Hospital, Vancouver, in 1982-83. After three years of service in the Canadian Forces Hospital, Cornwallis, Nova Scotia, he returned to the University of Western Ontario where he pursued a residency in radiology from 1986 to 1990, receiving his FRCS(C) in diagnostic radiology in 1990. Short and stocky, he always carried a military bearing. His stay in Moncton only lasted for three years. He resigned in August 1993 to take a position in Port Huron, Michigan.

Peter Grant Feero was born in Woodstock, New Brunswick, on March 11, 1956. He graduated in pharmacy from Dalhousie in 1978 but decided to write prescriptions rather than fill them and went off to receive a BSc in medical sciences in 1982 and an MD in 1984 from Memorial University. He did a rotating internship in the Dalhousie program from 1984 to 1985. After a year of general practice in Souris, Prince Edward Island, he got tired of writing prescriptions and took to the cutting field of medicine and did a residency in urology at Queen's University from 1986 to 1989 with another year at Memorial University (1989-90). He became certified by the Royal College in 1990 and then joined the staff of The Moncton Hospital.

Edmond Jones was born on September 24, 1955, received his MD from McGill in 1984 and then did a surgical internship in the McGill University program (1984-85). He then entered the McGill residency program in otolaryngology at the Royal Victoria, Montreal General, Jewish General and Montreal Children's hospitals. In 1989 he received his FRCS(C) and was certified as a specialist in otolaryngology by the Corporation professionelle des médicins du Québec. He also became a Diplomate of the American Board of Otolaryngology. He served as chief of his department in 1993.

At the beginning of the 1990s the miracle of the penicillin age began to give away to the emergence of resistant strains of bacteria producing new and more deadly and hard to control infections. The Department of Internal Medicine, with the enthusiastic support of their surgical colleagues, was able to recruit an infectious disease specialist. Guy William (Bill) Thompson was born in Southampton, England, on February 1, 1956, and received a BSc from the University of Waterloo in 1980 and an MD from the University of Western Ontario in 1985, followed by a medical internship at Victoria Hospital, London, from 1985 to 1986. From 1986 to 1988 he did a residency in internal medicine at Victoria Hospital, London, and went to the Health Sciences Centre, St. Boniface, Manitoba, for two years of residency in infectious diseases from 1988 to 1990. He received his FRCP(C) in internal medicine in 1990. One of the most difficult problems facing the infectious disease consultant since the mid-eighties has been the treatment of the AIDS patient and Dr. Thompson now operates the largest AIDS treatment facility in New Brunswick.

Vitia Kozel joined the Department of Family Practice but her work was confined to the geriatric department. She was born in Czechoslovakia and received her MD degree from Charles University in Prague in 1981. From 1979 to 1981 she did a residency in internal medicine at Ostrava General Hospital. After immigrating to Canada she worked as a lab technician in Toronto from 1981 to 1986 and from 1987 to 1988 she worked as a neonatal intensive- care assistant at Grace Maternity Hospital in Halifax. To get her LMCC she served a rotating internship at The Moncton Hospital from 1988 to 1989 and from 1989 to 1990 did a residency in geriatric medicine at Camp Hill Hospital in Halifax. She was appointed to the staff to practice geriatric medicine at The Moncton Hospital but stayed on staff only until 1992.

Patricia Thomas was born on December 8, 1950, graduated with an MD degree from Dalhousie in 1984 and then served a rotating internship in the Dalhousie program from 1984 to 1985. She served as a Military Medical Officer at Camp Gagetown from 1985 to 1988 and from 1988 to 1989 did a family practice in Oromocto before moving to Moncton in 1990.

During the 1990/91 fiscal year there were 15,068 adult and children admissions in addition to 1,642 newborns. There were 11,432 operations performed in the surgical suite, including 5,323 day surgery patients. Services provided included 24,445 electrocardiograms; 3,129 gastrointestinal procedures; 1.495 social service cases; 4,794 speech pathology; 90,997 radiological examinations; 7,238 CT scans; 5,470 nuclear medicine procedures; and 5,831 ultrasound examinations. In addition to 70,408 visits to the emergency room there were 26,158 clinic visits as follows: Arthritis—2,774; Chemotherapy—5,241; Chest—3,792; TB—508; Colposcopy—2,137; Diabetic Day Care—2,439; Diet Counselling—1,651; Weight Checks—1,038; Diagnostic—311;

Eye—676; Haemophiliac—174; Pain—2,940; Urodynamics—412; and Multiple Sclerosis—152.

A new era in the history of The Moncton Hospital began in 1991 as Bill Kilpatrick resigned as president after serving the hospital for 29 years. He moved to Peterborough, Ontario, where he became president of the Peterborough Civic Hospital. His place was taken by the medical director, Dr. Ginette Gagné-Koch, and so the century ends as it had begun, with a woman in charge of the hospital. On taking over the position of president, Dr. Gagné-Koch launched Vision 2000 as a statement of where the hospital was heading as it entered a new century. Input was sought from both the staff of the hospital and its users. On June 8, 1991, the term of Dr. Peter Gorman as chief of staff expired and he was succeeded by Dr. Preston Smith.

With the increase in single parent families and instances of both parents entering the workforce, the need for child care facilities increased and The Moncton Hospital rose to the challenge when it opened the "First Steps" child care centre in January. This was the first hospital-based child care centre in the province and is a co-operative effort between The Moncton Hospital and the Greater Moncton YMCA. It is administered by the Parents' Association and is open exclusively to the children of hospital employees.

This year the Friends of the Moncton Hospital undertook to equip the Medical-Surgical and Neurosciences Intensive Care Units with compact state-of-the-art monitoring equipment. The provincial government committed $288,000 towards the estimated total cost of $469,500 for the project and the Friends volunteered to raise the balance of $181,500. It was also during this year that the Friends of the Moncton Hospital had a doctor, Dr. Arthur Oatway, as its chairman. In 1987 the Friends had established an education fund and this year they decided to substantially increase this fund. The board voted to allocate unspecified bequests, 50 percent of interest earned on investments and donations from employees through payroll deduction to the Fund Committee, chaired by Gordon Sherrard, until a total of $100,000 was reached. The objective was to increase the interest income from this fund so that more staff education needs could be met.

Other major contributors to the hospital's welfare were also active during the year and there were also many individual contributions which are too numerous to mention. The Nurses' Auxiliary purchased a bed settee for the geriatric unit and a sum of money was donated for their use. Six defibrillators were purchased as well as a television and VCR for the Medical/Surgical Intensive Care Unit. They continued to sponsor a Well Women Clinic, in which six doctors were assisted by auxiliary members. Bursaries were given to two nursing students and sums of money were given to various employees to attend short educational courses. A contribution was made for the stained glass donor wall which was installed in the main lobby.

The School of Nursing Alumni provided more than $100,000 to the hospital to cover the cost of Life-Line units, equipment, furniture and books for the library, and construction and furnishing of the pastoral care department and chapel, now moved into new quarters on the first floor of the Parlee wing. Scholarships were awarded by the alumni to several alumni who were pursuing Baccalaureate or Masters education in either Nursing or Health Services Administration. Many more members were sponsored to attend short courses or conferences throughout Canada and the United Stares. Most of the money was raised through the operation of the coffee shop.

The Ladies' Auxiliary continued to support special projects for the hospital, such as the recreation activity program of the geriatric unit, the child-adolescent psychiatric unit and the donor wall. Fold away cots were donated to the hostel, as well as the usual annual contribution of gifts for patients and stockings for children in the pediatric unit at Christmas. The pediatric unit took on a new look this year as it moved to larger, more up-to-date quarters on the first floor.

The Leightons made an exit en masse from the staff in 1991, with Dr. Claude Leighton retiring and son, Ross, and daughter-in-law, Peggy, moving to Halifax. Several other members of the staff departed, including Dr. Roel Poblete, Dr. Tim Cooper, Dr. Aditya Mishra, Dr. Gilles Belisle and Dr. Bruce Bender. Several new members joined the staff, however, including Dr. Aditya Mishra, Dr. Vinod Sharma, Dr. Peter Docherty, Dr. Peter Clive, Dr. Lyle Weston, Dr. Byrne Harper, Dr. Dale Robinson, Dr. Vicki Taylor, Dr. Bill Rice, Dr. Andrew Clark, Dr. Susan Skanes, Dr. Fred Watkins, Dr. Terrence Trudeau, Dr. Ying Ying Ong and Dr. Jeanne McNeill. Dr. Luc Bourque joined the courtesy staff in orthopaedics.

Dr. Aditya Mishra made both an entrance and a departure in 1991. He was born on September 11, 1961, and was educated at Dalhousie University, receiving a BSc in 1980, and an MD in 1984. He did a rotating internship in the Dalhousie program from 1984 to 1985. From July to December 1985, he served in the emergency room of the Chaleur Regional Hospital and then did a general practice in Halifax for six months in 1986 before starting a residency in ophthalmology at the Halifax Infirmary in 1986, culminating in his receiving his FRCS(C) in Ophthalmology in 1990. He joined the staff in January 1991 but left to sub-specialize before the year was out.

Vinrod Sharma was born in India on February, 24, 1956, and received his MB, BS from SMS Medical College, University of Rajasthan, India. He interned at University of Rajasthan from 1978 to 1979 and then studied internal medicine at the same University from 1979 to 1982. After immigrating to Canada he did a rotating internship at Dalhousie from 1983 to 1984. He then went to the University of Western Ontario where he did a year of internal medicine from 1985 to 1986 with two years of residency in radiation oncology from 1984 to 1985 and 1986 to 1987. Apparently, radiation oncology did not suit his fancy and he returned to Dalhousie for another two years in internal medicine from 1987 to 1989 followed by a Fellowship in Gastroenterology from 1989 to 1991. He received his Fellowship in Internal Medicine in 1990 as well as his American Boards in Internal Medicine.

Dr. Peter Docherty came to Moncton with special training in rheumatology and fulfilled one of the needs of the Department of Internal Medicine. He was born on January 7, 1962, and received his MD from the University of Western Ontario in 1986. After an internship at the Victoria Hospital, London, Ontario, he remained for a residency in internal medicine from 1987 to 1989. He then travelled to Dalhousie University where he did a rheumatology residency from 1989 to 1991. In 1989, he received his Diplomate of the American Board of Internal Medicine and in 1990, his specialist certificate in internal medicine from the Royal College of Physicians and Surgeons of Canada. In August 1992 he was appointed to the board of Directors of the Arthritis Society.

Dr. Peter Clive became the latest addition to the Department of Medical Imaging, where he quickly earned a reputation for his skill in invasive procedures. He was born on July 1, 1958, and attended the University of Ottawa where he received a BSc in 1978 and an MD in 1982. He did a rotating internship in the Dalhousie program from 1982 to 1983. From 1985 to 1987, he did a residency in internal medicine at the University of Ottawa and then returned to Dalhousie for a residency in radiology from 1987 to 1991. He received his FRCP(C) in diagnostic radiology in 1991. He left Moncton in 1996.

The Department of Neurological Sciences was enriched by the appointment of three neurologists to the staff in 1991. Lyle E. Weston was born in Fredericton on July 13, 1959, received a BSc from the University of New Brunswick in 1981 and an MD from Dalhousie in 1985. After a rotating internship at Dalhousie, he did a neurology residency from 1986 to 1990 and became certified in neurology. Before coming to Moncton he did a year of clinical fellowship in neuroelectrophysiology at Dalhousie.

Byrne Harper was born on August 7, 1958, and received his MD from Dalhousie in 1984. He did a medical internship at the Victoria General Hospital from 1985 to 1986, followed by a residency in internal medicine from 1985 to 1986. He then moved on to the University of Western Ontario for a residency in neurology from 1986 to 1989 followed by a clinical fellowship and an EMG fellowship from 1989 to 1990. He received his FRCP(C) in neurology in 1990.

The third addition to the neurology staff, Dr. Dale Robinson, was appointed to the active staff of the Dr. Georges-L. Dumont Hospital and the courtesy staff of The Moncton Hospital. He was born on March 25, 1961, and received his MD from Dalhousie in 1985. He did a rotating internship at Victoria Hospital, London, Ontario, from 1985 to 1986 and returned to Dalhousie for a residency in internal medicine from 1986 to 1987. From 1987 to 1990 he was in Montreal for a residency in neurology at McGill, and he was certified by the Corporation professionelle des médicins du Québec in addition to receiving his FRCP(C) in Neurology.

Vicki Taylor was born in Doaktown on April 28, 1959, and after receiving a BSc from Mount Allison in 1979, she was awarded an MD degree from Memorial in 1983. She remained in Newfoundland for a family practice internship and residency from 1983 to 1985. From 1986 to 1989 she was a resident in ophthalmology at the University of Toronto followed by a fellowship in vitreo-retinal surgery from 1989 to 1990. She received her FRCS(C) in ophthalmology in 1989 and was on the staff of Princess Margaret Hospital, Toronto, as ocular oncologist in 1990 before returning to her native New Brunswick in 1991. Coming from the Miramichi, it is to be noted that during her student years she was a Miramichi salmon fishing guide in 1975 and 1976. From 1975 to 1980 she was also an equestrian instructor.

Two additions were made to the Department of Orthopaedics in 1991, Dr. Robert William Rice and Dr. Andrew Clark. Bill Rice was born on September 15, 1954, and received a BSc in 1978 from St. Mary's University and an MD from Dalhousie in 1982. After serving a rotating internship at Dalhousie from 1982 to 1983, he entered general practice before returning for postgraduate work in orthopaedics first at Memorial University from 1985 to 1987 and then at Dalhousie from 1987 to 1989. He did a further year of fellowship in spinal surgery at the University of Western Ontario in 1990. He received his FRCS(C) in orthopaedic surgery in 1990. He served as Chief of Orthopaedics in 1993 and 1994 but resigned from the staff in 1995, to seek his fortune in the United States going to Beckley, West Virginia.

Andrew Clark was born in Halifax on June 1, 1960, and received a BSc in 1980 and an MD from Dalhousie in 1984. After a year in the Dalhousie rotating internship program from 1984 to 1985, he began a residency in orthopaedics, spending 1985 to 1987 at Memorial University and 1987 to 1989 at Dalhousie University, receiving his FRCS(C) in orthopaedics in 1989. He did further training in total joint arthroplasty at the New England Baptist, Peter Bent Brigham and the Women's Hospital in Boston from January, 1990 until June 1991. After finishing this training he came to Moncton, taking over the practice of Dr. Ross Leighton who had departed for Halifax.

Dr. Luc Bourque, a Moncton native, made a third addition to the orthopaedic staff, although as a courtesy appointment. He was born on February 22, 1959, received a PSS degree from the Université de Moncton in 1979 and graduated with an MD from the University of Sherbrooke in 1983. After an internship at Notre Dame Hospital in Montreal from 1983 to 1984, he did a residency in orthopaedics in Montreal from 1984 to 1989, becoming certified by the Corporation professionelle des médicins du Québec and the Royal College of Physicians and Surgeons of Canada in 1989. He then joined the active staff of the Dr. Georges-L. Dumont Hospital.

Susan Skanes was born on July 17, 1960 and received her MD from Memorial University in 1983. She went to Montreal where she did a rotating internship at the Royal Victoria Hospital in 1983 to 1984, followed by a residency program in general surgery from 1984 to 1989 with her becoming certified in general surgery by the Royal College in 1989. She spent the next two years at the Lahey Clinic specializing in plastic and reconstructive surgery, was certified in plastic surgery in 1991 and in September of that year became the second female surgeon on the plastic surgery staff .

John Frederick Watkins was born in St. Stephen, New Brunswick, and received a BSc from Mount Allison in 1979 and an MD from Dalhousie in 1983. He served a rotating internship at the Royal Victoria Hospital in Victoria, British Columbia from 1983 to 1984 and then returned east to do residencies in general surgery from 1985 to 1985 and plastic surgery from 1987 to 1989 receiving his FRCS(C) in Plastic Surgery in 1989. This was followed by a clinical fellowship at the Victoria General and the Isaac Walton Killam Hospital from July to December 1989, followed by another clinical fellowship in plastic and maxillofacial and micro/hand surgery at the University of Toronto in 1990. He came to Moncton in January 1991, and served a locums for six months but was then off to Louisville, Kentucky, where he was a hand surgery fellow at the Christen Kleinert Institute for Hand and Microsurgery. He subsequently returned to Moncton to continue on the active staff. With his additional training in microvascular surgery, he added a new dimension to the plastic surgery service so that it was no longer necessary to send patients with large soft tissue defects to Saint John or Halifax for free flap grafts.

A new addition to the psychiatric service in 1991 was Dr. Terrence Trudeau. He received a BA in 1970 from Carleton University and then his MD from the University of Ottawa in 1975. After a rotating internship at the Jewish General Hospital in Montreal, he embarked on training in psychiatry, serving a psychiatric residency at Hôpital General, Dijon, France, from 1976 to 1978 and then returning to Montreal for a year at Hôpital Notre Dame from 1977 to 1978. He did a year of child psychiatry at Hôpital St. Justine, Montreal, from 1978 to 1979 and then another year at Hôpital de la Chartreuse, Dijon, France, from 1979 to 1980. He returned to Montreal for another year of residency at the Royal Victoria from 1980 to 1981 and received his FRCP(C) in Psychiatry in 1981 and was certified in psychiatry by the Corporation professionelle des médicins du Québec in 1982. From 1981 to 1986, he practised in Montreal at Hôpital Rivière-des-Prairies. He first came to Moncton in 1986, working at the Mental Health Clinic until 1989 when he was appointed psychiatrist at the Atlantic Child Guidance Centre, Halifax. He returned to Moncton in 1991, however, and has since restricted his practice to child psychiatry, serving on the newly-opened child and adolescent psychiatric unit.

Ying Ying Ong was born in the Philippines on April 10, 1947, and in 1972 received an MD degree from the University of Santo Tomas. She did a rotating internship at Santo Tomas University Hospital from 1972 to 1973 and from 1973 to 1975 took postgraduate work in anatomical pathology at the same institution. She travelled to the United States and served a residency in general pathology at Norwalk Hospital, Connecticut, from 1975 to 1979. She then came to Canada and did a residency in anatomical pathology at

Dalhousie University from 1979 to 1981. She became certified by the American Board of Pathology in 1982. From 1983 to 1987 she served as pathologist at the Sydney City Hospital. Following this, she started on the locums trail, working at the Queen Elizabeth Hospital in Charlottetown, the Saint John Regional and the Everett Chalmers Hospital during 1989-91. On coming to Moncton her only role was that of locums but she served for various periods in 1991, 1992 and 1993.

The only new family practitioners to be appointed to The Moncton Hospital in 1991 were Dr. Jeanne McNeill and Dr. Karen Silver. Jeanne McNeill was born on November 1, 1961, and received premedical training at the University of New Brunswick and her MD from the University of Alberta in 1985. After a family practice internship and residency at Edmonton General Hospital from 1985 to 1987, she remained in Edmonton where she did family practice from 1987 to 1990. She came to Moncton to take over the practice of Dr. Peggy Leighton who had moved to Halifax. Despite the fact that she was replacing a family physician, the Department of Health applied the rules that would only pay a doctor 75 percent of the fee schedule for three years when a doctor settled in an urban area deemed by the Professional Review Advisory Committee (PRAC) to be oversupplied.

Karen Silver was born on March 1, 1963, and received a BSc in 1984 and an MD from Dalhousie in 1989. She did an internship and family medicine residency at Dalhousie from 1989 to 1991. She came to Moncton to do a locums for Dr. Frank Kelly from 1991 to 1992 and has remained on staff since. In 1992 she became a part- time physician to the Diabetic Clinic.

Budget restrictions in 1991 were reflected in a slight decrease in adult and child admissions to 14,688, despite a reduction in the length of stay from 10.73 to 10.13 days. There were also fewer births recorded with 1,525 reported versus 1,642 in 1990/91 fiscal year. Operations performed were only down to 11,231 from 11,432 the previous year. Despite OR and bed closures during the year, the introduction of same day admission helped relieve the situation somewhat. There was also a substantial rise in day surgery to 6,580 from 5,323 the previous year. Except for speech pathology and social services, which showed slight reductions, all the other services showed slight increases in volume of work: audiogram—2,554; electrocardiograms—25,030; gastrointestinal unit procedures—3,539; social service cases—1,264; speech pathology—3,112; radiological examinations—94,190; CT scans—8,070; nuclear medicine procedures—5,311; ultrasound examinations—8,451. Emergency visits showed a decrease to 67,695 from 70,408 the previous year, but clinic visits showed an increase to 28,007 from 26,158 the previous year with the following recorded: Chemotherapy—6,364; Chest—4,316; TB—519; Colposcopy—2,151; Diabetic Day Care—2,456; Diet Counselling—1,502; Diagnostic—24; Eye—3,069; Haemophiliac—1,298; Pain—1,950; Reproductive Health—3,041; Urodynamics—421; and Multiple Sclerosis—0.

The year 1992 was one of transformation for The Moncton Hospital. Webster's Concise Dictionary defines hospital as "a medical institution for the care of the sick" and a corporation as "a legally formed business company." In keeping with a new reality, The Moncton Hospital became part of a business conglomerate by decree of the provincial government. In March 1992, New Brunswick's Minister of Health and Community Services introduced a bill in the legislature which resulted in significant changes in the structure and operations of the provincial health care system. Effective July 1, 1992, the existing boards of the 51 hospitals and health service centres in the province were replaced with 8 hospital corporations, each governed by a Board of Trustees and administered by a regional Chief Executive Officer. The Moncton Hospital therefore became a part of Region 1 Hospital Corporation (South-East), which included in addition to The Moncton Hospital, the Albert County Hospital, the Sackville Memorial Hospital, Health Services Centre, Rexton and the Petitcodiac Health Centre. All members of existing boards were replaced by government appointments, although some members of the old board were retained. To ensure that the large urban hospital would not be able to exert undue influence over issues and concerns that affected the smaller rural areas, the government decreed that no board would have more than 40 percent of its members from the urban area of the region. In order to preserve duality in the administration of health in the eastern part of the province, two separate corporations were formed in the south-east: Region 1 Hospital Corporation (South-East) and the Beausejour Hospital Corporation. Robert Radford remained as chairman of the new board. The only other members of the old board who remained were Allen McWilliams and Margaret Rideout. Dr. Ginette Gagné-Koch became CEO of the Corporation. Allen McWilliams became Chairman in 1994.

With this new structure the medical staff is now appointed to the Region 1 Hospital Corporation (South-East), combining staffs from all facilities but with privileges granted in one or several of the five facilities in the region. The medical staff by-laws were revised with the medical staff executive expanded to accommodate elected officers from both the urban and rural communities and the Medical Advisory Committee restructured to allow for additional members from the rural facilities. The medical staff would no longer appoint a member to the board of Trustees, but the president of the medical staff automatically became an ex-officio member of the board of trustees. In addition, the chief of staff, as part of senior management, attends the board meetings.

New additions to the staff in 1992 included Dr. Warren Giberson, Dr. James Crowley, Dr. Suzanne Hall Losier and Dr. Karen Hicks. Dr. Monique-Louise LeBlanc was appointed to the staff on joining the Petitcodiac Health Centre.

Warren Giberson was born on July 3, 1957, and before going into medicine decided on a career in botany receiving a BSc from Mount Allison in 1979 and an MSc in botany from the University of Alberta in 1982. He then entered Memorial University where he received a BMedSc in 1984 and an MD in 1986, receiving the gold medal and being the class valedictorian. After a rotating internship at St. Michael's Hospital, he took a year of general surgery at the Mayo Clinic from 1987 to 1988. From 1989 to 1991, he did a residency in otolaryngology at the University of Toronto and received his FRCS(C) in otolaryngology. He then came to Moncton to join his ophthalmologist wife, Dr. Vicki Taylor.

James Declara Crowley was born in Ireland on February 14, 1941, and took his premedical and medical education at the University of Cork, receiving his MB, BCh degrees in 1965. He interned at South Charlotte Infirmary, Cork, from 1965 to 1966. He was a resident in obstetrics at Erinville Maternity Hospital, Cork, from 1966 to 1967 and from 1967 to 1968 was a resident in obstetrics at Rotunda Hospital, Dublin, and in gynaecology at Hospital for Women in Leeds. He did a year of training in urology from 1968 to 1969 at Bradford Royal Infirmary, Bradford, England. After another year as a resident in obstetrics and gynaecology at the University of South Manchester, England, from 1969 to 1970, he entered private practice in England from 1970 to 1971. On coming to Canada in 1971, he repeated his training serving as a resident in obstetrics and gynaecology in Vancouver from 1971 to 1972 and at Mount Sinai in Toronto from 1972 to 1973 and then a year of general surgery at the University of Western Ontario from 1973 to 1974 and another year as chief resident in obstetrics and gynaecology at Memorial University from 1974 to 1975. After another two years as a fellow in the Department of Obstetrics and Gynaecology at Memorial from 1975 to 1977, he became a Diplomate of the American Board of Obstetrics and Gynaecology. From 1978 to 1991 he was the department head of obstetrics and gynaecology at Carbonear General Hospital, Newfoundland, serving as chief of staff in 1983 and 1984 and as president of the medical staff from 1988 to 1991. In 1980 he received his FRCS(C) in obstetrics and gynaecology and also became a Fellow of the American College of Obstetricians and Gynaecologists. In 1991 he moved to the mainland and after a year at the Miramichi Hospital, he transferred to Moncton.

Suzanne Hall Losier was born on October 4, 1960, and received a BSc from the University of Western Ontario in 1983 and an MD from Dalhousie in 1990. Following graduation she did the family medicine internship and residency program at Dalhousie from 1990 to 1992, becoming certified in family medicine by the College of Family Medicine of Canada. She also received her ACLS in 1991 and her ATLS in 1992. She joined the staff taking over the practice of Dr. Cathy MacLean at the Moncton Medical Clinic.

Karen Hicks born on March 21, 1962, received a BSc from Dalhousie in 1983 and a BEd in 1985, but then switched to Memorial where she graduated with an MD in 1990. She returned to Dalhousie for a family medicine internship and residency from 1990 to 1992. She came to Moncton in July 1992, to do a locums but stayed on staff and became a full-time emergency room physician in December 1993.

Dr. Monique-Louise LeBlanc was born on October 11, 1961, and received a DSS degree from the Université de Moncton in 1984 and an MD degree from Dalhousie in 1991. After serving a rotating internship in the Dalhousie program from 1991 to 1992, she did a locum at the Petitcodiac Health Centre from July-November and then joined the staff of the clinic. In the summer of 1993, she left the clinic and established a family practice in Moncton.

For only the second time in its history, an annual report was not forthcoming from The Moncton Hospital. An annual report for South-East Hospital Corporation for 1993 to 1994 was prepared, but never printed and distributed to the public, presumably due to financial restraints.

Financial restraint continued to plague the hospital and its management looked to innovative programs to cut down expenditures without cutting services. The Same Day Admissions Program, the Home Medication Program and the Rehabilitation Day Hospital are all examples of efforts to cut expenditures. The government acknowledged that an imbalance in funding for hospital corporations existed at the time with the South-East corporation being underfunded. This had been common knowledge for years, however, but at least the government was finally paying more than lip service when it said it was attempting to redesign the hospital funding distribution system within the province.

During the year, the government purchased a mobile Lithotripsy Unit to service The Moncton Hospital, as well as the Saint John Regional Hospital and the Everett Chalmers Hospital. As a result, it was no longer necessary to send patients to Halifax for this innovative treatment of kidney stones. The first treatments at The Moncton Hospital would not occur until March 1994. Dr. Gorman and the hospital had presented a brief to the Department of Health on the need of a Magnetic Imaging Unit for The Moncton Hospital and the government announced that mobile Magnetic Imaging Service would commence in 1995. "Better half a loaf than none at all." This was also the year that Dr. Gilbert Quartey, with his long-time interest in spine implants for pain control, implanted a titanium drug infusion pump in a young paraplegic giving him relief from painful muscle spasms and rigidity in his paralysed limbs. This was the first time such a pump had been inserted in a patient in New Brunswick and only the second time it was done east of Ottawa.

The Maritime Air Ambulance Interprovincial Steering Committee announced the selection of The Moncton Hospital as the location for the dispatch/flight co-ordination centre for the Maritime Air Ambulance with the flights originating out of Halifax but with Moncton providing a back-up air medical crew for the service. It was planned to have the service operational by the summer of 1994, but Nova Scotia had second thoughts. New Brunswick indicated a willingness to go it alone and subsequently implemented the service in 1996.

Eight nurses from The Moncton Hospital graduated this year from the province's first specialized education program for nurses working in the operating room environment. The program, which was designed by the hospital's staff educators, is called the Post Basic Perioperative Program. A self-directed learning modular program, it is the first of its kind in New Brunswick. It took the graduates 2,000 hours of study on their own time over a two to three-year period.

The neurosurgery department opened its first Spina Bifida Clinic under clinic co-ordinator, Clair Petitpas, RN, and this involved a multidisciplinary team of physicians, nurses, physiotherapists, occupational therapists, dieticians and other professional staff. With the clinic, the hospital is now able to provide comprehensive care, support and education which effectively interfaces with community-based care.

As a result of its strategic planning process, which included the Vision 2000 initiative and a careful analysis of hospital management literature, the South-East Hospital Corporation set up a steering committee to organize all clinical services along program management lines. Its main purpose was to produce a team of caregivers who would manage the resources provided to their service and thereby making better use of the resources, identifying areas of waste and then applying the savings to other areas of greater need. In reality it is decentralized management and it remains to be seen if management at the bottom is more successful that management from the top.

New additions to the staff in 1993 were mostly to the Department of Pathology: Dr. Rowan Shinder, Dr. Richard Fitzmaurice and Dr. Hamzch Tarabichi. Others included Dr. Mary Catherine MacSween, Dr. Victoria Manfredi, Dr. Timothy Stultz and Dr. Frank Lord. In July 1993 the government introduced PRAC and since then, the number of new additions to the staff have been severely curtailed. No longer does the staff decide its needs and then go out and try to recruit. Now, government has set guidelines for the number and type of each physician needed in each regional health district and no medicare billing numbers are given to physicians unless the region is below its quota. In Health District 1, this regional allotment is further complicated by the fact of trying to satisfy the needs of the two hospitals and language groups.

Rowen Shinder was born in Montreal on July 4, 1961. He received a BSc from McGill in 1983 and an MD from the University of Toronto in 1988. He did a rotating internship at Mount Sinai Hospital from 1988 to 1989 and a residency in pathology at the University of Toronto from 1989 to 1993, when he received his FRCP(C) in anatomical pathology as well as becoming a Diplomate of the American Board of Pathology in Anatomical Pathology.

Richard John Fitzmaurice was born in England on November 12, 1956, and received his MB, ChB degrees from Manchester University Medical School in 1981. He served as house officer at Royal Preston Hospital from 1981 to 1982. He started training in pathology at the University Hospital, Nottingham, from 1982 to 1983 and continued on at Royal Free Hospital, London, in 1983, Hope Hospital, Salford, 1983-84, Saint Mary's Hospital, Manchester, 1984-85, and North Manchester General Hospital, 1985-86, followed by a fellowship in osteoarticular pathology at the University of

Manchester from 1986 to 1989. He remained as a lecturer in pathology at the University of Manchester and director of pathology at Manchester Royal Infirmary from 1989 to 1992. He came to Canada in September 1992, as director of pathology at Grenfell Regional Health Services, Newfoundland. After joining the staff of The Moncton Hospital, he remained less than two years, resigning in September, 1995.

Dr. Hamzeh Tarabichi was born on July 20, 1962, in Damascus, Syria. He received his MD from the University of Aleppo in the Dominican Republic in 1985. He became an American citizen and then came to Canada. He interned from 1987 to 1988 in the McGill program and from 1988 to 1992 did a residency in pathology at Dalhousie University, receiving his FRCP(C) in anatomical pathology. He worked at Edmundston Regional Hospital in 1992-93 before coming to Moncton in August 1993. In 1993 he became a Diplomate of the American Board of Anatomical and Clinical Pathology.

Another doctor who appeared on the scene to join her husband on the staff was Mary Catherine McSween, the wife of Peter Docherty. She was born on October 23, 1961, and educated at Dalhousie, receiving her BSc in 1983 and her MD in 1987. She did a rotating internship at St. Joseph's Hospital, London, Ontario, in 1987-88, followed by a locum practice in Sarnia, Wallaceburg and Woodstock, Ontario. She then returned to Dalhousie where she did an internal medicine residency with a subspecialty of endocrinology from 1989 to 1993, and received her FRCP(C) in Internal Medicine in 1993.

Dr. Victoria Manfredi was born on July 9, 1957, and received a BA from Rutgers University in 1978. She came to Canada for her medical education and graduated from Dalhousie University in 1991. She did a straight medical internship in the Dalhousie program from 1991 to 1992 and then a rotating internship from 1992 to 1993. In October, 1993, she began working part-time on the staff of the Petitcodiac Health Centre and subsequently started a family practice in Riverview.

Timothy Stultz, a Riverview native, was born on June 7, 1966, and received a BSc from Mount Allison in 1988 and an MD from Dalhousie in 1992. He served a rotating internship in the Dalhousie program from 1992 to 1993 and joined the staff of the Albert County Hospital with privileges at The Moncton Hospital, where he frequently assists in the operating room.

Frank Lord was born on May 18, 1960 and received a BSc from the Université de Moncton in 1981 and his MD from the University of Sherbrooke in 1985. He served as an intern and resident in the family medicine program at the University of Sherbrooke from 1985 to 1987 and was certified in family medicine. He became an emergency room physician at the Dr. Georges-L. Dumont Hospital and physician to Dorchester Penitentiary and Westmorland Institution. His appointment to The Moncton Hospital is limited to caring for inmates admitted to the hospital.

Beginning on February 17, 1994, the Program Management Steering Committee began working on the implementation of Program Management at the South-East Hospital Corporation. The membership of the Committee were: Jim Clements, Dave Davidson, Ruth Dunnett, Ruth Duffy, Judy Hughes, Joan Lutes and Carroll Ann O'Leary. Also on the committee were the following members of the medical staff: Dr. Antoine Salloum, Dr. Preston Smith, Dr. Ken Mitton and Dr. Bob Trifts. The first work of the committee members was to educate themselves on program management and its implementation in various locations across Canada. The committee then went on to lay a critical path for implementation of program management. The committee finally wrote the following philosophy of Program Management:

Program Management is a structure which organizes the hospital into clinical programs and delegates the responsibility for their effective and efficient operation to the Program Team and its leadership. The philosophy of Program Management at South-East Hospital Corporation is that of a participatory type of management that promotes team building and collaboration amongst all members of the Patient Care Team. The program and its structures will be patient-focused and will promote community partnership. Physician involvement is an essential part of the philosophy of Program Management. Decision making in this organization will be decentralized. Empowerment will enable the Program Team to promote continuous improvement in the quality and efficiency of program delivery. This approach is proactive, flexible and responsive to changes in the health care environment. Program Management will promote mutual respect and support among all professions and all Programs in a manner that advances all of South-East Hospital Corporation.

By October, the Program Management Committee had completed a substantial part of the planning for implementation of program management. Eight programs were defined as follows:

1. Neuro/Orthopaedic/Rehab/Rheumatology;
2. Pediatrics/Obstetrics/Neonatology/Gynaecology;
3. Family Practice/Geriatrics;
4. Adult Psychiatry/Child & Adolescent Psychiatry;
5. Emergency;
6. General Surgery;
7. Plastics/Urology/Ophthalmology/Otorhinolaryngology; and
8. Medicine.

A decision was made to start all the programs at once rather than to use a gradual approach. Each program would have an administrative director and a medical director. Recruitment of the administrative directors would begin internally in the hospital and go external if no applications were found for the job. The medical staff would have representation on the committee that selects the administrative directors. The medical directors would be selected by the medical staff and the appointment would be confirmed by the vice-president responsible so that administration was comfortable working with these physicians. The medical director for each program was required to be a physician from that program. Money had been set aside to provide administrative training for those medical directors without administrative experience.

A budget crisis again confronted the staff in 1994. In March, the administration reported that there would be a budget deficit of $2.8 million. Savings in non-clinical areas, such as reduced heating costs, improved waste management, MedBuy, new materials management carousel, changing formula for meal cost, expansion of same day admissions surgery program, savings from early retirement packages and reduced management positions, together with anticipated changes in operating in Albert and Sackville reduced the budget deficit by 1.5 million, but 1.3 million of this deficit would have to come out of clinical programs. The medical staff was presented with two options. Option 1 was to keep five OR theatres (four general and one local) in use and close one medical unit in addition to the usual summer closures, plus a reduction in diagnostic and ambulatory care with normal operations to resume in October. Option 2 was to reduce to summer closure levels for two months until after Labour Day and to close the entire hospital for two weeks at the end of July except for emergency services. The Medical Advisory Committee passed a motion "that the Medical Advisory Committee does not support any further cuts, but if the board of Trustees feel that cuts must be made, then the least compromising to patient care is felt to be Option 2, provided this is extended Corporation wide and affects all facilities." By May the board notified the staff that even with summer closures there would be a budget shortfall of 1.3 million dollars and the board had requested a balanced budget. The Medical Advisory Committee then passed another motion: "that prior to any reduction in clinical services, the Medical Advisory Committee insists Administration review in detail the operating budget to explore all possible areas of cost reduction that will not affect clinical services." Subsequently, a special task force was set up comprising senior management plus four physicians, Dr. Bond, Dr. Gorman, Dr. John Murphy and Dr. Rubin, and they reviewed the budget line by line. They were able to produce proposed savings in the non-clinical field of $618,000 by reducing stationary and supply usage, reducing administrative positions and deleting on call costs for ECG's by reassigning through the nursing office. In the clinical area, savings of $412,000 were proposed by:

1. changing rehabilitation services so that there would be ten inpatient beds, including four rheumatology beds and providing a day program for eight to ten patients;
2. sick time on day shift would not be replaced unless dictated by exceptional circumstances;

3. eleven beds would be closed on geriatrics, seven of which would be acute care family practice beds; and
4. day patients would be increased by two.

These changes would bring the shortfall down to $393,646. After the summer closures, the new financial officer for the hospital, Gitta Kulczycki, who replaced William King on his retirement, reported that the hospital had saved a considerable amount of money with the summer closures but still faced a projected shortfall of $350,000 to $400,000 and must remain vigilant. One bright spot on the horizon was the announcement by the government that a new funding formula would be coming into place in February of 1995. The basic intent would be to provide hospitals with funding based on what they do and there would be an allocation using Case Mix Groups (CMG) and Resource Intensity Weights (RIW). Tertiary care for all programs would be funded on a line-by-line basis reflecting workload and acuity and these would become protected budgets. It was therefore important that all tertiary care and elevated secondary services be clearly identified as these would obviously receive more protection. It was thought that the hospital might do quite well once funded under this basis and that all complaints of inadequate funding in the past would be vindicated.

The reality of PRAC (Professional Review Advisory Committee) came into full focus in 1994 when the recruitment of new physicians to the staff came to a virtual standstill. At the request of the Medical Advisory Committee, all departments were asked to bring forward their medical manpower requirements with the following requests resulting:

- Anaesthesia—1 or 2 in addition to a replacement for Dr. Armstrong;
- Family Practice felt their department should remain open for several new physicians;
- General Surgery—a general surgeon with emphasis on a surgical oncologist or surgical intensivist;
- Medicine—2 cardiologists, 1 infectious disease consultant, 1 hematologist/oncologist, 1 rheumatologist, 1 physiatrist;
- Medical Imaging—1 replacement for Dr. Coop;
- Obstetrics and Gynaecology—1;
- Ophthalmology—1;
- Orthopaedics—1;
- Pathology—1 anatomical pathologist in addition to a new laboratory director; Pediatrics—1;
- Psychiatry—1 child and adolescent psychiatrist.

Because of PRAC, the executive of the medical staff was mandated to examine manpower issues not related to credentialing. The needs of the medical staff to provide optimal care to the citizens it serves, however, are not quite the same as those mandated by government and it was necessary for the

Medical Advisory Committee to priorize its wish list for 1994/95 as follows:

1. ophthalmology;
2. infectious diseases;
3. cardiology;
4. anaesthesia;
5. general surgery;
6. pathology;
7. orthopaedics; and
8. oncology.

The only new additions to the staff in 1994 were Dr. Malcolm MacAuley, who assumed the position of Director of Laboratories for Region 1 Hospital Corporation, and Dr. Charles Duffy to serve the Albert County Hospital, but with privileges also at The Moncton Hospital.

Dr. MacAuley was no stranger to Moncton, having served briefly as a pathologist at The Moncton Hospital from 1968-69. Malcolm was born on October 19, 1934, in Yarmouth, Nova Scotia, and received his MD from Dalhousie in 1958 after serving a rotating internship in the Dalhousie program from 1958 to 1958. He served as a resident in anatomic pathology at the Western Infirmary, University of Glasgow (1958-59), followed by a year at the Victoria General Hospital from 1959 to 1960. From 1960 to 1963 he did a general pathology residency at Kansas University Medical Centre, Kansas City, and in 1964 he was certified in anatomical and clinical pathology by the American Board of Pathology and the Royal College of Physicians and Surgeons of Canada. From 1964 to 1968 he served as pathologist at Magee Women's Hospital and Allegheny General, Pittsburgh, and was an Assistant Professor at the University of Pittsburgh. He returned to Canada and served as pathologist at The Moncton Hospital from 1968 to 1970. He then went to Halifax where he remained as pathologist at the Victoria General Hospital in Halifax from 1970 to 1994 and rose to the position of full professor at Dalhousie. He returned to Moncton in September, 1994, to assume the position of Director of Laboratories for Region 1 Hospital Corporation. He keeps in touch with his Scottish background, wearing a kilt and playing the bagpipes at numerous medical events.

Charles Henry Duffy was born on July 4, 1965, and received his premedical training at the University of Prince Edward Island. He received his medical education at Memorial, receiving a BMSc. and an MD in 1990. He then did the family medicine program at Dalhousie from 1990 to 1992, receiving certification from the Canadian College of Family Practice in 1992. From 1992 to 1994, he served locums in family medicine in Prince Edward Island and Campbell River, British Columbia. His stays at the Albert County Hospital and in Moncton were short, as he departed in July 1995, for Montague, Prince Edward Island.

The number one priority which had been listed by the Medical Advisory Committee was ophthalmology, but attempts to add to the ophthalmology staff in 1994 proved to be a frustrating affair. At this time The Moncton Hospital had only two ophthalmologists on staff, Dr. Vicky Taylor and Dr. Eric Stevens. Dr. Stevens had reached 60 years of age and could cease taking emergency calls. Both Dr. Cobb and Dr. Britton had resigned from the hospital staff in 1987 and ceased doing surgery but remained on the staff of the Dr. Georges-L. Dumont Hospital even though they did not take emergency calls. This left the Dr. Georges-L. Dumont Hospital with five ophthalmologists on staff and only two at The Moncton Hospital. The Moncton Hospital had sponsored Dr. Lynn Brewer to take postgraduate work in ophthalmology, but when she was ready to join the staff in 1994, there was not an opening authorized by PRAC. Negotiations were entered into with the Minister of Health and he came up with a solution in which Dr. Brewer would be given a number on condition that a cap at $2.7 million would be placed on Medicare payments to the ophthalmologists in Moncton. This solution was felt to set a dangerous precedent in Medicare funding and the ophthalmologists at the Dr. Georges-L. Dumont Hospital stated that they would give no co-operation to The Moncton Hospital in the future if this was accepted. Consequently, Dr. Brewer moved west and the ophthalmology manpower shortage at The Moncton Hospital remained unresolved.

As a special project for the hospital's approaching Centennial year, the Friends of the Moncton Hospital decided they would take on the huge task of raising $2.7 million dollars with the objective of updating the hospital's neurosciences service making it a Neurosciences Centre of Excellence. The funds raised were to be distributed as follows:

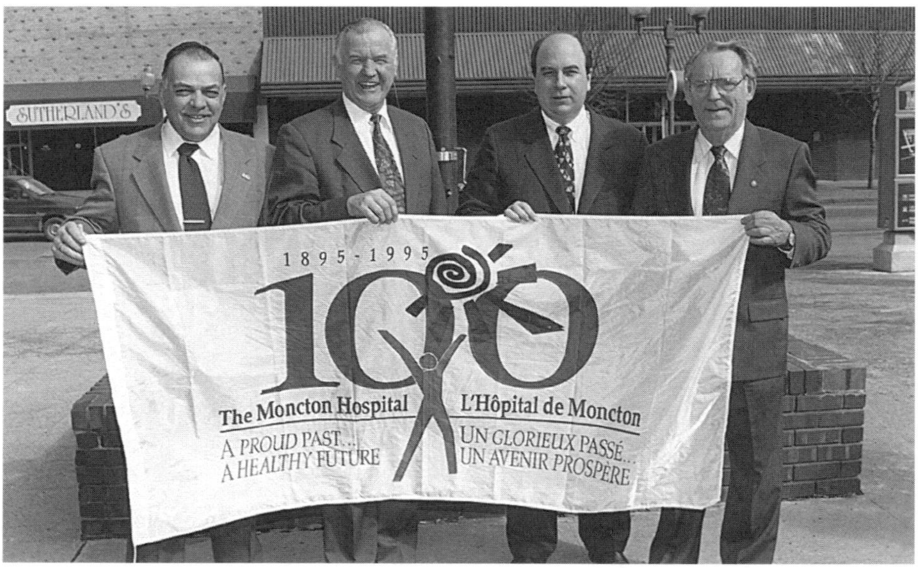

The beginning of the Centennial Campaign started with the raising of the Centennial Flag in downtown Moncton. From left toright: D. Johnson, representing the Mayor of Riverview; Leopold Belliveau, Mayor of Moncton; Mr. Robert Irving, Campaign Chairman; and Mr. W. Malenfant, Mayor of Dieppe.

Neurosurgery	$776,000
1. Viewing wand System	
2. Intraoperative Angiography	
3. Support equipment	
Neurointensive Care Unit	$300,000
Neuro-electro Diagnostics	$307,000
1. Electromyograph (EMG) Machine Upgrading	
2. Evoked Potentials Machine	
3. Digital Electroencephalograph (EEG)	
Radiology	$672,000
1. S.P.E.C.T. Gamma Camera	
2. Laser Camera	
Gastroenterology—G.I. Equipment	$223,000
Laboratory—New Equipment	$125,000
Anaesthesia—New Equipment	$115,000
Rehabilitation—Improved Equipment	$99,000
Orthopaedics—Spinal Table	$43,000
Urology—Improved Equipment	$36,000

Although the focus of the fund raising project was on Neurosciences, it was apparent that all departments would benefit from the campaign.

A fund-raising organization was hired and Robert Irving agreed to serve as chairman of the Centennial Capital Campaign under Les Parrott, the president of The Friends of the Moncton Hospital Foundation. Dr. Kim DeWare

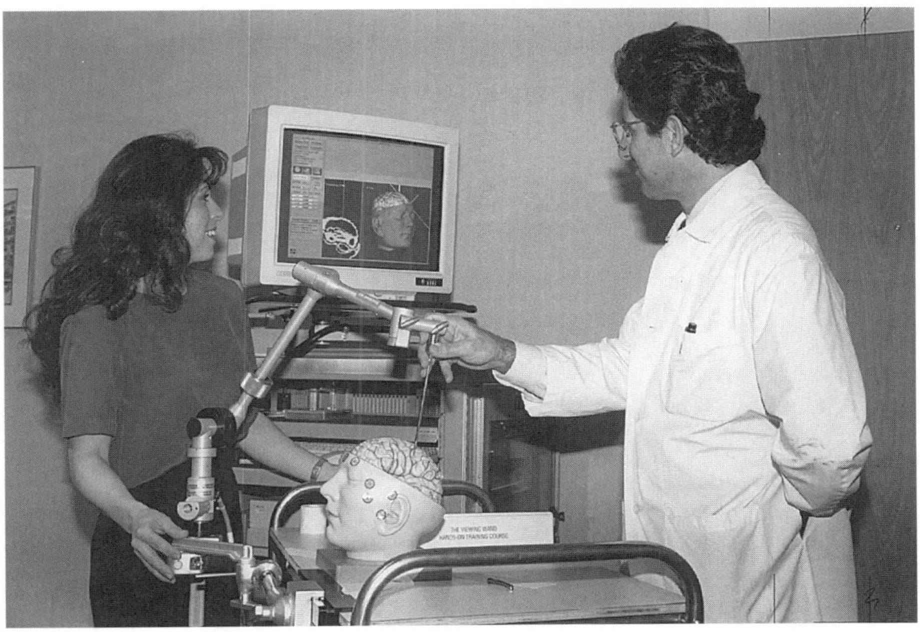

Nurse Carla Dubois and Dr. A. Salloum demonstrate the wand purchased with funds raised by the Centennial Campaign.

headed up the drive for contributions from the medical staff. Dr. Peter Gorman and Dr. Antoine Salloum played major roles in the campaign, addressing numerous service clubs and organizations over the next year in the quest for donated funds.

With this centennial year of incorporation of the hospital in 1995 it was also felt that such a significant event in the life of The Moncton Hospital should be celebrated. Dr. Victor McLaughlin was appointed Chairman of the hospital's Centennial Committee and the first planning session was held on March 17, 1994, with the following members present:

Dr. V. McLaughlin, Chairman
Dr. G. Gagné-Koch, CEO
Miss R. Duffy, Vice President
Miss M. MacLeod, Administrative Assistant
Ms. S. Soucoup, Media Co-ordinator
Mr. R. Holmes, Friends of the Moncton Hospital
Mrs. E. Fair weather, Nurses' Hospital Auxiliary
Mrs. C. Straight, The Moncton Hospital Nurses' Alumnae

This meeting was primarily organizational and it was felt that the committee should have broad representation from all the various hospital departments and organizations and individuals were subsequently approached for involvement and the first meeting of the committee was held on April 7, 1994 with the following representatives:

Chairman	Victor McLaughlin
Assistant	Marlene MacLeod
Public Relations	Susan Soucoup
The Moncton Hospital Nurses' Alumnae	Cathy Straight
The Moncton Hospital Nurses' Auxiliary	Edith Fairweather
Friends of the Moncton Hospital	Robert Holmes
Volunteers	Dawn MacPherson
Board of Trustees	Margaret Rideout
FM. Management	John Sanford
Nurse Managers	Jean MacKeigan
Regional Directors	Connie Colpitts
Medical Staff	Donald MacLellan
Senior Management	Carroll Ann O'Leary
Employee Recognition Committee	Lydia Underhill
The Moncton Hospital Ladies' Auxiliary	Kay McCartney

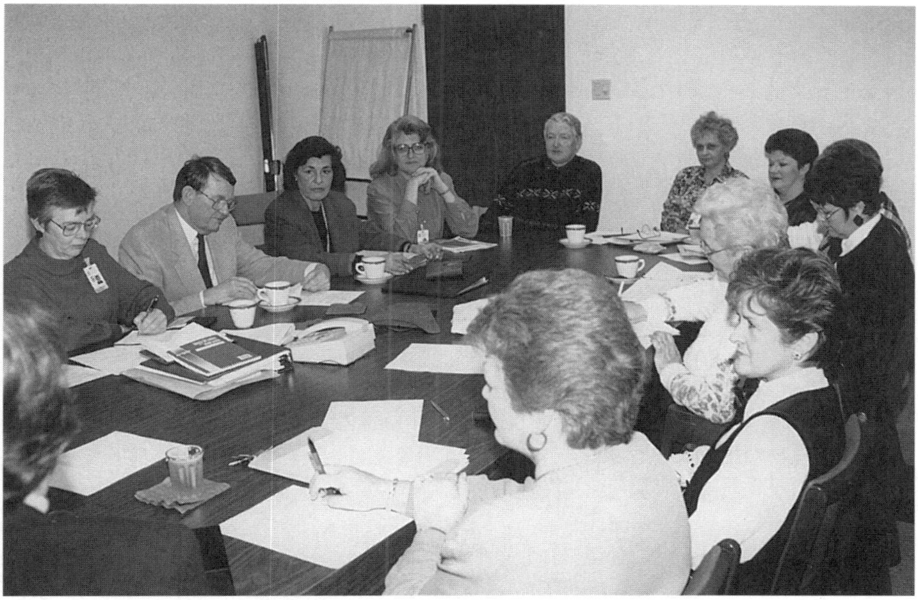

The Committee meeting for the planning of the Centennial celebrations. Clockwise from left: Jean MacKeigan, Dr. D.I. MacLellan, Carroll Ann O'Leary, Susan Soucoup, Robert Holmes, Cathy Straight, Lydia Underhill, Vana Hooper, Edith Fairweather, Dr. Ginette Gagné-Koch, and Dawn MacPherson.

These people would meet regularly, over the next twenty-one months to plan for celebrations during the centennial year. As the hospital received its charter on March 5, 1895, but did not treat the first patient until 1898, it was decided that the conception of the hospital should be celebrated rather than its birth. It was also decided to adopt the logo of the Friends of the Moncton Hospital Capital Campaign for the Centennial celebrations: "A Proud Past, A Healthy Future." It was agreed that it would not be prudent to use hospital funds in these times of financial restraint and going to the corporate sector and competing with the Friends for funds was not an option. While many of the activities planned would be self-financing, in the longer term it was necessary to have some seed money and this was provided by the Friends, the Ladies' Auxiliary, the Nurses' Auxiliary and the Nurses' Alumnae. Committees were formed for publicity, special events, history and memorabilia, as well as various subcommittees, as planning for special events took place. During the rest of 1994, planning progressed so that by the beginning of 1995 everything was in place to start the celebrations in March. The chairman felt that some administrative assistance was necessary in achieving the various tasks throughout the year if our celebrations were to be successful. It was agreed that a team from the education department comprised of Jim Clements, Joan Allain and Shirley Ross would be appointed to act as liaison, with committee members providing assistance as required.

The year 1995 was not just a year of celebrations. There were still the day-to-day tasks of running the hospital. It had been able to maintain a balanced budget during the year, and received assurances from the government of a new funding formula. This would take into consideration the acuity of the cases admitted to an institution. This would be an advantage to a hospital like The Moncton Hospital which served as a referral centre for complicated cases requiring treatment resulting in higher costs. After much public outcry because of extensive waiting lists for elective surgery through the province, the government, in April, gave a one time grant of $800,000 to be used to help reduce waiting lists.

Program Management became a reality on April 1, 1995, when the Program Administrative Directors and Medical Directors were announced by Vice-presidents Ruth Duffy and Carroll Ann O'Leary.

1. Neuro/Orthopaedic/Rehab/Rheumatology—Marilyn Babineau and Dr. Michael Forsythe;
2. Pediatrics/Obstetrics/Neonatology/Gynaecology—Cathy Straight and Dr. Glen Brodie;
3. Family Practice/Geriatrics—Valerie Hussey and Dr. Ken Mitton;
4. Adult Psychiatry/Child and Adolescent Psychiatry—Marilyn Bishop and Dr. Mary Mitton;
5. Emergency—Joan Lutes and Dr. Peter O'Hanley;
6. General Surgery—Lydia Underhill and Dr. Fred Murphy;
7. Plastics/Urology/Ophthalmology/Otorhinolaryngology—Lydia Underhill and Dr. Douglas Inglis;
8. Medicine—Ruth Dunnett and Dr. Bill Thompson;

Within each program, advisory committees were created to ensure representation from all the disciplines and medical specialities that contribute to patient care in their specific areas. The program directors meet once a month and the program administrative directors met twice daily during the summer to review the bed situation, patients waiting in emergency for admission, and to ensure continuous vigilance of patient care. To the program directors fell the task of making arrangements for bed and OR closures during the March and Christmas breaks, as well as during summer vacations.

The program directors became responsible for deciding on the renovations that could be carried out with the limited dollars available. Among changes proposed was the relocation of the Neurosurgery ICU from 3,600 to 4,100 floor and the relocation of 4100 to the renovated space on 3,600. Clinical engineering was relocated to 5,500 so that the pre-admission clinic/day of surgery admission unit currently on 6,600 could move closer to the surgical suite. Renovations were carried out on 4,200 to make it more suitable for the care of burn patients and work was done on 6600 to ensure good facilities for the care of infectious diseases patients.

The senior advisor-nursing position was filled by Catherine Aquino-Russell while Marilyn MacDonald was appointed Clinical Nurse Specialist. Judith Hughs performed a senior advisor role in physiotherapy as well as being manager of outpatient therapy (OT & PT).

When the South Tower was opened in 1987, it was hoped that Phase Two of the redevelopment plan of The Moncton Hospital would begin but financial restraints prevented it from getting off the ground. In the meantime, a new master program/master plan for the continuing development of The Moncton Hospital was being prepared during the year from a program perspective.

With the emphasis placed in the centennial campaign on the neurosciences program, a plan for a Neurosciences Centre of Excellence was developed by the neuro/ortho/rehab program and presented to the board of trustees and the Minister of Health. In addition, the general surgery and surgical specialties programs prepared position papers on trauma care and burn care for presentation to the provincial government.

The directors of the programs relating to surgery, with the help of others, grappled with the fair distribution of operating room time, resulting from the $800,000 grant from government to reduce the waiting list. They decided that those waiting the longest should have priority. An innovation in the operating suite was the appointment of Dr. Tony Bond to serve as Medical Director.

It had been the policy of the hospital that interns would pronounce a patient dead in the absence of the attending physician from the hospital but this became a problem in 1995 with the demise of the intern program. A new policy was introduced so that nurses could make the pronouncement in cases of expected death. In unexpected deaths, the pronouncement still remained the responsibility of a physician.

Although the hospital had proposed in a brief to government an MRI for The Moncton Hospital, the government instead purchased a mobile MRI to be used by both The Moncton Hospital and the Saint John Regional Hospital. After a coin toss, won by The Moncton Hospital, the MRI was unveiled at a special ceremony at The Moncton Hospital attended by Premier Frank McKenna, and the Hon. Dr. Russell King, minister of health. In addition, a new CT Scanner was installed at the hospital. Although the hospital had a computer system it lagged behind the Saint John Regional and the Dr. Georges-L. Dumont hospitals in the use of computers. This, however, was about to change with the signing of a contract at the end of the year for a new state of the art $6-7 million computer system which would place it in the forefront of hospital computerization in North America.

For several years, the hospital had sponsored Well Women's Clinics with the help of the Nurses' Auxiliary. In 1995 a Well Women's Clinic was established off site and not only offered advice but also mammograms. This clinic was named "The Katherine Wright Wellness Centre," in honour of the many years of her service to The Moncton Hospital.

In common with other hospitals in North America, the hospital was seeing increased resistance of bacteria to antibiotics, with some bacteria cultured in our intensive care unit that were resistant to all antibiotics. In order to help alleviate the problem, or at best slow down the process of resistant bacteria,

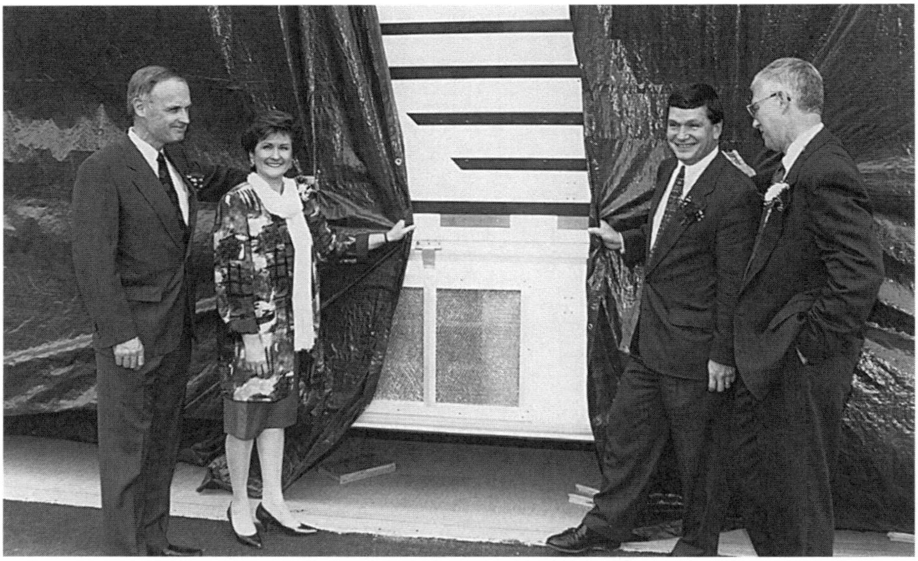

The inauguration of Mobile MRI Service in New Brunswick. From left to right: Hon. Dr. Russell King, Minister of Health; Dr. Ginette Gagné-Koch, CEO of South-East Health Care Corporation; Hon. Frank McKenna, Premier of New Brunswick; and Mr. David Carlin, CEO of the Saint John Regional Hospital.

Dr. Thompson, infectious diseases specialist, proposed an antimicrobial restriction policy.

Although PRAC still had a stranglehold on the ability to fulfil the needs of medical staffing, five doctors were added to the staff in 1995. PRAC had proposed that manpower staffing be conducted along linguistic lines but this would present hardship, especially in bringing in new family physicians. At a meeting of the board of trustees on June 21, 1995, the board reconfirmed its position in medical manpower planning in Region 1 by unanimously passing the following motion:

> That it is very important that medical manpower planning be jointly done by the two hospital corporations without interference from the Department of Health and Community Services; and that necessary steps be taken by the board Chairman to ensure that the formula proposed by the Minister of Health and Community Services be removed in order to allow for productive manpower planning in an environment of trust and co-operation between the medical staff of the two hospital corporations.

Dr. Bill Rice resigned from the Department of Orthopaedics in September 1995 which presented a manpower problem in orthopaedics. In the summer of 1994 a joint call schedule was developed in orthopaedics between the Dr. Georges-L. Dumont and The Moncton Hospital. With retirements, sickness and resignations, the orthopaedic department was reduced to two men on the call roster for orthopaedics. The orthopaedic staffs of the two hospitals decided that they should only be on call one night in six, and hence every sixth night or weekend there would be no one on call for emergencies. This meant the patient would have to be transferred to Fredericton or Saint John.

The five new additions to the staff in 1995 were Dr. Chantel Trudeau, Dr. Gordon Dow, Dr. Brian Davidson, Dr. Jamie Penfold and Dr. Raymond Braun.

Chantel Trudeau was born in France on September 30, 1953, and received her MD from the Université de Dijon, France, in 1984. She came to Canada in 1987 and served a rotating internship in the Dalhousie Program from 1987 to 1988. She did a residency in internal medicine at the Victoria General in Halifax from 1988 to 1989 and the Saint John Regional Hospital from 1989 to 1991. She pursued further studies in cardiology at the Montreal Heart Institute, Notre Dame Hospital and Saint Justine Hospital in Montreal from 1992 to 1994 and received her FRCP(C) in Internal Medicine in 1994. In February 1995, she began a locum at The Moncton Hospital and in September 1995 was appointed full-time to the internal medicine staff with the subspecialty of cardiology.

The Moncton Hospital was in great need of a second specialist in infectious diseases. The increased importance of treatment for these was recognized, with 75 percent of AIDS cases in New Brunswick being treated at The Moncton Hospital. Also a large number of oncology patients are rendered immunocompromised as a result of chemotherapy treatment. PRAC recognized this need by the hospital, and allowed Dr. Gordon Dow to join the staff. He was born on March 15, 1962, and received a BSc from the University of New Brunswick in 1985 and an MD from Dalhousie in 1987. He served a rotating internship at Dalhousie from 1987 to 1988. This was followed by a residency in internal medicine at the Vancouver General Hospital and University Hospital, Vancouver, from 1988 to 1991. From 1991 to 1993, he did a residency in infectious diseases at St. Boniface General Hospital and the Health Sciences Centre in Winnipeg. He was certified by the Royal College of Physicians and Surgeons of Canada in internal medicine in 1992 and in the subspecialty of infectious diseases in 1993.

Brian Davidson is a Riverview native, born on January 21, 1969. He received his BSc in 1989 and his MD in 1993 from Dalhousie. He took the two-year intern and residency program in family medicine at Memorial University from 1993 to 1995, receiving certification in family medicine from the College of Family Physicians. On completion of his residency, he joined the Moncton Medical Clinic, taking over the practice of Dr. William Dennis who retired in June 1995.

Jamie Penfold was born on September 26, 1961, and received a BSc in 1983 and an MD in 1987 from the University of British Columbia. In her senior year she served as editor of the class newspaper, *The Functional Inquirer*. She had her first taste of medicine in the Maritimes when she served a rotating internship in the Dalhousie Program from 1987 to 1988. After a year of doing locums in general practice in British Columbia, she returned to

Halifax for a residency in anaesthesia at the Victoria General Hospital from 1989 to 1993, followed by a year of fellowship in clinical pediatric anaesthesia at the Izaak Walton Killam Hospital from 1993 to 1994. She received her FRCP(C) in anaesthesia in 1994. Before coming to Moncton in July 1995, she spent another fellowship year in anaesthesia pain management at Harvard Medical School. With this extra training she naturally joined the Pain Clinic at The Moncton Hospital as well as being a member of the anaesthetic staff.

The South-East Hospital Corporation, which is responsible for staffing the Albert County Hospital, found itself in a dilemma with the resignation of Dr. Charles Duffy, but solved the problem with the recruitment of Dr. Raymond Braun. Braun was born on June 18, 1956, and received a BA in 1981 and an MD in 1984 from the University of Saskatchewan. He interned at St. Paul's Hospital, Saskatoon, from 1985 to 1986 and then took one year in an obstetric and gynaecology residency at the Royal University Hospital, University of Saskatchewan, from 1985 to 1986. He became certified in family medicine by the Canadian College in 1986 and practised family medicine in Saskatoon from 1986 until he came to the Albert County Hospital and The Moncton Hospital in 1995.

In 1995 this saga draws to an end as we begin to celebrate 100 years of The Moncton Hospital. March 5, 1895, marked the day of incorporation and, at first, this was naturally selected as the day to begin our celebrations. Unlike one hundred years ago, however, there was now a March Break in the school system so it was felt appropriate to put the birthday party off until March 17,

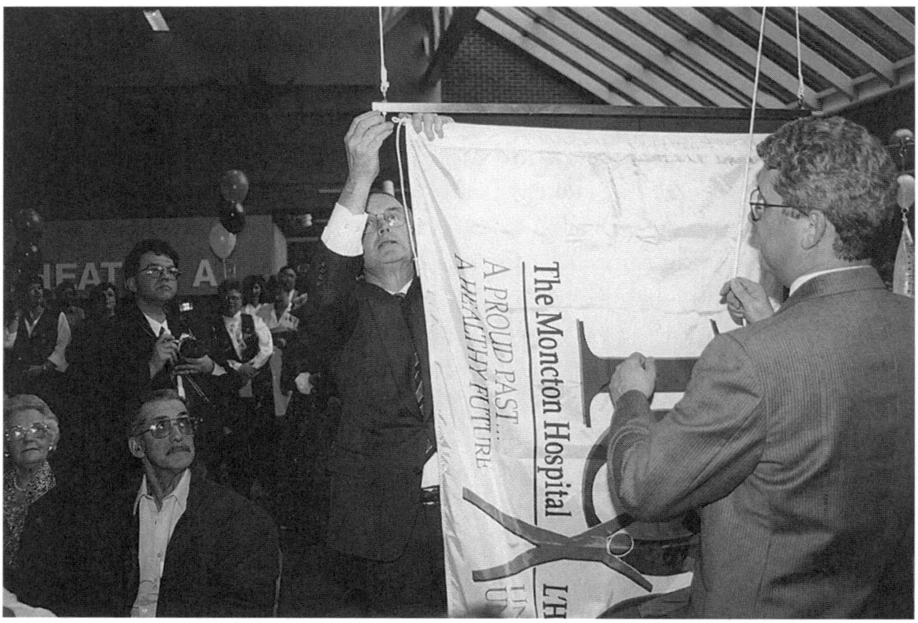

Hon. Dr. Russell King, Minister of Health, and Mr. A. MacWilliams, Chairman of the Board, raising a Centennial flag in the lobby of The Moncton Hospital in March 1995.

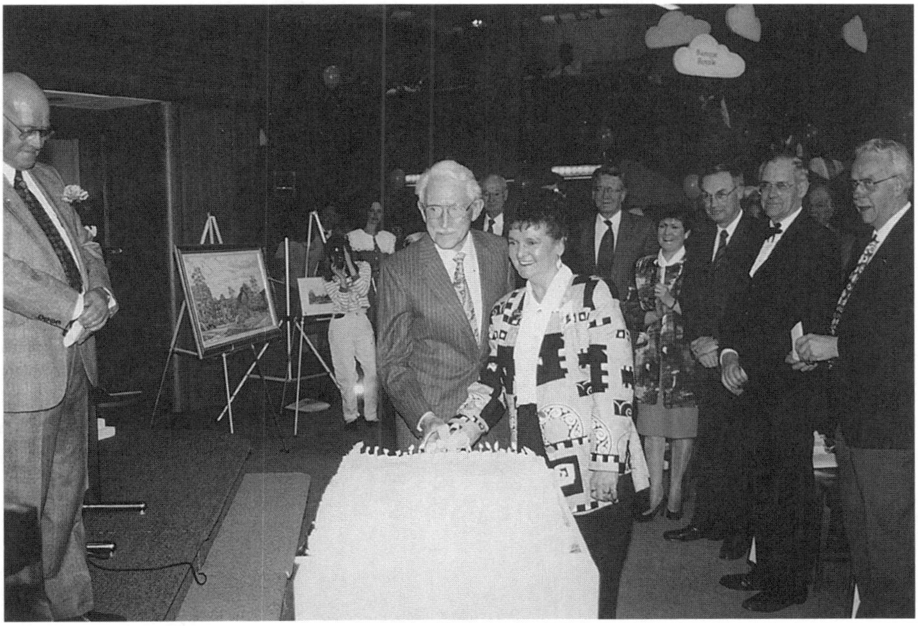

The opening ceremonies for Centennial Year with Dr. J.C. MacCrea and Mary LeBlanc cutting the birthday cake in March 1995.

1995. On March 16, 1995, the *Moncton Times–Transcript* put out a special supplement to mark the occasion. The opening ceremony was held in the lobby of the hospital with Dr. James Noonan acting as master of ceremonies and, as usual, the audience of hospital staff and invited dignitaries was kept in stitches with his repertoire of one-liners. The minister of health, the Hon. Dr. Russell King, was in attendance and when he was donning a sweatshirt with the centennial logo, Jim remarked that this was the first time he had seen the minister pull the wool over his own eyes. A centennial flag was raised in the lobby by the chairman of the board, Allen McWilliams, and the Minister of Health. The Centennial Committee had commissioned Barbara Saffron to produce a painting of the Old Moncton Hospital on King Street and one hundred limited edition prints were to be made available to the public. The original painting was purchased by the accounting firm, Doane Raymond, and one of the partners, John Sanford, also a member of the Centennial Committee, presented the painting to the hospital and limited edition prints were given to all the board chairmen, past and present. A giant birthday cake was cut by two of the longest serving members of the hospital staff, Dr. James C. McCrea and Mary LeBlanc, to go along with other refreshments served in the basement. A collection of photos covering hospital events over the past one hundred years was displayed. Edith Fairweather set up a booth and sold memorabilia on this occasion, as well as during other events throughout the year.

Under the chairmanship of Connie Colpitts and the Rev. Ronald Maund, hospital chaplain, a rededication service was held in the auditorium on March 19, 1995, with a capacity crowd in attendance. Since the clergy had played

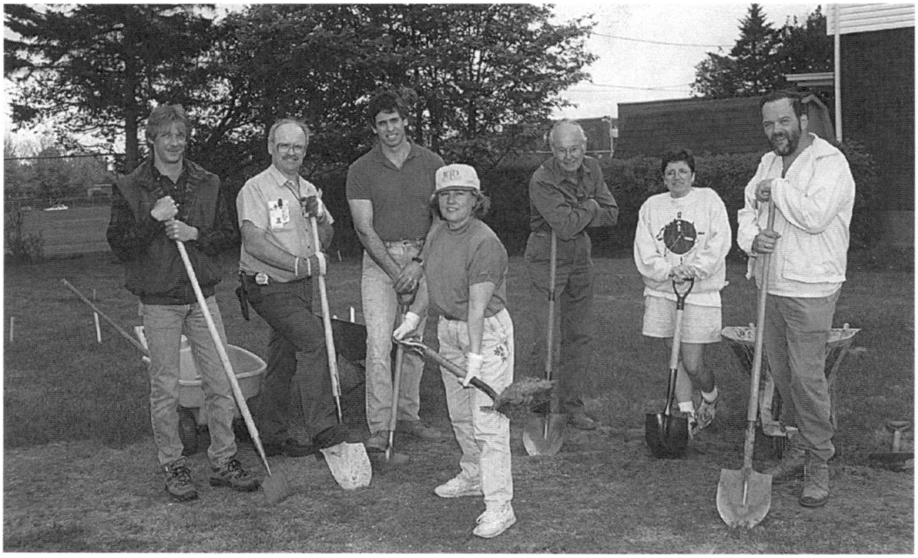

The crew creating Centennial Park at the hospital site. From left to right: Jamie Harrison, Bernie LeBlanc, Alfred Babineau, Jessie Gaudet, Dr. Victor McLaughlin, Janice Langelin, and Dennis Schaffer.

such a large role in initiating plans for the first hospital, this was, indeed, a very appropriate way to start the second hundred years. Besides Rev. Maund who delivered the homily/meditation "A Healthy Future," various local clergymen took part in the service; Rev. Dr. Doug MacEachern, St. John's United Church; Rabbi Davis Ellis, Tiferes Synagogue; Rev. Wally Corey, St. George's Anglican Church; Fr. Bernard Sloan, St. Bernards Roman Catholic Church and Fr. B. Boudreau, Roman Catholic chaplain to the hospital. Mrs. W.J. Milliea gave the Lord's Prayer in Micmac. Charlie Munroe Jr. and Ray Doucet opened the service with a fanfare of trumpets, and music for the service was provided by Dr. Bob Caddick on the organ and Dr. Peter Lightfoot on the piano with a choir of hospital staff lead by Clair Petitpas. During the service, Dr. MacLellan gave an historic reflection with slides produced by Stephen Herc and Shirley Dobson gave a talk on the women who figured so prominently in the early development of the hospital.

On April 29, 1995, the Capitol Theatre was packed to capacity as "Spring Thaw" was again presented after an absence of a few years, and highlighted the large pool of talent that exists in the hospital. The program committee consisted of Lydia Underhill and Susan Libby with Dr. Kim DeWare and Dr. Billy Harper serving as MCs for the evening. At the end of the evening, Billy removed his black tuxedo to don black tights and participate in the Ballet de Bouctouche with Gary Chesser, Glen Brodie, Greg Donald and John Steeves, as the medical staff's contribution to the evening's entertainment. They were such a hit that they were asked to perform again at the annual meeting of the New Brunswick Medical Society held in Moncton in September.

In May of each year the hospital holds employee recognition day in which pins are presented to employees recognizing their years of service to the hospital. On May 12, 1995, every employee of the hospital was presented with a special lapel pin bearing the centennial logo.

To have something of lasting value to mark the centennial year, it was decided to establish a small park on MacBeath Avenue and a planting party was held on June 10 to get the project underway. Special thanks go to Dr. Victor McLaughlin, Alfred Babineau, Jessie Gaudet and Joan Allain for bringing this project to a successful conclusion.

Under the chairmanship of Jean MacKeigan, a hospital picnic was to be held at Centennial Park in conjunction with Canada Day celebrations. A great day was planned, but the weather, unfortunately, did not cooperate and the event had to be moved indoors to the Dud James Arena.

During the Centennial Committee's deliberations it was felt that the old hospital property on King Street should be properly recognized as a historic property, having served the citizens of Moncton for almost fifty years. With the permission of the present owners of the building, Les Réligieuses de Notre Dame du Sacré Coeur, a ceremony was held on August 21, 1995, chaired by Dr. A. Salloum and a plaque (14 x 44 inches) was unveiled on a large stone in front of the oldest section of the building. At a reception after the ceremony, the Sisters took the guests on a tour of the old hospital, bringing back fond memories to those who had served in it. Especially gratifying was the excellent condition of the old building.

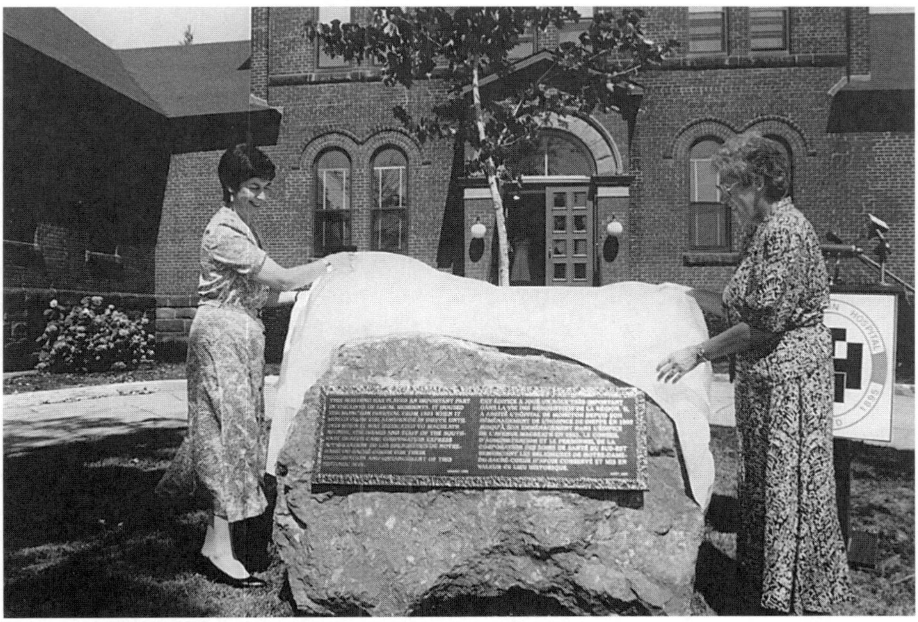

Ruth Duffy and Sr. Bernice Gaudet unveil an historic plaque in front of the old Moncton Hospital on King Street.

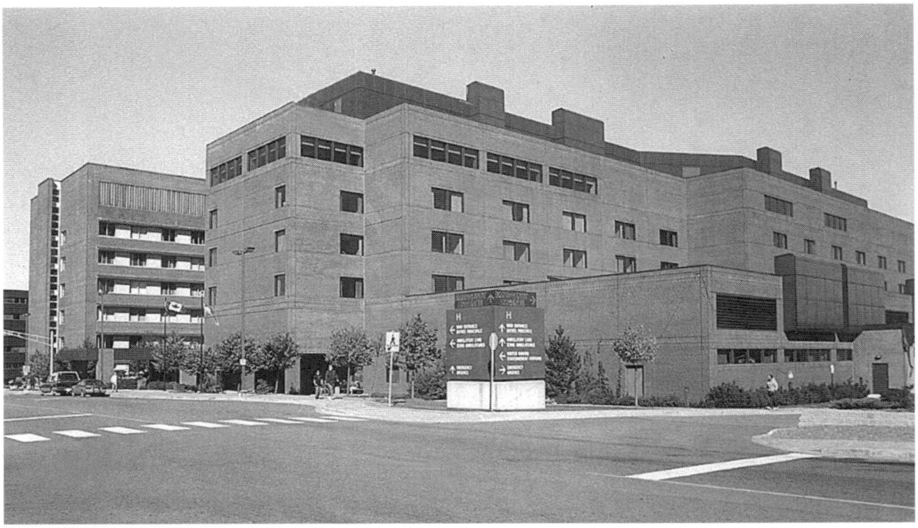

The Moncton Hospital, as it appears today.

As their own project for raising funds for the centennial events, Victor and Peggy McLaughlin grew 500 chrysanthemum plants during the summer and these went on sale on September 8, 1995. The other main event for September was a Health Fair organized by Lydia Underhill, and this was held in the hospital cafeteria on September 30, with 36 booths set up as well as a blood pressure clinic and a teddy bear picnic.

Between October 23 and October 27, a craft fair organized under a committee chaired by Mrs. V. Hopper was held, with 22 groups participating, including the Ladies' Auxiliary.

As part of the Centennial celebration, Radio Canada telecast a mass on October 28, 1995, to commemorate the Centennial Anniversary of The Moncton Hospital. This was held in the auditorium of the hospital and was telecast on November 12. The homily was given by Father Ernest Leger with Father Benoit Boudreau and Rev. Ronald Maund, the hospital chaplains, participating. Once again, the hospital choir had a chance to show off their talents by combining with the choir of Notre Dame de Grace.

To conclude the year of celebrations, a dinner, followed by a dance, was held at the Beausejour Hotel, where members of the community joined with members of the medical staff. Dr. McLaughlin gave a slide show reviewing all the events of the year. Dr. Ginette Gagné-Koch announced at this dinner that the board had authorized that the Centennial Park, created on the hospital grounds, would henceforth be called "The Dr. Victor McLaughlin Centennial Park" in honour of all the work Dr. McLaughlin had done in connection with the year's celebrations. In the afternoon before the dinner, a dessert party had also been held for the hospital staff, in the cafeteria, and also for the staff, there was a skating party at the Coliseum on Sunday afternoon, December 3.

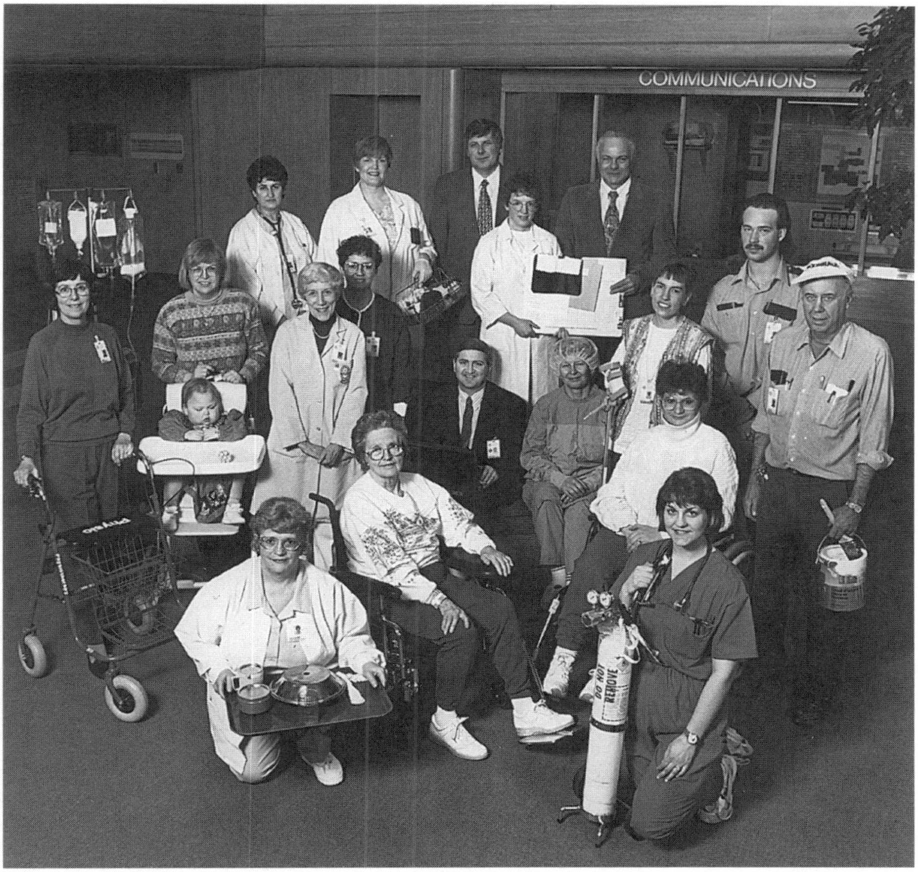

Representatives from all departments are necessary to make a modern hospital run.

During the year it became apparent that items of historical interest were scattered throughout the hospital and a proper archives centre was needed. The creation of such a centre was authorized by the board, and architects drew up plans to build such a centre on the second floor adjacent to the library. It is hoped that this will become a reality in the near future.

Appendices

APPENDIX A

Chairmen of The Board

1895-1901	Mr. George B. Willett
1901-1905	Mr. J.M. Ross
1905-1908	Mr. J.S. Rayworth
1908-1916	Mr. F.W. Sumner
1916-1917	Mr. James Doyle
1917-1943	Mr. A. Cavour Chapman
1943-1947	Mr. Ambrose Wheeler
1947-1959	Mr. Leonard Lockhart
1959-1960	Mr. Harold Tait
1960-1963	Mr. Leonard Lockhart
1963-1973	Mr. Ralph Belyea
1973-1976	Mr. Howard Grayston
1976-1983	Mr. Robert A. MacQuade
1983-1988	Mr. Ralph Black
1988-1994	Mr. Robert Radford
1994	Mr. Allen McWilliams

Superintendents, Executive Directors, Presidents and CEOs

1898-1904	Miss M.C.Grant
1904-1909	Miss Janet MacEachern
1909-1911	Miss Sophie MacDonald
1912-1915	Miss Blanche MacDonald
1916-1918	Miss Lottie E. Corbett
1918-1919	Miss Adele MacDonald
1919-1947	Miss Alena J. MacMaster
1947-1948	Dr. John MacKenzie
1948-1949	Mr. George Filliter
1949-1955	Dr. Donald F.W. Porter
1955-1970	Dr. Austin M. Clarke
1970-1991	Mr. William A. Kilpatrick
1991	Dr. Ginette Gagné-Koch

APPENDIX B

Superintendents and Directors of Nursing

1906-1909	Miss Janet MacEachern
1909-1911	Miss Sophie MacDonald
1912-1916	Miss Blanche MacDonald
1916-1917	Miss Lottie E. Corbett
1918-1919	Miss Adele MacDonald
1919-1945	Miss Alena J. MacMaster
1945-1950	Miss Barbara Beattie
1951-1953	Miss Florence Breau
1953-1975	Mrs. Katherine Wright
1975-1982	Miss Myrna Sherrard
1982-1986	Mrs. Katherine Wright
1986	Mrs. Carroll Ann O'Leary

N.B.: In 1975 The Moncton Hospital School of Nursing closed, to be replaced by the A.J. MacMaster School of Nursing. The Director of Nursing of The Moncton Hospital ceased to be the Director of The Nursing School.

APPENDIX C

Presidents of the Medical Staff

1930	Dr. A.R. Myers
1931	Dr. W.P. Kirby
1932	Dr. C.R. Baxter
1933	Dr. L.H. Price
1934	Dr. A.E. Forbes
1935	Dr. H. E. Britton
1936	Dr. A.R. Landry
1937	Dr. A.R. Landry
1938	Dr. G. Lyons
1939	Dr. W.S. Fitzpatrick
1940	Dr. W.S. Fitzpatrick
1941	Dr. R.D. Roach
1942	Dr. J.W. Dobson
1943	Dr. K.W. MacKenzie
1963	Dr. R. Fitch
1964	Dr. V. McLaughlin
1965	Dr. E.D. Levittan
1966	Dr. W.G. Allanach
1967	Dr. R.M. Dysart
1968	Dr. L. Ramsay
1969	Dr. D.I. MacLellan
1970	Dr. R. I. McKenna
1971	Dr. G.V. Parsons
1972	Dr. J.C. McCrea
1973, 1974	Dr. P.G. Lyons
1975, 1976	Dr. E. MacLeod
1977, 1978	Dr. J.H. Rich
1979, 1980	Dr. W.A. Oatway
1981, 1982	Dr. D. H. Hiltz
1983, 1984	Dr. T.E. Edgett
1985, 1986	Dr. D. I. MacLellan
1987, 1988	Dr. O. Audain
1989, 1990	Dr. R. Roberge
1991, 1992	Dr. R. Trifts
1993, 1994	Dr. J. S. Noonan
1995, 1996	Dr. R. Caddick

APPENDIX D

Medical Staff Representatives to the Board of Trustees

1914-1933	Dr. H.H. Coleman
1933-1942	Dr. J.A. McNaughton
1943-1946	Dr. R.D. Roach
1947	Dr. E.W. Ewart
1957-1960	Dr. G.V. Parsons
1960-1965	Dr. S.A. Hopper
1965-1971	Dr. J.A. Dobson
1971-1972	Dr. W.A. Oatway
1972-1976	Dr. J.H. Rich
1976-1981	Dr. E.A. MacLeod
1981-1984	Dr. Grant Llewellyn
1984-1985	Dr. W.A. Oatway
1985-1991	Dr. K.J. Deware
1991-1992	Dr. R.A. Trifts

N.B.: In addition to the Medical Staff Representative, the Moncton Medical Society appointed additional members to the board in some years as follows:

1934-1937	Dr. H.H. Coleman
1937-1940	Dr. C.R. Baxter
1940-1946	Dr. J.W. Dobson

In 1921 Dr. L.N. Bourque served as a representative of the City of Moncton. From 1949-1960 Dr. A.L. Richardson served as a representative for the County of Westmorland

With the formation of the South-East Health Care Corporation in 1992, the medical staff no longer had the privilege of electing a member to the board of trustees.

APPENDIX E

Milestones

1894	First citizens' meeting on December 31
1895	Act of Incorporation of hospital on March 5
1898	Ladies' Auxiliary formed on June 10
1898	First hospital opened in almshouse on June 11
1903	Cornerstone laid for new hospital by Lieutenant Governor Snowball on October 29

(cont'd p. 308)

Milestones (cont'd)

1903	New hospital opened on King Street on November 11
1905	ENT Department formed
1906	First School of Nursing formed
1909	First graduates of School of Nursing
1912	First X-ray machine installed
1919	First motorized Studebaker ambulance
1921	Annex to hospital opened
	First laboratory opened
	First medical staff association
1922	First accreditation by American College of Surgeons
1924	First use of insulin
	School clinics for T&As
1930	New wing opened
1932	First Department of Urology
1934	First hospital pharmacy formed
1939	New Ambulance
	First Department of Orthopaedics
1940	First Electrocardiographic Service
1945	Dr. Parsons, the first fully trained anaesthetist, joins staff
1947	Hospital Board and Miss MacMaster resign on May 14
1948	New working hours for nurses
1948	First Pap smears
1950	Construction begins for new hospital on November 30
1952	First Department of Psychiatry
1953	New Hospital opened on MacBeath Ave. on August 21
1954	Cottage at Shediac Cape donated by Mr. and Mrs. Leonard W. Lockhart
1955	First obstetrician, Dr. J.A. Delaney, joins staff
1956	Fire in medical library of hospital
1957	New nurses' residence opened on December 11
1959	Government Hospital Insurance begins on July 1
1960	Moncton Hospital Annex opens on January 1
1961	Medical Advisory Committee formed
1962	Joyce Wing opened on September 12
1964	Opening of Department of Inhalation Therapy
1966	Friends of the Moncton Hospital Foundation Incorporated
1968	New X-ray Department and Radioisotope Lab opened
	First Coronary Intensive Care Unit opened
1970	Pulmonary Function Lab opened
1971	Opening of Clark Wing
	First total hip arthroplasties performed
1972	Opening of Department of Neurosurgery
	Professional Arts Building erected

1973	Agnew Peckham & Associates present master plan for new construction
1974	First Chief of Medical Staff
1976	First Chemotherapy Clinic
	Fire at Nurses' Cottage
	First Thoracic Surgeon, Dr. Orville Messenger
	First Christmas appeal of Friends of the Moncton Hospital Foundation
	First annual medical staff dinner
1977	Clergy organized
	First neonatology unit
1978	First CAT scanner obtained
	Burn unit opened on May 5, 1978
1979	Remodelled coronary care unit opened
	Day Surgery Unit opened
	Neonatology unit opened
1980	Construction project announced by Hon. Brenda Robertson in June
1981	First ER Physicians
	New 12-bed intensive care unit opened
	First respirologist, Dr. Acres, joins staff
1982	Sod turned for new south tower by Premier Hatfield on September 24
	Vascular laboratory opened
	Pain Clinic formed
	Proposal for Cardiac Surgery Unit
1983	Presentation of brief to government on radiotherapy
1984	Pastoral Care Department formed
	YAG Laser obtained
1986	New CAT Scanner obtained
	Brief presented to government on Cardiac Surgery Service
1988	Haemophiliac Clinic opened
1989	New South Tower opens
1990	Hugh T. Reardon Eye Clinic opens
	Child/Adolescent Psychiatric Unit opens
	Infectious Disease Service opens with Dr. Thompson joining staff
1991	Same day admission policy instituted
1992	Mobile Lithotripsy Unit becomes available
	Air ambulance, Dispatch/flight co-ordination centre opens
1995	Program Management instituted.
	Friends of the Moncton Hospital Centennial Campaign
1995	Centennial Celebrations
	Mobile MRI service opened

INDEX